The Michigan Manual of Clinical Diagnosis

The Basis of Cost-Effective Medical Practice

The Michigan Manual of Clinical Diagnosis

The Basis of Cost-Effective Medical Practice

Edited by

Richard D. Judge, MD
Clinical Professor of Internal Medicine
Assistant Dean for Student Affairs
University of Michigan Medical School
Ann Arbor, Michigan
Senior Cardiologist
Michigan Heart and Vascular Institute
Ann Arbor, Michigan

James O. Woolliscroft, MD
Professor of Internal Medicine
University of Michigan
Ann Arbor, Michigan

Gerald B. Zelenock, MD
Professor of Surgery
Section of Vascular Surgery
The University of Michigan Medical Center
Ann Arbor, Michigan

George D. Zuidema, MD
Professor of Surgery (Emeritus)
and Vice Provost for Medical Affairs
University of Michigan Medical Center
Ann Arbor, Michigan

With

Patricia Barr
Office of Educational Resources and Research
University of Michigan Medical Center
Ann Arbor, Michigan

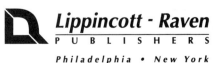
Lippincott - Raven
PUBLISHERS
Philadelphia • New York

Acquisitions Editor: Richard Winters
Developmental Editor: Mary Beth Murphy
Manufacturing Manager: Dennis Teston
Production Manager: Kathleen Bubbeo
Production Editor: Xenia Golovchenko
Indexer: Anne Cope
Compositor: Compset
Printer: RR Donnelley

Printed in the United States of America

9   8   7   6   5   4   3   2   1

Library of Congress Cataloging-in-Publication Data
The Michigan manual of clinical diagnosis: the basis of cost-effective medical practice/edited by Richard D. Judge . . . [et al.].
      p.   cm.
    ISBN 0-316-47581-5
    1. Diagnosis—Handbooks, manuals, etc.   2. Physical diagnosis-Handbooks, manuals, etc.
I. Judge, Richard D.
    [DNLM: 1. Diagnosis—handbooks.   2. Clinical Medicine—economics—handbooks.
3. Clinical Medicine—organization & administration—handbooks.   4. Attitude of Health Personnel.   5. Quality of Health Care.   6. Physician-Patient Relations.
WB 39 M624 1997]
RC71.3.M467   1997
616.07'5—dc21
DNLM/DLC
for Library of Congress

Contents

Contributors

Paul T. Adams, MD
Clinical Assistant Professor of Internal Medicine, University of Michigan Medical Center, 1500 East Medical Center Drive, Ann Arbor, Michigan 48109

Christopher J. Andershock, MD
Section of Emergency Services, University of Michigan Medical Center, 1500 East Medical Center Drive, Ann Arbor, Michigan 48109

Mel L. Barclay, MD
Associate Professor, Division of Maternal-Fetal Medicine, Department of Obstetrics and Gynecology, University of Michigan, Mott Hospital, 1500 East Medical Center Drive, Ann Arbor, Michigan 48109

William G. Barsan, MD
Professor of Emergency Medicine, University of Michigan Medical Center, 1500 East Medical Center Drive, Ann Arbor, Michigan, 48109

William D. Belville, MD
Associate Professor of Surgery, Department of Urology, University of Michigan Medical Center, 1500 East Medical Center Drive, Ann Arbor, Michigan 48109

Terry J. Bergstrom, MD
Professor of Ophthalmology, Kellogg Eye Center, University of Michigan Medical Center, 1500 East Medical Center Drive, Ann Arbor, Michigan 48105

Carol R. Bradford, MD
Assistant Professor of Otolaryngology, University of Michigan Medical Center, 1500 East Medical Center Drive, Ann Arbor, Michigan 48109

Lisa M. Colletti, MD
Associate Professor of Surgery, University of Michigan Medical Center, 1500 East Medical Center Drive, Ann Arbor, Michigan 48109

Michael T. Goldfarb, MD
Lecturer, Department of Dermatology, University of Michigan Medical Center, 1500 East Medical Center Drive, Ann Arbor, Michigan 48109

Roger J. Grekin, MD
Professor of Internal Medicine, Ann Arbor Veterans Administration Medical Center, University of Michigan, 2215 Fuller Road, Ann Arbor, Michigan 48105

Cyril M. Grum, MD
Professor of Internal Medicine, 3110 Taubman Center, Box 0368, University of Michigan Medical Center, Ann Arbor, Michigan 48109

Ronald D. Holmes, MD
David G. Dickinson Professor of Pediatrics, Department of Pediatrics, University of Michigan Medical Center, 1500 East Medical Center Drive, Ann Arbor, Michigan 48116

Carolyn M. Johnston, MD
Assistant Professor of Obstetrics and Gynecology, University of Michigan Medical Center, 1500 East Medical Center Drive, Ann Arbor, Michigan 48109

Richard D. Judge, BSEE, AA, MD
Clinical Professor of Internal Medicine and Assistant Dean for Student Programs, Department of Internal Medicine, Division of Cardiology, University of Michigan, 1301 Catherine Street, Ann Arbor, Michigan 48109

Joseph C. Kolars, BA, MD
Associate Professor of Internal Medicine, University of Michigan Medical Center, 1500 East Medical Center Drive, Ann Arbor, Michigan 48109

Mark A. McQuillan, MD
Clinical Assistant Professor, Internal Medicine, University of Michigan Medical Center, 1500 East Medical Center Drive, Ann Arbor, Michigan 48109-0376

Linda M. Selwa, MD
Clinical Assistant Professor of Neurology, University of Michigan Medical Center, 1500 East Medical Center Drive, Ann Arbor, Michigan 48105

Michael J. Shea, MD
Associate Professor of Internal Medicine, University of Michigan Medical Center, 1500 East Medical Center Drive, Ann Arbor, Michigan 48109

Vernon K. Sondak, MD
Associate Professor of Surgery, University of Michigan Medical Center, 1500 East Medical Center Drive, Ann Arbor, Michigan 48109

James O. Woolliscroft, MD
Professor of Internal Medicine, University of Michigan, 1500 East Medical Center Drive, Ann Arbor, Michigan 48109

Gerald B. Zelenock, MD
Vice Provost for Medical Affairs and Professor of Surgery, Emeritus, University of Michigan Medical Center, 1500 East Medical Center Drive, Ann Arbor, Michigan 48109

Preface

In 1961, the year of publication of the first edition of this book, medical diagnosis was largely clinical and technology was usually confirmatory. As we approach the 21st century, medical diagnosis is largely technologic and clinical assessment functions more to direct the physician to the best diagnostic laboratory study or procedure. Despite this role reversal, the importance of clinical examination continues to be preeminent for several reasons.

The physician is, by far, the least expensive and/or most cost-effective factor in the modern health care equation, and accurate clinical evaluation at the time of first contact allows more selective use of expensive diagnostic technology. This is appropriate and optimal care. The uncertain physician more often turns to multiple tests and multiple consultations in his/her search for an answer to the patient's problem. This is invariably more expensive, and often one study or consultation begets another, setting off a technologic cascade. When this occurs, costs escalate rapidly. Good clinical medicine is also cost-effective medicine.

But there is more to doctoring than diagnosis. In following the course of a patient's illness, whether acute or long term, the clinician can no longer rely on serial technology. No more daily chest x-rays or semiannual exercise tests. Adjustments in management must be made (and rightly so) on the basis of clinical observation. Changes in weight, venous distention, and crackles direct adjustments in the treatment of congestive heart failure. Symptoms and patient examination, not annual echocardiograms, are the basis for following mitral valve prolapse long term. Follow-up technology is vital, but it must be used selectively and judiciously.

A third reason for the preeminence of clinical skills in the process of doctoring is humanistic. The term "clinical" comes from the Greek word for bed, $\kappa \lambda \iota \nu \iota \kappa o \delta$. It is at the bedside and in the examination room that crucial medical decisions are made and care is directed. Here is where the art of medicine finds its expression.

In his commencement address, Adam Goldstein, a 1995 graduate of the University of Michigan Medical School who had experienced serious illness during his fourth year of medical school, had some compelling things to say to his classmates. He gave them six tips that he called "hidden lessons."

Lesson #1: *Pain is real*—. . . my advice is not to ignore the situation. Don't be afraid to be the one who lends the hand to squeeze, or to be the one with the comforting voice. Let your patient know that he/she is not alone.

Lesson #2: *See each patient every day*—. . . even if it is just for one minute; even if it is just to say, "Hi, there's nothing new but I was thinking of you. Do you have any questions?' And take an extra five seconds to pull up a chair and sit down.

Lesson #3: *Friends, family, and significant others are an important part of the healing process*—. . . try to include them in discussions that include such topics as diagnosis, treatment, and prognosis. Often your patient is in no position mentally or physically to make important decisions on his/her own.

Lesson #4: *Know what you know and know what you don't know*—. . . patients appreciate and expect honesty. Don't be afraid to say, "I don't know." I developed more respect for my cardiologist when he admitted he did not completely understand some aspects of my cancer. . . .

Lesson #5: *Patients express similar illness in different ways*—. . . treat each patient according to his/her needs, not the diagnosis. Make every effort to treat each patient as an individual.

Lesson #6: *Open your ears and mind, not just your mouth, when talking to your patients*—. . . THEY possess all the needed information.

Amen, Adam.

Introduction

The influence of technologic advancements on the practice of medicine is enormous. The ability of physicians to accurately diagnose and treat disease conditions is greater now than ever in history. However, technology has also fundamentally altered the practice of medicine. Rather than using the history and a finely honed physical examination to make the correct diagnosis, increasingly the role of the physician is to determine the differential and then utilize technology to confirm the correct diagnosis. This does not diminish the role of the physician's clinical examination skills. We postulate that the frequently encountered overreliance on technology reflects poorly developed examination skills in which the physician has little confidence. The modern practice of medicine requires an integration of traditional physical examination skills with technology.

However, despite the dramatic changes in medicine, there also are constants that have remained essentially unchanged for centuries. The interaction of an individual seeking help with a care provider, the physician, remains basically the same. As such, it is befitting for students to focus on the fundamentals, the immutable aspects of physicianhood that will endure throughout their careers. The patient/physician interaction, verbal and nonverbal communication skills, knowledge about disease presentation, and skill in examining patients to detect the telltale signs of disease are among these constants.

In *The Michigan Manual* we present the physiologic approach to the clinical examination and provide examples of how the examination is augmented by technology, the majority of which was not widely available when the first edition of the precursor to this manual was published in 1963. We seek to focus on the constants as practiced in the context of modern medicine.

James O. Woolliscroft, MD

The Michigan Manual of Clinical Diagnosis

The Basis of Cost-Effective Medical Practice

1. MEDICAL HISTORY

James O. Woolliscroft

I. General Considerations

The medical history is the most frequently used and arguably the most powerful diagnostic tool possessed by clinicians. The interview forms the basis for initiating, developing, and sustaining the patient-physician relationship, and it defines the roles and responsibilities of the patient and physician.

A. The clinician obtains information that does the following:

1. Focuses the diagnostic workup and allows the clinician to determine the probability that a patient is suffering from a disease
2. Helps assess the therapeutic efficacy of interventions and monitor the progress of illness
3. Allows assessment of the risk for the development of disease
4. Provides the opportunity to develop an understanding of the unique characteristics and social supports of the person who is the patient

B. The patient has an opportunity to tell what is wrong with him or her and to be reassured that you are listening and will try to help. Don't let the mechanics of how you are going to organize things or the pressure of time keep you from hearing what your patient is saying.

II. Medical Knowledge

A. Diagnosis

1. Presenting signs and symptoms. There are very few pathognomonic signs or symptoms. Most patients present with nonspecific complaints. Knowledge of the constellation of symptoms that various diseases present allows you to actively process the verbal and nonverbal information the patient provides. Symptoms associated with diseases you are considering are specifically sought to confirm or dispel your suspicions. The traditional review of systems categorizes complaints by the organ system usually involved. As you work through this manual, you will become familiar with key presenting signs and symptoms and the most common underlying pathophysiologic abnormalities.
2. Epidemiology in your setting. Depending on the location and type of your practice, the probability of a specific sign or symptom indicating a given disease changes. For example, a patient presenting with a high fever in Utah is much less likely to have malaria than is a similar patient in Nigeria. Understanding signs and symptoms in the context of disease prevalence allows the interview process to narrow the list of likely disease candidates and develop the differential diagnosis.

B. Therapeutic monitoring: natural history of disease. Most of your practice will consist of seeing patients with already established diseases whose progress and response to therapy are being determined. To assess the efficacy of your interventions accurately, knowledge of the natural history of the disease and the potential side effects from therapy is required.

C. Prevention: risk for disease. Primary and secondary prevention is based on knowledge of risk factors for disease. In addition to age and sex, there are multiple categories of risk factors that should be pursued during the interview with each patient (Table 1-1). Determining each patient's risk profile provides the opportunity for behavioral modifications or appropriate therapy and screening programs to decrease the risk for subsequent disease.

III. Interviewing Skills

A. Well-developed interviewing skills allow you to apply your knowledge base.

B. Cultural diversity. The diversity of cultures in most metropolitan areas virtu-

Table 1-1. Disease Risk Factors

Category of risk factor	Examples
Genetic	Family history of breast cancer, colon cancer, non–insulin-dependent diabetes mellitus
Disease-associated	Risk for colon cancer in patient with longstanding ulcerative colitis
Treatment-associated	Chronic corticosteroid therapy and risk for osteoporosis; risk for pneumococcal septicemia in patient with splenectomy
Environmental	Lead exposure through job restoring old houses
Lifestyle/behavioral	Smoking, substance abuse, sexual behavior

ally assures that you will care for patients from a different culture than your own. Remember that mores for appropriate patient and physician conduct as well as communication patterns are culturally determined. Developing the ability to interact with your patients in a culturally appropriate manner will facilitate your care and enhance your understanding of what could be mistaken for noncompliant behavior. Basic principles to guide your interaction follow:

1. What is the person's understanding regarding the meaning of his or her illness? Is it fate? A curse? Penance for past misdeeds?
2. What is the patient's expectation from the physician? Should dietary and physical "prescriptions" be part of the therapeutic plan?
3. What are the social norms for illness behavior and how should concerned family and friends respond?
4. Who is the ultimate decision-maker? The patient? An elder? A spouse?

IV. Social Support Systems

A. Only through continued effort will you develop your knowledge and skills to use the interview fully as a diagnostic and therapeutic tool. It is an active process, calling on your best synthesis abilities in true Sherlock Holmes fashion. However, you can learn about your patients as individuals, each with a unique story, while your other skills are still rudimentary.

B. Understanding the social supports and personal strengths each patient possesses will allow you to tailor your therapeutic interventions appropriately. Continue to see your patients as the unique individuals they are, and it will enrich your professional life and enhance your ability to provide the best care possible for them.

V. The Medical Write-up

A. The medical write-up summarizes, integrates, and synthesizes information obtained through the interview, physical examination, and available laboratory studies. The write-up must reflect active thought and synthesis and include only the data that are germane to the patient's care. Flexibility in approach is needed; the focus may be on an acute disease, a chronic disease, or health maintenance.

B. Components of a write-up. It is rare for all components to be completed with any patient at a given interaction; you must pick and choose the appropriate sections to develop a functional, thoughtful summary of your patient's condition at the time.

1. Identification data
    a. The patient's name and registration number
    b. Date and time the data were collected. The time that the history and physical examination were performed is important if clinical events change.
2. Source of history and reliability

   a. Generally, the informant is the patient. Occasionally, information may be gathered from family, friends, paramedical personnel, or even "old records" if no other sources are available.
   b. Your impression of the reliability of the information obtained should also be stated.
3. Chief complaint (CC). The CC reflects the problem or problems for which the patient is seeking help. There are three general types of CCs: problem-related, administrative, and preventive.
   a. The *problem-related CC* documents the symptom that the patient noted and that led him or her to seek your assistance. It is best framed in the patient's own words. Avoid inserting a premature diagnosis in the CC. Report symptoms rather than your opinion or someone else's opinion of what is wrong. Think of the problem-related CC as the "lead-in" to a short story in which positive and negative clues contribute to a total understanding of the events that have led to the patient's coming to you.
   b. The *administrative CC* describes a patient visit in the course of *an already known illness,* for example, "CC: Third course of chemotherapy for small cell carcinoma of the lung diagnosed 4 months ago."
   c. The *preventive CC* describes the reason for a clinical visit by a patient who feels well. Examples include prenatal examination or simply a patient's desire to optimize his or her health status (check-up examinations).
4. History of present illness (HPI)
   a. The *problem-related HPI.* This type of HPI is a concise, well-organized, chronologically correct description of the features of the illness that led to the CC. The CC raises several hypotheses, and you are making a case for the most likely diagnosis.
      (1) Begin with genetic (family) and acquired risk factors for the problem (disease) being described.
      (2) Next, present the chronologic sequence of the events leading to the patient's presentation.
      (3) Weave "pertinent negatives" into the narrative at the following points in the history:
         (a) A given symptom or event suggests a point of differential diagnosis.
         (b) A classic part of a symptom complex is absent.
      (4) If a patient has multiple active problems that appear to be unrelated and that together led to the visit, you might wish to describe them under separate problem headings. Such an approach is generally easier than trying to integrate apparently independent problems into one section.
   b. The *administrative HPI.* Here, the disease is already known, and all that is required is a brief, well-organized summary of the patient's status between the last visit and the present. Data to include are the patient's functional status and complications either of disease progression or therapy.
   c. The *preventive HPI.* This should be very brief or nonexistent since there is no "present illness." Relevant historical data are recorded in the Risk Factor Assessment section of the write-up.
5. Risk factor assessment. This section is used to characterize the patient's risk for future diseases or complications from current disease. It is useful to consider the specific types of risk factors that a patient may have.
   a. Fixed risks
      (1) Demographic risks: age, sex, and ethnicity. On occasion, race, religion, or country of origin are of importance.
      (2) Genetic risks (often referred to as the family history): age, health status, or cause of death of the patient's close blood relations (first-degree relative: mother, father, siblings) and family of marriage

(spouse, children). At a minimum, inquiry should be made about a family history of breast cancer, colon cancer, and myocardial infarction under the age of 60. Any disease that "runs in the family" should be characterized.

   b. Acquired risks. These are generally of greater importance than fixed risks.

   (1) Environmental risks

   (a) Exposure and occupational history. A plethora of risk factors are encountered in the working environment as well as in certain hobbies. Examples are silica (in miners and sandblasters), blood products, organic solvents (in hospital laboratory workers), potentially harmful chemicals (in woodworking, ceramics).

   (b) Travel history. Note only travel to other countries or specific regions of the United States where contact with different infectious diseases is possible.

   (2) Lifestyle/behavioral risks

   (a) Substance use/abuse. Note the substance, and quantify the amount of intake (e.g., number of packs of cigarettes per day, number of cans of beer or glasses of wine per week or day). Most important, describe the impact of the substance use on the patient's life.

   (b) Sexual history. Transmission of serious infectious diseases and the development of cervical cancer are related to sexual behavior. Sexual preference, practices, and activity level are relevant to determining the risk for developing these problems.

   (c) Health maintenance habits. These habits include diet, exercise routine, automobile seat belt use, monthly breast self-examination for women, and testicle self-examination for men.

   (3) Disease-associated risks. Past illnesses may put a patient at increased risk for developing associated disease. Traditionally, much of this information resides in the past medical history. In this section, only record specific disease states that increase a patient's risk for other diseases (e.g., ulcerative colitis and the risk for subsequent colon cancer).

   (4) Treatment-associated risks

   (a) Surgical procedures. Examples include splenectomy (increases the risk for subsequent bacteremia with encapsulated bacteria), terminal ileum resection (increases the risk for the development of B_{12} deficiency and anemia).

   (b) Transfusions. The receipt of blood products should be noted and dated.

   (c) Medications. Certain medications are capable of producing undesirable side effects and may increase the risk for development of specific diseases or clinical syndromes. The risks associated with each medication that a patient is taking should be considered.

   (d) Allergies and adverse reactions. The *exact* symptoms and manifestations related to an allergy or an adverse reaction must be clarified and recorded. Often what is thought by the patient to be an allergy is an adverse reaction, such as diarrhea in association with antibiotics.

   (e) Immunizations. The immunization status of each patient should be documented. All adult patients should have their tetanus status ascertained, and depending on the patient, rubella, influenza, hepatitis, and pneumonia status recorded.

6. Past medical history. The past medical history is a survey of all of a patient's previous illnesses and contacts with physicians that are not directly pertinent to the history of the present illness.

    a. Childhood illnesses. Document only diseases that are of potential importance.

    b. Adult illnesses.

        (1) Active illness. Include active illnesses not directly related to the present illness in the past medical history.

        (2) Inactive illness. Note inactive disease and affirm the "inactivity" (i.e., no active disease process). Examples are past episodes of hepatitis or peptic ulcer disease. Again, record only illnesses that are potentially important for current or future events.

    c. Surgical procedures. Record surgical procedures and any untoward events such as excessive bleeding, or anesthetic complications.

    d. Trauma history. List accidents and injuries sequentially, including the name of the hospital if hospitalization was required. (A history of recurrent trauma should prompt further inquiry into possible predisposing conditions as abuse or alcoholism).

    e. Medications. Catalogue the patient's current medications, dosage, and schedule including an assessment of the patient's adherence to the prescribed regimen. Use of nonprescription, over-the-counter medication should be specifically determined.

7. Social history. The goal of the social history is to define the patient as a person, including the nature of the patient's environment and his or her reaction to it.

    a. Personal profile. Key facts include occupation, marital status, recreational pursuits, and financial status. In some cases, cultural background and spiritual beliefs may be relevant.

    b. Support systems. The existence and strength of social support networks such as those provided by family, friends, and church may influence the patient's ability and motivation to adhere to the treatment regimen.

8. Review of systems (ROS). Include all important, but not immediately applicable, data about organ system functions and malfunctions in the ROS. This will be easier if you have properly covered all the questions that ought to have been asked in the HPI, including both positive and negative replies. Because patients may not know which complaints are or are not related to the HPI, it is your job to weave all relevant symptoms into the fabric of the HPI, no matter when during the interview you hear about them.

9. Physical examination. The examination should be directed toward elucidating and confirming hypotheses developed during the history.

    a. Document findings (or the absence thereof) in the write-up. Knowing which physical features correlate with your diagnostic suspicions makes the physical more than a routine and will help to bolster your diagnostic acumen.

    b. Each area should be specifically identified as follows:

        i. General Appearance
        ii. Vital Signs
        iii. Skin
        iv. Head
        v. Eyes
        vi. Ears
        vii. Nose/Mouth/Throat
        viii. Lymph Nodes
        ix. Neck
        x. Pulmonary
        xi. Cardiovascular
        xii. Breasts
        xiii. Abdomen
        xiv. Rectal

xv. Extremities

xvi. Neurologic (include mental status as a subsection)

10. Laboratory. Laboratory data generally serve only to confirm or deny what you hypothesized from the history and found on the physical examination. Include only those laboratory data that are pertinent to your patient.

11. Problem list. Take the information that you identified in the data base and synthesize a prioritized list of problems.

2. CUTANEOUS SYSTEM (SKIN)

Michael T. Goldfarb

I. Glossary

Albinism: a disease of generalized hypopigmentation in which little or no melanin is formed.

Alopecia: absence of hair from location where it usually grows.

Bulla, pl. *bullae*: loculated fluid in the skin; a large blister.

Café au lait spots: sharply marginated brown patches. The presence of one of two such spots is normal.

Carotene: a yellow-orange pigment found in many foods.

Crusts: Dried or hardened serum proteins on the surface of the skin.

Erosion: a superficial loss of skin.

Erythema: redness.

Freckles: sharply circumscribed small brown macules.

Keratin: the protein product of skin metabolism. Scale is formed by the macroscopic accumulation of keratin.

Lentigo, pl. *lentigines*: sharply circumscribed small brown macules that appear late in life after years of sun exposure.

Macule: a circumscribed area of color change.

Melanin: the brown pigment of the skin that is made by melanocytes.

Nodule: a large palpable mass, usually elevated above the skin surface.

Papule: a small palpable mass, usually elevated above the skin surface.

Plaque: a flat elevated mass, the confluence of papules.

Pruritus: itching.

Pustule: a cloudy or white vesicle, the color of which is due to the presence of polymorphonuclear leukocytes.

Scale: the macroscopic accumulation of keratin; light gray flakes.

Scleroderma: a disease in which the dermal component of the skin is thickened.

Seborrhea: oiliness of the skin due to lipids that originate in the sebaceous gland.

Ulcer: as applied to the skin, a deep loss of tissue or large erosion.

Urticaria: the presence of edema in the skin secondary to histamine release.

Vesicle: a small loculation of fluid in the skin; a small blister.

Vitiligo: circumscribed areas of pigment loss.

Wheal: an edematous papule, the primary lesion of urticaria, a "hive."

Xerosis: dryness of the skin.

II. Techniques of Examination and Normal Findings

A. Important factors and considerations. Differentiating important from unimportant information is critical.

    1. Lighting. Bright, overhead fluorescent light is best.

    2. Exposure. Appropriate handling of the gown and drape allows for thorough examination of all areas of the skin.

B. Techniques of doing a directed physical

    1. Inspection and palpation

        a. With patient sitting, examine exposed areas first (scalp, hair, face, mouth, neck, arms, hands, and fingernails) (Fig. 2-1).

        b. With patient supine and gown covering breasts and sheet covering groin area, examine the abdomen, lower chest, anterior surface of lower legs, feet, and toenails. Examine breasts, if appropriate.

        c. With patient sitting and gown open in back, examine the back, shoulders, and upper chest.

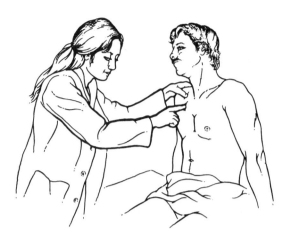

Fig. 2-1. First, with the patient sitting on the edge of the examining table, examine the exposed areas including the scalp, hair, face, mouth, neck, arms, hands, and fingernails.

       d. Examination of the buttocks, posterior legs, and genitalia may not be needed in the absence of known cutaneous disease (Fig. 2-2).

  C. Expected findings in a normal adult (Fig. 2-3)

    1. Color. Range of normal is great and depends on race, nationality, and degree of sun exposure. Color is derived from three sources, and color changes are related to changes in the balance of the following:

      a. Red erythematous hues from oxygenated hemoglobin within the cutaneous vasculature

      b. Brown hues from melanin in the epidermis

      c. Yellow hues from nonvascularized collagen, bile, carotene pigments

    2. Texture. Skin texture depends on age, sex, and region of skin being examined.

      a. *Softness* from layer of fat cells under the dermis

      b. *Moisture* from water diffusion through skin, and by sweating on surface

      c. *Lubrication* from sebaceous glands

      d. *Warmth* from circulation of blood

      e. *Roughness* from keratin produced by epidermal cells

    3. Mucous membranes. These are characteristically pink and moist. Mottled brown or black melanin pigmentation on oral mucous membranes may be present in black patients.

    4. Hair. Normal distribution is well known.

      a. Facial, axillary, and pubic hair depend on presence of sex hormones.

      b. Scalp hair (normally grows about 0.3 mm/day or about ½ inch/month). Examine for length, texture, fragility, sheen, and ease with which hairs can be manually removed from follicles.

    5. Nails (normally grow about 0.1 mm/day)

      a. Fingernails should be smooth, translucent, evenly attached to nail bed.

      b. Paronychial tissue should be intact.

  D. Expected findings in elderly (age >75 years)

    1. Appearance

      a. Skin is thinner, less elastic, and wrinkled with mottled pigmentation. Subcutaneous fat is also diminished.

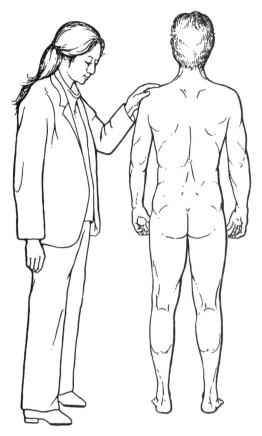

Fig. 2-2. Next, ask the patient to stand facing away from you and examine the back, buttocks, and posterior legs.

  b. Hair is thinner owing to involutional as well as genetic alopecia. Also, more hair will become gray with advancing age.

  c. All the nails grow at a slower rate. Fingernails often become brittle and ridged. Toenails tend to become thick and dystrophic.

 2. Function

  a. The skin of the elderly is more susceptible to trauma, heals more slowly, and is less of a barrier to the environment. The melanocytes do not function as well and may not be able to tan the skin adequately to protect it from ultraviolet exposure. The skin also is less efficient at responding to an allergic stimulus and possibly less able to protect it from a neoplastic development. Also, because of the loss of subcutaneous fat, the body is not able to keep itself as warm and many elderly people are easily chilled.

  b. Because of decreased activity of sweat (eccrine) glands, the elderly person is more susceptible to hyperthermia. Also, owing to decreased function of sebaceous glands, dry skin is a common problem.

III. Cardinal Symptoms. Pain and pruritus sensations are both carried by the cutaneous branches of the peripheral nervous system.

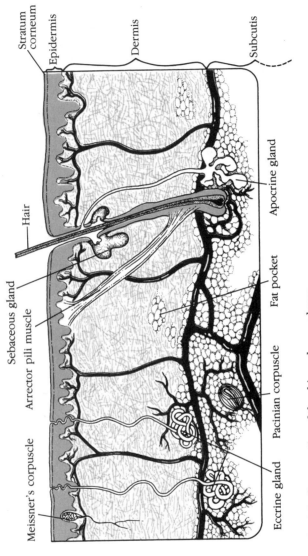

Fig. 2-3. Cross-section of the skin and appendages.

A. Causes of pain are usually apparent.
  1. Skin around nerves is no longer intact; nerves are exposed to dry, hostile environment.
  2. Cutaneous inflammatory reaction
  3. External trauma
B. Pruritus sensation carried by small nerve fibers of skin; causes may not be clear.
  1. Generalized pruritus
    a. Systemic diseases, such as chronic disease of thyroid, pancreas, liver, kidneys; or hematopoietic system disease such as Hodgkins's disease, polycythemia vera.
    b. Cause unexplained—possible psychiatric cause
  2. Localized pruritus (often a difficult therapeutic problem)
    a. Associated with visible cutaneous disease. Itching may interfere with patient's ability to function; scratching may exacerbate the skin disease.
    b. If no associated skin disease is present, pruritus may have no pathologic meaning.
IV. Abnormal Findings
  A. Change in color. Although the range of normal is great, changes from previous skin color are important. *Macules* are small, localized areas of color change; *patches* are larger areas.
    1. Brown (melanin pigmentation)
      a. Generalized increase may be caused by pituitary, adrenal (Fig. 2-4), or liver disease.
      b. Localized increase is seen in *café au lait* spots, freckles, lentigines, nevi, and areas of postinflammatory hyperpigmentation.
    2. White (absence of melanin)
      a. Generalized hypopigmentation seen in albinism

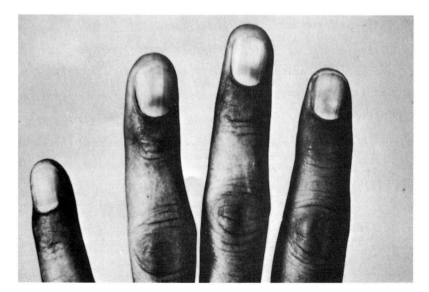

Fig. 2-4. Hyperpgimentation of the fingers and nails in adrenal insufficiency (Addison's disease). Note accentuation of pigmentation at the knuckle folds.

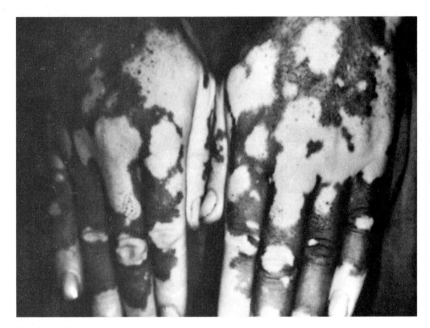

Fig. 2-5. Vitiligo of the hands.

   b. Localized hypopigmentation seen in macules or patches of vitiligo
       (Fig. 2-5), scars, postinflammatory hypopigmentation, other cuta-
       neous diseases
 3. Yellow
   a. Generalized yellowness caused by increased bile pigment is seen in
       liver failure (jaundice).
   b. Generalized diffuse yellowness caused by increased carotene pigmen-
       tation is sometimes seen in vegetarians and persons with diabetes.
   c. Generalized pale yellow color of normal collagen may be seen in ane-
       mia (particularly pernicious anemia and that of chronic renal disease)
       and is caused by changes in the color of less well-oxygenated blood.
 4. Erythema (redness caused by increased cutaneous blood flow)
   a. Generalized erythema usually caused by inflammation and may occur
       with drug eruptions, viral exanthemas, or urticaria.
   b. Localized erythema and inflammation are seen in a vast array of cu-
       taneous diseases.
   c. Noninflammatory redness may be due to increased number of in-
       travascular red blood cells (polycythemia) or extravascular red blood
       cells (petechiae, purpura).
 5. Other colors. Ingested or injected medications may color skin (e.g., slate
     gray from silver salts, yellow from quinacrine).
B. Change in texture
 1. Softness. Skin may lose elasticity when cutaneous fat is replaced by col-
     lagen (scleroderma), when collagen is replaced by scar tissue, or when
     distended by edema.
 2. Moisture. Thermal stimuli (fever, room heat) cause generalized sweating;
     emotional stimuli cause localized sweating (forehead, palms, soles, ax-

illa, groin). Moist skin may rarely be caused by the increased metabolic rate of hyperthyroidism.

3. Lubrication. Oily skin is normal in most people after puberty; no pathologic states are associated with increased sebaceous secretion. Decreased lubrication (dryness, chapping, xerosis) is common after age 60 years and may also be caused at any age by too-frequent bathing. Xerosis (abnormal dryness of the eye) may be caused by a deficiency of thyroid or sex hormones.

4. Warmth. Generalized increased warmth is due to increased cutaneous blood flow delivering body heat to the surface of skin where it is lost by convection, conduction, radiation; this may be caused by fever or exercise. Localized areas of warmth may be seen with cutaneous inflammation. Coolness reflects decreased blood flow, as seen in the lower legs of patients with peripheral arteriovascular disease.

C. Specific cutaneous lesions. Lesions represent structural changes in the skin and are always pathologic, although sometimes of little significance. Determining which can be ignored is a matter of experience (Fig. 2-6).

1. Palpable lesions have substance and mass and are usually elevated above the surface of the skin.

   a. Definitions

   (1) A *papule* is a small palpable lesion

   (2) A *nodule* is a large papule

   (3) A *plaque* is a confluence of papules or nodules forming a large· flat-topped lesion.

   b. Causes

   (1) Proliferation of cells found in skin (inflammatory cells, metastatic tumor cells, and leukemic cells).

   (2) Accumulation of fluid within skin, either diffuse (*hive* or *wheal*) or loculated (blister). Small blisters are called *vesicles*, large blisters are called *bullae*, cloudy or white blisters containing many polymorphonuclear leukocytes are called *pustules*.

2. Erosions and ulcers represent loss of skin permitting serum and inflammatory cells to exude (*weeping, oozing*). When this exudate dries, *crusts* (yellow-brown friable granules) form. It is important to distinguish between crusts (epithelial loss) and *scale* (epithelial proliferation manifested by light gray flakes).

   a. Definitions: an *erosion* is superficial loss of skin; an *ulcer* is deep loss of skin.

   b. Causes (determination of cause greatly simplifies differential diagnosis)

   (1) External trauma, most commonly scratching

   (2) Unroofing of vesicular or bullous lesions

   (3) Necrotic effect of vascular ischemia

V. Common Clinical Disorders

A. Eczema. Eczema and dermatitis are synonymous terms that imply inflammation of the skin from a variety of different causes.

1. Acute: vesicles, bullae, crusting, erythema; possibly pruritus and even tenderness

2. Chronic: scaling, exaggeration of normal skin markings, lichenification

3. Causes

   a. Irritant (various chemicals)

   b. Allergic contact (poison ivy, nickel)

   c. Noncontact (atopic dermatitis, neurodermatitis or lichen simplex chronicus, stasis dermatitis (Fig. 2-7), nummular [coin-shaped] dermatitis, dyshidrosis, or hand dermatitis)

4. Treatment

   a. Topical corticosteroids (hydrocortisone) can hasten improvement for all of these conditions; oral corticosteroids may be necessary in recalcitrant cases.

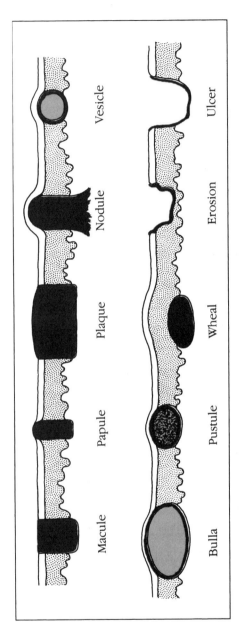

Fig. 2-6. Most common structural changes in the skin.

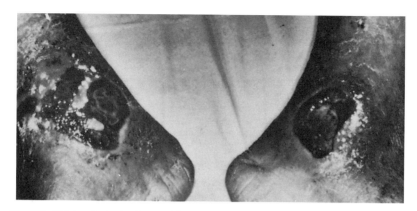

Fig. 2-7. Bilateral stasis ulcers with surrounding dermatitis.

     b. Contact dermatitis. It is important to remove the offending agent from the patient's environment.
     c. Dryness of the skin. Apply a suitable emollient (petrolatum).
 B. Papulosquamous diseases. These diseases are characterized by scaly papules that may coalesce into plaques.
    1. Psoriasis: erythematous plaques with a silvery scale most commonly on the scalp and extensor surfaces of the extremities; pitting of the nails is a common finding (Fig. 2-8)
    2. Lichen planus: flat-topped, violaceous polygonal papules with minimal scales of the wrist and thighs and an even white, lacy network on the buccal mucosa
    3. Pityriasis rosea: a self-limited eruption of erythematous, thin, oval plaques with a collarette of scales oriented along the skin lines of the trunk
    4. Seborrheic dermatitis: erythema with greasy scale of the face and scalp

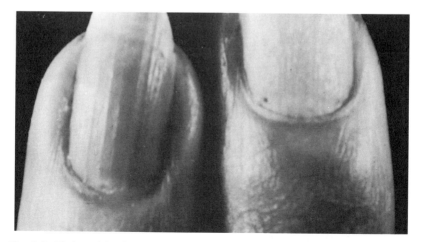

Fig. 2-8. Pitting of the fingernails in psoriasis.

5. Treatment
   a. Topical corticosteroids (hydrocortisone) will help clear all these conditions.
   b. For psoriasis, numerous therapies have been used including ultraviolet light and a new topical vitamin D (calcipotriene).
   c. For seborrheic dermatitis, *Pityrosporum ovale* may have a role in the cause of the disease, and the use of a topical antifungal agent (ketoconazole) has been helpful.

C. Hair loss
   1. Causes. Hair loss is due to a wide variety of causes.
      a. Genetic hair loss or androgenetic alopecia is the most common cause. The result ranges from baldness in men to hair thinning in women.
      b. Telogen effluvium: resting hair that is lost temporarily at a greater rate approximately 3 months after a stressful event (physical or emotional).
      c. Anagen effluvium: growing hair that is lost temporarily due to chemotherapy
      d. Alopecia areata: usually patchy but may be complete hair loss, which is thought to be an autoimmune process (Fig. 2-9)
      e. Trauma: trichotillamania (deliberate plucking) and traction alopecia
      f. Scarring alopecia: can follow episodes of radiation therapy, trauma, fungal infections, discoid lupus, and lichen planus
   2. Treatment. Treatment of hair loss is usually treating the underlying disease or removing the stress that caused the problem.
      a. Topical minoxidil has been used for treating androgenetic alopecia.
      b. Topical and intralesional corticosteroids have proved efficacious for hair loss from alopecia areata, discoid lupus, and lichen planus.

D. Acneiform eruptions

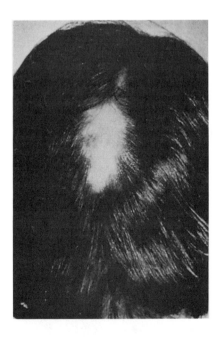

Fig. 2-9. Alopecia areata. The area of hair loss is sharply marginated, and the exposed scalp appears normal.

1. Acne vulgaris. One of the most common problems in dermatology, this disease affects most adolescents.
   a. Cause. Diseases of the pilosebaceous unit cause acne vulgaris. The primary lesion is a comedo; with inflammation it develops into an inflammatory papule, then a pustule, then even a cyst. These lesions are located on the face, chest, and back.
   b. Treatment. Therapy may include topical antibiotics (benzoyl peroxide, clindamycin), topical tretinoin (helps eliminate the primary lesion, the comedo), and oral antibiotics (tetracycline). Recalcitrant cystic acne may even be treated with oral isotretinoin, but numerous precautions are necessary because it is a potent teratogen.
2. Acne rosacea is a similar condition involving erythema of the central face with papules and pustules. It is found usually after age 30 years.
   a. Cause. A number of factors seem to be involved with the etiology of acne rosacea, including endocrine changes, vasomotor lability, and *Demodex folliculorum*.
   b. Treatment. Therapy may include topical antibiotics (metronidazole) and oral antibiotics (tetracycline). Patients should be told to avoid various factors that can cause flushing of the face (extreme temperature changes, hot oral liquids, alcohol).

E. Vesiculobullous diseases: characterized by a vesicle or bullae as the primary lesion. Skin biopsies are essential in diagnosis. A biopsy of involved skin should be stained with hematoxylin and eosin to determine the exact location of the blister (within the dermis, dermal-epidermal junction, or upper dermis). A biopsy of perilesional skin observed with direct immunofluorescence will determine pattern and types of immunoglobulins in the skin and lead to the correct diagnosis, in most cases.

1. Pemphigus vulgaris is a chronic bullous disorder that affects primarily middle-aged adults. It is characterized by oral blisters and erosions as well as diffuse flaccid bullae on the skin. It is fatal if not treated, and treatment involves oral immunosuppressive agents (corticosteroids, azathioprine).
2. Bullous pemphigoid is a nonfatal blistering disease of the elderly. It is characterized by tense bullae on an urticarial base. Treatment is similar to that for pemphigus vulgaris, but lower doses of immunosuppressive agents are usually adequate.
3. Dermatitis herpetiformis involves small pruritic vesicles in a group distribution in young and middle-aged adults. Patients can be successfully treated with dapsone or a gluten-free diet.
4. Epidermolysis bullosa, comprising a group of inherent disorders, is characterized by the development of blisters after a minimal trauma. This condition may range from mild discomfort to extreme disability and disfigurement, depending on the location of the blister on the skin. Exact classification of the disease may require electron microscopic evaluation of the skin biopsy.

F. Superficial fungal infections: the most common types of cutaneous infection. Correct diagnosis of fungal disease is accomplished with KOH examination and fungal cultures.
   1. Causes
      a. Dermatophyte or the classic "ringworm." This infection is characterized by well-demarcated, slightly erythematous, and scaly annular eruption. Infection may involve the feet (tinea pedis), hands (tinea manuum), body (tinea corporis), and groin (tinea cruris). When the dermatophyte involves the nails (onychomycosis, tinea unguium), it is characterized by nail separation, subungual debris, and dystrophy. When infection involves the scalp (tinea capitis), it is characterized by hair loss with or without inflammation (Fig. 2-10).
      b. Candidiasis. Cutaneous infection from candidiasis often involves moist areas (intertriginous, mucosal). Classic skin presentation is

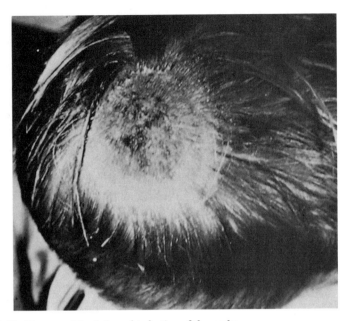

Fig. 2-10. Tinea capitis. A fungal infection of the scalp.

brightly erythematous patches with satellite lesions that may range from papules to even pustules.

 c. Yeast. *Pityrosporum obiculare* can lead to tinea versicolor. It is characterized by white to brown, well-demarcated patches with a superficial fine scale that involves primarily the torso.

 2. Treatment

  a. Topical antifungal agents (azoles, allylamines)

  b. Systemic agents when the infection is widespread or deep-seated (oral griseofulvin, oral azoles)

G. Cutaneous bacterial infections. For the correct diagnosis of any of these infections, culture of the pus or crust is in order. Treatment involves the correct selection of an appropriate topical or systemic antibiotic (often a penicillinase-resistant penicillin).

 1. Impetigo is the most common bacterial infection of the skin (Fig. 2-11). It is caused by a streptococcus or staphylococcus organism. It presents most commonly on the face or shoulder, but may involve any area of the body or any age group. The classic presentation is erythematous papules with erosions and honey-yellow crust. The eruption can be bullous; if so, the pathogen is staphylococcus. Treatment is with an appropriate topical antibiotic (mupurocin ointment) or oral antibiotic (penicillinase-resistant penicillin).

 2. Furuncle or boil is another common infection, often from a staphylococcus organism, which presents as a painful, erythematous nodule. Drainage of the boil is often necessary for rapid resolution.

 3. Cellulitis is a diffuse bacterial infection presenting as deeply indurated, erythematous, tender skin, which may be associated with systemic signs (e.g., fever, lymphadenopathy).

H. Cutaneous viral infections

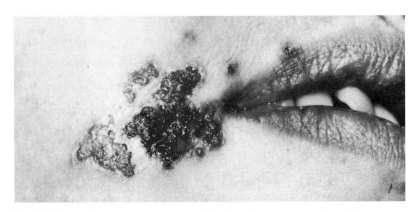

Fig. 2-11. Impetigo. A crusted weeping, infectious lesion common in children.

1. Herpes simplex is the most common cutaneous viral infection. Affected patients usually present with group vesicles on the lips or genitals, which proceed to pustules and crusting, and finally heal. The initial episode is the most severe with milder recurrences every few months in many cases. Oral antiviral therapy (acyclovir) can be used to treat more serious herpes simplex infections.

2. Herpes zoster, also called shingles, is caused by the chickenpox virus (varicella). It is a recurrence of the viral infection that was acquired usually in childhood and had been dormant for years. Presentation often is initially pain in a dermatome that becomes a vesicular eruption. In older patients, postherpetic neuralgia is a common long-term complication. Treatment most often involves oral antiviral therapy (acyclovir).

3. Warts constitute one of the most challenging problems in dermatology. They are caused by the human papillomavirus and can affect almost any skin surface. Presentation is usually an elevated, hyperkeratotic papule that can grow and spread if not treated. Treatment involves a host of destructive methods (cryosurgery, salicylic acid, electrosurgery, laser) with none of them being effective in all cases.

4. Molluscum contagiosum is a similar problem, with presentation of multiple, small, umbilicated papules on the skin. This disease often resolves with simple curet removal or a light liquid nitrogen freeze.

I. Benign tumors. Tumors of the skin, especially benign tumors, are by far the most common human neoplasms.

1. Seborrheic keratosis is a common epidermal growth often found in middle-aged to older people. It is a well-circumscribed, tan to brown lesion with a roughened surface.

2. Epidermal cysts are subepidermal dome-shaped growths that range from a few millimeters to many centimeters.

3. Nevi or moles are fleshy, tan to dark brown papules that usually begin to form during childhood.

4. Cherry angiomas are extremely common lesions, bright red in color, and 1 to 5 mm. These lesions usually form after age 30 years.

5. Skin tags are fleshy, pedunculated lesions found most commonly in areas of skin folds. These benign lesions do not have to be excised unless they are cosmetically disturbing to the patient, become irritated or they interfere with the function of a nearby organ (in the field of vision), or there are concerns about the exact diagnoses (benign versus malignant). After

excision, the specimen obtained should be sent for histologic evaluation to confirm that the lesion was benign and that a premalignant or malignant growth was not missed.

J. Nonpigmented premalignant and malignant tumors. Because of chronic exposure of the skin to the sun, premalignant or malignant skin lesions are commonly found in fair-skinned, middle-aged to older people. The diagnosis of all these tumors should be made with a skin biopsy. Treatment involves removal of the lesion with a variety of techniques including cryosurgery, electrodesiccation and curettage, excision surgery with documented clear margins on pathology, and radiation.

   1. Actinic keratoses are the most common premalignant tumors. They are indistinctly marginated, erythematous lesions, with an adherent scale. Actinic keratoses may evolve into squamous cell carcinoma over a period of years.

   2. Basal cell carcinoma is the most common malignant tumor. This tumor most often presents as a pearly lesion with telangiectasias and has a tendency to ulcerate. However, a basal cell carcinoma may present as a fibrotic plaque (morphea-like basal cell carcinoma) or an erythematous plaque (superficial basal cell carcinoma). Basal cell carcinomas usually do not metastasize.

   3. Squamous cell carcinoma often presents as an erythematous nodule that may become ulcerated and crusted. This tumor has a limited ability to metastasize.

K. Pigmented premalignant and malignant tumors. Pigmented malignant tumors are a great concern in dermatology owing to the metastatic potential of these lesions.

   1. Congenital nevi affect practically 1% of newborns, and the larger the lesion the greater the chance of malignant transformation (about 15% to 20% in giant congenital nevi). Therefore, removal of large congenital nevi is indicated when possible, and some physicians even remove the smaller ones.

   2. Dysplastic nevi are acquired nevi often characterized by irregular pigmentation. There is frequently a genetic predisposition to developing these lesions. A patient with dysplastic nevi is at higher risk for developing malignant melanoma in one of these lesions or in normal skin. The degree of risk in a person with dysplastic nevi increases with the number of pigmented lesions and with a strong family history of dysplastic nevi or melanoma.

   3. Malignant melanoma is the most dangerous of the skin lesions because of its ability to metastasize to almost any site in the body (Fig. 2-12). The earlier the melanoma is detected, the better the prognosis. On histology, the vertical thickness of the tumor gives key prognostic insight, with thin lesions (1 mm or less) associated with an excellent prognosis and thick lesions (3 mm or greater) with a poor prognosis. After a melanoma has metastasized, therapy is usually ineffective. Therefore, excisional biopsy of suspected pigmented lesions is usually in order with wider reexcision if the lesion is a melanoma. There are four types of malignant melanoma.

   a. Superficial spreading melanoma (most common, found in middle-aged persons)

   b. Nodular melanoma (poor prognosis)

   c. Lentigo maligna melanoma (elderly persons; starts years earlier as an irregular, hyperpigmented macule called a *lentigo maligna*)

   d. Acral lentiginous melanoma (found on the palms, soles, and the nail beds)

L. Drug eruptions. With the numerous drugs currently used in medicine, drug eruptions are commonly seen in both the outpatient and inpatient settings.

   1. Cause. Determination of the offending agent is not always clearcut, since patients may be on more than one drug. By knowing which drugs cause which skin eruptions most commonly, the physician will have a better

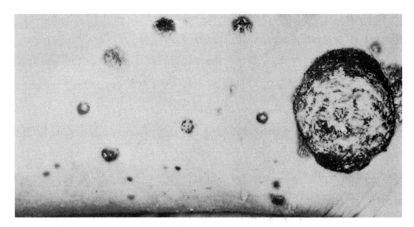

Fig. 2-12. Malignant melanoma with satellite cutaneous metastases.

idea of which drug or drugs to discontinue first. The *Physicians' Desk Reference* is often an excellent place to start when trying to decide what agent is causing the drug eruption.

2. Most common drug eruptions. Some drug reactions have causes other than drug exposure (e.g., various foods, infectious disease), and this should be considered.
   a. Morbilliform (maculopapular eruption)
   b. Urticaria (hives)
   c. Erythema multiforme (target lesions)
   d. Vasculitis (palpable purpura) (Fig. 2-13)
   e. Erythema nodosum (tender nodules on the legs)
   f. Toxic epidermal necrolysis (life-threatening desquamation of the skin)
   g. Fixed drug eruption (recurrent plaque in same area with each exposure to the drug)
   h. Photosensitive reaction (resembles an exaggerated sunburn in light-exposed areas)
3. The treatment of choice for a drug eruption is discontinuation of the offending agent, but therapy to hasten the resolution of this problem has included topical and systemic corticosteroids, systemic antihistamines, and even life support measures in severe cases.

VI. **Available Technology**
   A. Skin biopsy: the most important diagnostic technique in dermatology
   1. Types
      a. Shave biopsy. A shaving of involved skin, usually epidermis and partial-thickness dermis, is obtained with a scalpel or curet. No suture is necessary.
      b. Punch biopsy. Epidermis and full-thickness dermis of involved skin is obtained usually using either a 2-, 3-, or 4-mm skin punch. Suture closure is usually used.
      c. Excisional biopsy. Complete removal of the involved skin with scalpel excision through epidermis and full-thickness dermis. Suture closure is used.
   2. Types of dermatologic disorders in which skin biopsies are useful
      a. Skin neoplasms

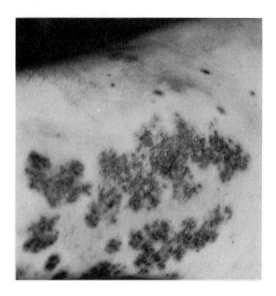

Fig. 2-13. Purpura of the foot in vasculitis.

     (1) Determine the exact diagnosis and nature of the neoplasm (benign or malignant).
     (2) Determine whether the lesion is completely excised.
    b. Other dermatologic conditions
     (1) Inflammatory diseases (psoriasis, lichen planus, connective tissue disorder, eczema, drug eruptions)
     (2) Vesiculobullous diseases (bullous pemphigoid, pemphigus vulgaris, dermatitis herpetiformis)
     (3) Infectious diseases (deep fungal diseases, acid-fast bacilli)
  3. Processing and interpretation
    a. The specimen is initially placed in formalin immediately after the specimen is obtained.
    b. The specimen is then embedded in paraffin.
    c. Suitable staining is then performed.
     (1) Hematoxylin and eosin is the most commonly used stain for most skin biopsies.
     (2) Special stains can be used for specific diseases (periodic acid-Schiff [PAS] for fungal diseases).
    d. Interpretation of the finished slide is usually done by a dermatopathologist using a light microscope.
    e. Special processing and interpretation are necessary for some of the more specific tests that can be performed on the skin biopsy.
     (1) Direct immunofluorescence for various vesiculobullous diseases and connective tissue diseases
     (2) Electron microscopy for epidermolysis bullosa
B. Potassium hydroxide (KOH) examination
  1. Diagnosis of fungal diseases
    a. Dermatophyte appears as long-branched hyphae.
    b. *Candida* appears as pseudohyphae.
    c. *Pityrosporum* or tinea versicolor infection appears as short hyphae with groups of small spores (often termed "spaghetti and meatballs").
  2. Technique

a. Specimen is obtained by scraping or clipping suspected fungal infection of skin, hair, or nails.
b. Specimen is placed on a slide; 1 drop of 10% KOH is added and then heated for a few seconds over an alcohol flame.
c. This leads to separation of the epithelial cells and enhances the ability to interpret the slide.
d. Light microscope is then used to find the hyphae or spores.
C. Microbial culture (for pathologic bacteria, fungi, viruses)
  1. Cultures obtained and transported to the laboratory in a suitable medium for the type of pathogen suspected
  2. Useful for diagnosing various viral, bacterial and fungal diseases
D. Patch test
  1. Diagnosis of allergic contact dermatitis
  2. Technique
    a. Suspected allergen is placed on skin in a semi-occluded fashion.
    b. It is left in place for 48 hours.
    c. Reading is done 24 hours after the patch is removed; a positive test result is an inflammatory reaction.
E. The cost figures cited in this table are **basic direct costs**. The figures are difficult to obtain and change quickly. They include *only* the cost of the test itself (technician, equipment, time, materials). No professional costs (interpretation) are included. Costs vary from region to region based on differences in some components such as labor. However, the relative cost ranking should remain similar.

Procedure	Code
Skin biopsy	
Shave biopsy	$$
Punch biopsy	$$
Excisional biopsy	$$
Potassium hydroxide (KOH) examination	$
Microbial culture	$$
Patch test	$$

$ = $0–$50; $$ = $50–$100.

VII. Bibliography

Arndt KA. *Manual of Dermatologic Therapeutics,* 5th ed. Boston: Little, Brown, 1995.
Arnold HL Jr, Odon RB, James WD. In: *Andrews' Diseases of the Skin. Clinical Dermatology,* 8th ed. Philadelphia: WB Saunders, 1990.
Champion RH, Burton JL, Eblina FJ. *Rook / Wilkinson / Ebling Textbook of Dermatology,* 5th ed. Oxford: Blackwell Scientific Publications, 1992.
Fitzpatrick TB. *Color Atlas and Synopsis of Clinical Dermatology. Common and Serious Diseases,* 2nd ed. New York: McGraw-Hill, 1992.
Fitzpatrick TB, Eisen AZ, Wolff K, Freedberg IM, Austen KF. *Dermatology in General Medicine,* 4th ed. New York: McGraw-Hill, 1993.
Sawyer GC, et al. *Manual of Skin Diseases,* 6th ed. Philadelphia: JB Lippincott, 1991.

VIII. Key Search Words
The following key words reflect the content of this chapter. They are provided to assist with an on-line search of computer databases, such as MEDLINE, if you wish to further pursue the topic of this chapter.

Acne rosacea
Alopecia areata
Carcinoma, basal cell
Carcinoma, squamous cell
Dermatitis
Dermatitis, allergic contact
Dermatitis, atopic
Dermatitis, contact
Dermatitis, irritant
Dermatitis, seborrheic
Dysplastic nevus syndrome
Eczema
Eczema, dyshidrotic
Erythema multiforme
Erythema nodosum
Herpes simplex
Herpes zoster
Keratosis
Keratosis, seborrheic
Lichen planus
Melanoma
Morbilliform
Neurodermatitis
Onychomycosis
Pemphigoid, bullous
Pityriasis rosea
Psoriasis
Skin aging
Tinea
Tinea capitis
Tinea pedis
Vasculitis

3. ENDOCRINE SYSTEM

Roger J. Grekin

I. Glossary

Acromegaly: a disorder in the adult resulting from excess secretion of growth hormone by the pituitary gland, characterized by overgrowth of bony, cartilaginous, and soft tissues, especially noticeable in acral parts.

Addison's disease: a disorder resulting from chronic underproduction of cortisol and aldosterone by the adrenal cortex, characterized by hyperpigmentation, asthenia, and low blood pressure.

Cushing's syndrome: a disorder resulting from chronic overproduction of cortisol by the adrenal cortex, characterized by thinned skin and wasted muscles, accumulation of fat on the trunk, easy bruising, plethora, and high blood pressure.

Exophthalmos: prominence or protuberance of the eyes, frequently associated with Graves' disease.

Goiter: enlargement of the thyroid gland.

Graves' disease: a disorder characterized by exophthalmos, goiter, and hyperthyroidism.

Gynecomastia: abnormal breast development in men.

Hirsutism: a state of increased amounts of body and facial hair, especially in the female.

Hypogonadism: absence or reduced function of the testis or ovary, characterized by diminished germ cell production and/or maturation, and by decreased production of sex hormones. Underdevelopment of secondary sexual characteristics or regression of developed secondary sexual characteristics results.

Myxedema: a disorder resulting from underproduction of thyroid hormone, characterized by puffiness of soft tissues, slowing of body movements, and deepening of the voice.

Virilism: a state of masculinization in the female characterized by frontal balding, hirsutism, increased muscle bulk, and clitoromegaly.

II. Techniques of Examination and Normal Findings

  A. General endocrine assessment

    1. Overall appearance

      a. Appropriateness of appearance for age and sex

      b. Growth and maturation

      c. Vital signs: blood pressure, pulse, respiration, and temperature

    2. General techniques

      a. Inspection

        (1) Patient sits erect, hands in lap, head, back, and chest exposed.

        (2) Note size and configuration of the following:

          (a) Skull, facial and jaw bones, facies, preauricular and supraclavicular areas, scalp, ears, nose, lips, tongue, teeth

          (b) Skin and its appendages

            (i) Color

            (ii) Pigmentation

            (iii) Texture and thickness

            (iv) Amounts and distribution of hair: scalp, facial, body

            (v) Distribution of subcutaneous fat

            (vi) Secondary sex characteristics

          (c) Eyes, particularly cornea and lens

          (d) Genitalia and breasts (see Chapters 11, 13, and 14)

    b. Palpation
      (1) Thickening or thinning of the skin. Pick up skin on dorsum of hand.
      (2) Muscle size. Palpate biceps and quadriceps as patient contracts the muscle.
  3. Habitus. Three basic body types can be recognized:
    a. Asthenic (ectomorph)
      (1) Slender, underweight
      (2) Narrow shoulders and anteroposterior chest diameter
      (3) Acute costal angle
      (4) Delicate bone structure, light musculature
      (5) Long hands and feet
      (6) Flat abdomen and small buttocks
    b. Sthenic (mesomorph)
      (1) Square, athletic
      (2) Heavy bone structure
      (3) Large, heavy musculature
      (4) Large buttocks
    c. Pyknic (endomorph)
      (1) Heavy, soft, rounded (owing to fat)
      (2) Bone structure may or may not be heavy
      (3) Protuberant abdomen
      (4) Wide costal angle
      (5) Short arms, legs, and fingers
      (6) Heavy, fat buttocks and thighs
  4. Skeletal proportions
    a. Aids in evaluating growth and development
    b. Commonly determined skeletal measurements:
      (1) Span of fingertip to fingertip (arms abducted)
      (2) Lower skeletal segment—floor to top of symphysis pubis
      (3) Upper skeletal segment—height minus lower segment
      (4) Skeletal or body ratio—upper divided by lower skeletal segment
      (5) Normal values
        (a) Span equals height (ratio is 1.0).
        (b) Skeletal ratio is 1.0 after age 10.
  5. Body weight
    a. Desirable weight correlates with reduced mortality rate.
    b. Table 1 lists metropolitan height and weight of adults.
  6. Special considerations
    a. Lack of facial hair is common in most Native American and some Chinese men and does not reflect a lack of testicular androgen.
    b. Some women with normal androgen levels manifest hirsutism as a familial or ethnic characteristic.
B. Thyroid
  1. Technique of examination. Patient should be sitting; provide a cup of water.
    a. Inspection
      (1) Face the patient, and have the patient extend the neck slightly.
      (2) Ask patient to swallow several sips of water.
      (3) Observe base of neck as patient swallows. Illuminate the neck obliquely with pen light to appreciate any subtle enlargement that rises during swallowing.
    b. Palpation
      (1) Posterior approach
        (a) Simultaneous palpation of both lobes (Fig. 3-1). Place tips of first two fingers of both hands on either side of the trachea, slightly below the thyroid cartilage.
        (b) The thyroid is near the surface and often is soft in texture. Use a *gentle*, light rotary motion to delineate nodules. Have

Table 3-1. Metropolitan Height—Weight Tables, 1983 (lb)

Men Height Feet	Inches	Small	Medium	Large	Women Height Feet	Inches	Small	Medium	Large
5	2	128–134	131–141	138–150	4	10	102–111	109–121	118–131
5	3	130–136	133–143	140–153	4	11	103–113	111–123	120–134
5	4	132–138	135–145	142–156	5	0	104–115	113–126	122–137
5	5	134–140	137–146	144–160	5	1	106–118	115–129	123–140
5	6	136–142	139–151	140–164	5	2	108–121	118–132	128–143
5	7	138–145	142–154	149–168	5	3	111–124	121–135	131–147
5	8	140–148	145–157	152–172	5	4	114–127	124–138	134–151
5	9	142–151	148–160	155–176	5	5	117–130	127–141	137–155
5	10	144–154	151–163	156–180	5	6	120–133	130–144	140–159
5	11	146–157	154–166	161–184	5	7	123–136	133–147	143–163
6	0	149–160	157–170	164–188	5	8	126–139	136–150	146–167
6	1	152–164	160–174	168–192	5	9	129–142	139–153	149–170
6	2	155–168	164–178	172–197	5	10	132–145	142–156	152–173
6	3	158–172	167–182	176–202	5	11	132–148	145–159	155–176
6	4	162–176	171–187	181–207	6	0	138–151	148–162	158–179

Weight according to frame (ages 25–59) for men wearing indoor clothing weighing 5 lb. and shoes with heels; for women, indoor clothing weight 3 lb. Reprinted with permission from the Metropolitan Life Insurance Company, New York.

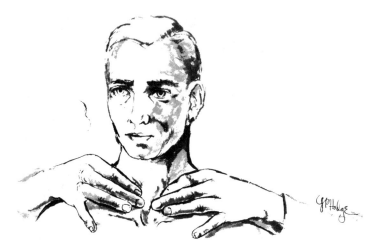

Fig. 3-1. Examination of the thyroid gland: posterior.

the patient swallow while holding fingers in one position to feel movement of thyroid.

(c) Left lobe palpation (Fig. 3-2). Flex neck to left to relax the sternocleidomastoid muscle. Palpate left lobe with right hand; place left hand behind sternocleidomastoid muscle to evert the gland; have patient swallow.

(d) Right lobe palpation. Flex neck to right to relax the sternocleidomastoid muscle. Palpate right lobe with left hand; place right hand behind sternocleidomastoid muscle to evert the gland; have patient swallow.

(2) Anterior approach

(a) Right lobe (Fig. 3-3). Flex neck to right. Use right thumb to displace larynx and thyroid gland. Palpate with thumb and

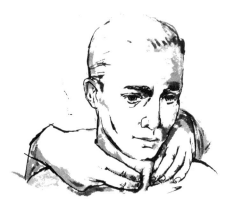

Fig. 3-2. Examination of the thyroid gland: lateral deviation posterior.

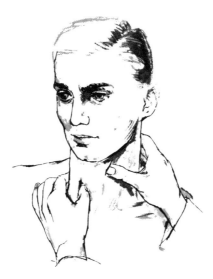

Fig. 3-3. Examination of the thyroid gland: anterior (lateral deviation to the right).

first two fingers of left hand behind the sternocleidomastoid muscle. Have patient swallow.

(b) Left lobe (Fig. 3-4). Flex neck to left. Use left thumb to displace gland. Palpate with thumb and first two fingers of right hand. Have patient swallow.

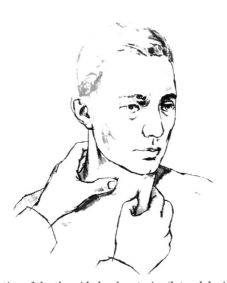

Fig. 3-4. Examination of the thyroid gland: anterior (lateral deviation to the left).

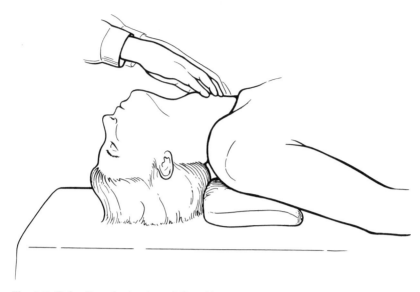

Fig. 3-5. Palpation of retrosternal thyroid.

      (3) Palpation of retrosternal thyroid
        (a) Some or all of the thyroid may descend into the chest.
        (b) Substernal glands can sometimes be palpated by placing a pillow under the patient's shoulders while in the supine position, allowing the head to fall back (Fig. 3-5).
  2. Normal findings
    a. The thyroid gland is usually not visible and often not (or only vaguely) palpable.
    b. Thyroid function is indirectly mirrored by general appearance, body weight, mental acuity, blood pressure, pulse rate, body temperature, appearance of the skin, muscle strength, eye findings, tremor, and deep tendon reflexes.
C. Gonads
  1. Technique of examination
    a. Male. Male genital examination is covered in Chapter 11.
    b. Female. Female genital examination is covered in Chapter 13.
  2. Normal findings
    a. Male
      (1) External genitalia
        (a) Adult male phallus demonstrates completed pubertal growth and development of the glans.
        (b) Adult male testis is 4 × 3 × 2.5 cm and is normally sensitive to pressure.
        (c) Scrotal skin is darkened with rugal folds.
      (2) Secondary sex characteristics
        (a) Male escutcheon (Fig. 3-6)
        (b) Facial and body hair
        (c) Frontal pattern baldness
        (d) Enlarged thyroid cartilage
        (e) Habitus
          (i) Shoulders broader than hips

            (ii) Less fat and more muscle
            (iii) Space between thighs
            (iv) Inward-curving calves
  b. Female
     (1) Pubertal development of internal genitalia
     (2) External genitalia
        (a) Pubertal development of labia majora and labia minora
        (b) Female escutcheon (see Fig. 3-6)
     (3) Adult breast development
     (4) Habitus
        (a) Hips broader than shoulders
        (b) More fat and less muscle
        (c) No space between thighs
        (d) Outward-curving calves
D. Pituitary, adrenal, pancreatic islets, parathyroid glands
  1. Technique of examination
    a. These glands are not accessible to physical examination.
    b. Imaging methods are necessary to evaluate the structure of these glands.
  2. Normal findings
    a. Assessment of adrenal function
      (1) Blood pressure and pulse (recumbent and upright positions)
      (2) Skin pigmentation and color
      (3) Weight
      (4) Presence of body hair (particularly in women)
      (5) Distribution of body fat
    b. Assessment of pituitary function
      (1) Assessed by addressing individual target gland function
        (a) Adrenal cortex
        (b) Thyroid
        (c) Gonad
      (2) Assessment of growth parameters
      (3) Visual field assessment (see Chapter 5)
    c. Assessment of parathyroid function

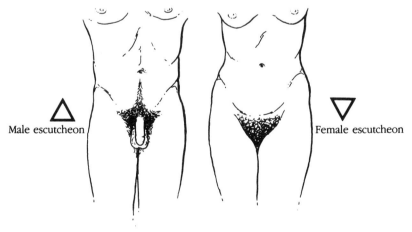

Fig. 3-6. Normal sexual hair distribution in adult men and women. Changes may signal hormonal abnormalities.

(1) Musculoskeletal irritability
(2) Mental status
(3) Hydration
   d. Pancreatic islets
     (1) Vital signs
     (2) Mental status

III. Cardinal Symptoms. Many of the following symptoms are also important objective physical findings.

  A. *Headache.* As a symptom caused by a pituitary tumor, the headache is often frontal or bitemporal in location.

  B. *Impairment of peripheral vision.* This symptom is produced when the optic chiasm is compromised by a pituitary tumor.

  C. *Increased perspiration.* This may be associated with excess growth hormone, thyroid hormone, or epinephrine, and with excess insulin activity causing hypoglycemia. *Decreased perspiration* is associated with deficient thyroid activity.

  D. *Hand tremor or sensation of tremulousness.* This is associated with excess thyroid hormone or epinephrine, or excess insulin activity with hypoglycemia.

  E. *Excess dark body hair in women.* Disorders of ovary or adrenal cortex result in excessive androgenic hormone production.

  F. *Temporal and vertex hair loss.* This hair loss may be associated with more profound degrees of excess androgenic activity in the female.

  G. *Loss of axillary and pubic hair.* This may be associated with decreased production of androgenic hormone classically associated with panhypopituitarism in either sex.

  H. *Fatigue and weakness.* Fatigue is associated with a large number of endocrine disorders, including Addison's and Cushing's diseases, primary aldosteronism, hyperparathyroidism, hyper- and hypothyroidism, and testicular and pituitary failure.

  I. *Light-headedness* or faintness, especially upon sudden standing. This is a frequent complaint in Addison's disease.

  J. *Excess pigmentation (darkening) of the skin and mucous membranes.* This commonly occurs in persons with Addison's disease.

  K. *Muscle cramps, spasm.* Cramping or spasm may be associated with hypoparathyroidism and primary aldosteronism.

  L. *Intolerance to heat or cold.* The former is associated with hyperthyroidism, and the latter with hypothyroidism.

  M. *Excess volume of urination.* Hyperparathyroidism, primary aldosteronism, diabetes mellitus, and diabetes insipidus may cause excess urination.

  N. *Protrusion of the eyes.* This is often associated with hyperthyroidism.

  O. *Weight loss.* Hyperthyroidism and Addison's disease often result in weight loss.

  P. *Amenorrhea.* This is associated with hypopituitarism, Cushing's disease, hyperprolactinemia, and ovarian failure.

  Q. *Irregular menses.* This is often associated with androgen excess.

IV. Abnormal Findings (Physical Signs of Endocrine Disease)

  A. Thyroid
    1. Enlargement or nodularity without clinical evidence of thyroid dysfunction. (Thyroid hyper- or hypofunction *can* accompany enlargement or nodularity, but usually does not.)
     a. Iodine deficiency
     b. Action of goitrogens
     c. Thyroid nodules or cysts
     d. Inflammation
    2. Hyperthyroidism
     a. Thyroid enlargement (usually)
     b. Signs of weight loss
     c. Fine tremor
     d. Warm, moist skin

   e. Brisk tendon reflexes
   f. Muscle weakness (proximal worse than distal)
   g. Rapid, bounding arterial pulses
   h. Wide pulse pressure (e.g., 180/70)
   i. Loud heart sounds
   j. Systolic ejection murmur, sinus tachycardia
   k. Atrial tachyarrhythmias (e.g., atrial fibrillation)
   l. Retraction of lids (stare, lid lag)
   m. Onycholysis (spooning or separation of nail from nail bed)
   n. Signs of Graves' disease (not related to hyperthyroidism)
      (1) Swelling of orbital contents
      (2) Swelling of conjunctivae (chemosis)
      (3) Weakness of extraocular muscles with limitation of upward gaze
         (late findings include loss of convergence and lateral movement)
      (4) Pretibial myxedema (darkening and thickening of skin)
      (5) Clubbing (thyroid acropachy)
3. Hypothyroidism
   a. Facial edema (puffiness of eyes)
   b. Thickening of lids and tongue
   c. Deepening of voice
   d. Slowness of speech and mentation
   e. Thickening and dryness of skin
   f. Coarsening and brittleness of hair
   g. Thinning of scalp hair and eyebrows (lateral)
   h. Subnormal body temperature
   i. Bradycardia
   j. Hypoactive reflexes with slow recovery phase
   k. Swelling of hands
   l. Muscle weakness
   m. Advanced disease—possible cardiac enlargement, pericardial and
      pleural effusion, hypertension, and coronary disease.
B. Gonads
   1. Male
      a. Prepubertal hypogonadism
         (1) Underdeveloped genitalia
         (2) Sparse body hair
         (3) Absent beard (juvenile facies)
         (4) Eunuchoid proportions (eunuchoidism)
            (a) Increased lower skeletal segment (relative)
            (b) Increased span (greater than height)
            (c) Tall stature with narrow hands and feet
            (d) Female-type fat distribution
      b. Adult hypogonadism (onset after completion of puberty)
         (1) Partial regression of secondary sex characteristics
         (2) Decreased facial and body hair
         (3) Decreased erection, potency, and libido, but no change in penile
            size
         (4) Decreased muscle strength
         (5) Softening of skin
      c. Estrogen excess
         (1) Gynecomastia
         (2) Decreased libido
   2. Female
      a. Prepubertal hypogonadism
         (1) Primary amenorrhea
         (2) Infantile genitalia
         (3) Sparse pubic and axillary hair
         (4) Failure of breast development
         (5) Eunuchoid proportions

           (a) Tall stature
           (b) Narrow hands and feet
           (c) Increased span and lower skeletal segment
      b. Adult hypogonadism
          (1) Secondary amenorrhea
          (2) Decreased breast size
          (3) Atrophy of external genitalia
      c. Androgen excess
          (1) Hirsutism
           (a) Coarse facial and body hair
           (b) Male pattern escutcheon
          (2) Virilism
           (a) Frontal balding
           (b) Increased muscle bulk and strength
           (c) Clitoromegaly
C. Adrenal glands
    1. Medullary hyperfunction (pheochromocytoma)
      a. Increased circulating epinephrine and norepinephrine account for all symptoms
      b. Paroxysmal or sustained hypertension
      c. Tremor
      d. Blanching of skin
      e. Tachycardia
      f. Sweating
    2. Cortex
      a. Cortical hyperfunction
          (1) Glucocorticoid excess (Cushing's syndrome)
           (a) Redistribution of fat
               (i) Fat accumulation in face, neck, supraclavicular, and cervicodorsal (buffalo hump) regions
               (ii) Facial changes
                  (a) Rounded face (moon facies)
                  (b) Bulging cheeks
                  (c) Preauricular fullness
                  (d) Plethoric appearance (polycythemia)
                  (e) Pouting lips
               (iii) Loss of fat over extremities and buttocks
           (b) Protein loss
               (i) Thin skin
               (ii) Easy bruising
               (iii) Stria
               (iv) Bone tenderness
               (v) Muscle atrophy
           (c) Wasted abdominal and extremity musculature
           (d) Hirsutism (fine, downy lanugo hair)
          (2) Mineralocorticoid excess (primary aldosteronism)
           (a) Hypertension
           (b) Muscle weakness due to potassium depletion
           (c) Alkalosis may cause tetany
          (3) Androgen excess (adrenogenital syndrome or adrenal tumor)
           (a) Hirsutism
               (i) Coarse facial and body hair
               (ii) Male pattern escutcheon
           (b) Virilism
               (i) Frontal balding
               (ii) Increased muscle bulk and strength
               (iii) Clitoromegaly
      b. Cortical hypofunction (Addison's disease)
          (1) Acute

  (a) Nausea, vomiting, and abdominal pain
  (b) Severe hypotension (shock)
  (c) Dehydration
  (d) Prostration
  (2) Chronic
  (a) Increased skin pigmentation
    (i) Exposed surfaces: distal extremities
    (ii) Pressure points: wrist, knees, elbows
    (iii) Scars, body folds, nipples
    (iv) Where garments exert pressure: belt, brassiere straps
  (b) Mucosal pigmentation
    (i) Blue-gray
    (ii) Buccal mucosa, tongue, gums
  (c) Possible vitiligo within pigmented areas
  (d) Muscle weakness and asthenia
  (e) Hypotension or orthostasis
  (f) Tachycardia
  (g) Decreased axillary and pubic hair in women
  (h) Weight loss
D. Parathyroid
  1. Hyperparathyroidism—physical signs due to accompanying hypercalcemia:
    a. Asymptomatic and normal physical examination (most patients)
    b. Muscle hypotonia and weakness
    c. Depression, mental confusion, obtundation, coma
    d. Corneal calcium deposits seen as faint white bands principally at 3 o'clock and 9 o'clock (band keratopathy)
    e. Calcium deposits (white flecks) on tarsal plates of eyelids and on eardrum
  2. Hypoparathyroidism—physical signs due to accompanying hypocalcemia:
    a. Tetany. Flexion of elbows, wrists, and metacarpophalangeal joints with extension of fingers; turning down of toes; arching of plantar surface of foot.
    b. Trousseau's sign. Apply a blood pressure cuff to forearm; inflate above systolic pressure for 3 minutes. Carpal spasm is positive sign.
    c. Chvostek's sign. Tap facial nerve. Contraction of facial muscles and orbicularis oculi is a positive sign (also positive in 10% of normal adults).
    d. Additional signs are cataracts, papilledema, dry skin, brittle nails, and thin patchy body hair.
E. Pancreatic islets
  1. Hypoglycemia
    a. Physical signs due to low blood sugar (hypoglycemia)
      (1) Diplopia
      (2) Mental confusion
      (3) Convulsions
      (4) Coma
    b. Physical signs due to secondary release of catecholamine
      (1) Tremor
      (2) Perspiration
      (3) Tachycardia
      (4) Anxiety
      (5) Papillary dilatation
      (6) Hunger
  2. Insulin deficiency
    a. Physical signs of moderate to severe hyperglycemia
      (1) Muscle weakness
      (2) Dehydration
        (a) Loss of skin turgor
        (b) Decreased tongue volume
        (c) Dry mucous membranes

          (d) Tachycardia
          (e) Hypotension
      (3) Evidence of weight loss
      (4) Drowsiness, confusion, stupor, coma
   b. Physical signs of ketoacidosis: tachypnea and deep respirations (Kussmaul respiration)
  3. Chronic diabetes mellitus (Signs are considered in Chapters 5, 8, 11, and 15.)
F. Anterior pituitary gland
  1. Giantism: abnormal body height due to prepubertal hypersecretion of growth hormone
  2. Acromegaly: postpubertal hypersecretion of growth hormone
   a. Early changes
      (1) Subtle coarsening of facial appearance
      (2) Prominent, moist, spongy soft tissues
   b. Later changes
      (1) Prominent forehead, coarse facial features, deep wrinkles
      (2) Mandibular elongation with overbite of lower incisors and separation of teeth
      (3) Thyroid enlargement
      (4) Dorsal kyphosis and degenerative arthritis
      (5) Large hands and feet
      (6) Husky voice due to enlargement of tongue and vocal cords
      (7) Enlargement of viscera, especially heart, liver, and spleen
      (8) Bitemporal field loss from compression of optic chiasm
  3. Dwarfism
   a. Pituitary dwarfism—prepubertal
      (1) Normal body proportions
      (2) Childlike features
  4. Hypopituitarism: reduced adenocorticotropic, thyrotropic, gonadotropic, melanotropic, and growth hormone in varying degree
   a. Features of mild hypothyroidism
   b. Loss of body hair (adrenal and gonadal deficiency)
   c. Asthenia, weight loss, and postural hypotension (adrenocortical deficiency)
   d. Depigmentation of areolar, skin, and genital regions (melanocyte-stimulating hormone deficiency)
   e. Hairless, pallid, smooth, dry, "alabaster" appearance
V. Available Technology
 A. Hormone analysis
  1. Immunoassays can be used to measure most clinically important hormone levels in blood.
  2. Primary organ failure is characterized by low levels of hormone secretion combined with elevated levels of tropic hormone that would normally be expected to stimulate hormone production.
   a. Adrenal insufficiency is characterized by low levels of cortisol and aldosterone and increased levels of adrenocorticotropic hormone (ACTH) and renin.
   b. Hypothyroidism is characterized by low levels of thyroxine and triiodothyronine and increased levels of thyroid stimulating hormone (TSH).
   c. Hypogonadism is characterized by low levels of estrogen or testosterone and increased levels of luteinizing hormone (LH) and follicle-stimulating hormone (FSH).
   d. Hypoparathyroidism is characterized by low levels of parathyroid hormone despite hypocalcemia.
  3. Secondary organ failure (hypopituitarism) is associated with low levels of both the tropic and the target hormones.

4. Primary hypersecretion syndromes are characterized by elevated target hormone levels associated with suppressed levels of tropic agents.

   a. Cushing's syndrome due to a hyperfunctioning adrenal tumor is characterized by elevated cortisol and suppressed ACTH.

   b. Primary aldosteronism is associated with elevated aldosterone and suppressed renin activity.

   c. Hyperthyroidism is associated with elevated thyroxine and triiodothyronine and suppressed TSH.

   d. Insulinoma is characterized by elevated insulin levels despite hypoglycemia.

5. Hypersecretion of tropic hormones is associated with continued oversecretion of the hormone despite suppressive levels of feedback agents.

   a. Cushing's syndrome due to hypersecretion of ACTH is characterized by increased ACTH despite increased cortisol.

   b. Hyperparathyroidism is characterized by increased parathyroid hormone despite elevated calcium levels.

B. Dynamic testing

   1. Diagnosis of hormone deficiency may require stimulation testing to confirm the diagnosis.

      a. ACTH stimulation is used to establish adrenal insufficiency.

      b. Insulin-induced hypoglycemia is used to establish deficiency of ACTH and growth hormone.

   2. Diagnosis of hypersecretion of hormones may require suppression testing.

      a. Dexamethasone suppression is used to diagnose Cushing's syndrome.

      b. Saline suppression may be used to diagnose primary aldosteronism.

C. Imaging studies

   1. Pituitary imaging is best performed with magnetic resonance imaging (MRI); computed tomography (CT) also usually provides adequate visualization.

   2. Thyroid visualization

      a. Thyroid ultrasonography is often used to characterize the nature of thyroid nodules. Simple cysts are unlikely to be malignant.

      b. Substernal thyroid glands may require radiographic characterization.

         (1) Chest radiograph will identify large substernal thyroid glands and indicate presence of tracheal deviation.

         (2) Chest CT provides better delineation of the size and extent of substernal goiters.

   3. Pancreatic islet cell anatomy can be difficult to assess.

      a. Abdominal CT scanning will demonstrate large islet cell tumors.

      b. Endoscopic ultrasonography provides better definition of small tumors.

   4. Adrenal CT scanning is routinely used for determining adrenal anatomy.

D. Radioisotope studies

   1. Radioiodine and technetium thyroid scans are commonly used to determine thyroid function and structure.

      a. Scanning may be of value in characterizing thyroid nodules. Autonomously functioning nodules are unlikely to be malignant.

      b. Isotope uptake is particularly helpful in characterizing the cause of hyperthyroidism.

   2. Parathyroid scanning is occasionally used to identify the location of hyperplastic or tumorous glands.

   3. Adrenal scanning

      a. Adrenal cortical scanning: iodocholesterol scan for identification of unilateral or bilateral function. Scans done during dexamethasone treatment can indicate mineralocorticoid activity.

      b. Adrenal medullary scanning: MIBG (radioiodinated metaiodobenzylguanidine) scans effectively identify active catecholamine-secreting tissue.

E. The cost figures cited in this table are **basic direct costs**. The figures are difficult to obtain and change quickly. They include **only** the cost of the test itself (technician, equipment, time, and materials). No professional costs (interpretation) are included. Costs vary from region to region based on differences in some components such as labor. However, the relative cost ranking should remain similar.

Procedure	Code
Hormone analysis; immunoassays	$$$$
Dynamic testing	
Stimulation testing	$$$$
Suppression testing	$$$$
Imaging studies	
Magnetic resonance imaging (MRI)	$$$$
Thyroid visualization	$$
Ultrasonography	$$
Chest x-ray	$
Computed tomography (CT)—chest	$$$
Pancreatic islet cell anatomy	*
CT—abdomen	$$$
Endoscopic ultrasonography	$$$
CT—adrenal	$$$
Radioisotope studies	
Thyroid	$$$$$
Parathyroid	$$$$$
Adrenal scanning	$$$$$$

$ = $0–$50; $$ = $50–$100; $$$ = $100–$200; $$$$ = $200–$500; $$$$$ = $500–$1000; $$$$$$ = >$1000; * = highly variable or not available.

VI. Bibliography

Daniels GH. Physical examination of the thyroid gland. In: Braverman LE, Utiger RD, eds. *The Thyroid.* Philadelphia: JB Lippincott, 1991:572–577.

Heshka S, Buhl K, Heynsfield SB. Obesity: clinical evaluation of body composition and energy expenditure. In: Blackburn GL, Kanders BS, eds. *Obesity: Pathophysiology, Psychology and Treatment.* New York: Chapman & Hall, 1994:39–79.

Molitch M. Clinical manifestations of acromegaly. *Endocrinol Metab Clin North Am* 1992;27:597–621.

Muir A, Maclaren NK. Autoimmune diseases of the adrenal glands, parathyroid glands, gonads, and hypothalamic-pituitary axis. *Endocrinol Metab Clin North Am* 1991;20:619–644.

Nordyke RA, Gilbert FI Jr, Harada ASM. Graves' disease: influence of age on clinical findings. *Arch Intern Med* 1988;148:626.

Oddie TH, Boyd CM, Fisher DA, Hales IR. Incidence of signs and symptoms in thyroid disease. *Med J Aust* 1972;2:981.

Plymate S. Hypogonadism. *Endocrinol Clin North Am* 1994;213:749–772.

Rosenfield RL, Lucky AW. Acne, hirsutism, and alopecia in adolescent girls: clinical expressions of androgen excess. *Endocrinol Metab Clin North Am* 1993;22: 507–532.

Silverberg J, Gharib H. Evaluation and diagnosis of nodular thyroid disease. In: Mazzaferri EL, Samaan NA, eds. *Endocrine Tumors* Boston: Blackwell Scientific Publications, 1993:233–242.

Yanovski JA, Cutler GB Jr. Glucocorticoid action and the clinical features of Cushing's syndrome. *Endocrinol Metab Clin North Am* 1994;23:487–509.

VII. Key Search Words

The following key words reflect the content of this chapter. They are provided to assist with an on-line search of computer databases, such as MEDLINE, if you wish to pursue the topic of this chapter further.

Acromegaly
Addison's disease
Adrenal glands
Adrenal gland diseases
Body constitution
Cushing's syndrome
Goiter
Hirsutism
Hyperthyroidism
Hypogonadism
Hypopituitarism
Hypothyroidism
Ovary
Parathyroid glands
Pituitary gland
Testis
Thyroid diseases
Thyroid gland
Thyroid hormones
Virilism

4. HEMATOPOIETIC SYSTEM

Paul T. Adams

I. Glossary

Agranulocytosis: absence of circulating polymorphonuclear leukocytes.

Anemia: reduction in the number of circulating red blood cells or hemoglobin or both with respect to age and sex.

Epistaxis: nosebleeds.

Erythrocytosis: increase in the number of circulating red blood cells with respect to age and sex.

Hematopoietic: blood-forming.

Hemolysis: accelerated dissolution or destruction of red blood cells *in vivo*.

Infectious mononucleosis: systemic infection associated with enlargement of lymph nodes and spleen and with eliciting an atypical lymphocytosis.

Leukemias: a group of disorders of the bone marrow characterized by excessive proliferation or failure of differentiation of one of the types of white blood cells.

Leukocytosis: increase in the white blood cell count above normal.

Leukopenia: decrease in the white blood cell count below normal.

Lymphadenitis: inflammation of one or more lymph nodes.

Lymphadenopathy: any lymph node enlargement.

Lymphoma: general term for neoplasms originating from the lymphoid reticulum.

Myeloid: pertaining to the granulocytic cell lines.

Neutropenia: an absolute decrease in the number of circulating granulocytic cells.

Petechiae: pinpoint-sized hemorrhages.

Polycythemia: erythrocytosis.

Polycythemia, secondary: erythrocytosis secondary to chronic hypoxia and other rarer causes such as renal tumors.

Polycythemia vera: primary or idiopathic erythrocytosis, often accompanied by leukocytosis, thrombocytosis, and splenomegaly.

Pruritus: itching.

Purpura: purplish discolorations caused by bleeding into the skin and visible mucous membranes, that is, "black and blue spots."

Shotty: descriptive term applied to lymph nodes meaning firm, freely movable, and nontender.

Splenomegaly: enlargement of the spleen.

Thrombocytopenia: reduction below normal in the number of circulating platelets.

Thrombocytosis: increase above normal in the number of circulating platelets.

II. Techniques of Examination and Normal Findings.

The physical signs associated with hematologic disorders are due either to changes in the reticulum of the lymph nodes, spleen, or liver, or to indirect manifestations involving the skin, mucous membranes, ocular fundi, or bone.

A. Lymph nodes

1. Examination techniques

   a. Important factors and considerations. Normal lymph nodes are not palpable, but nodes enlarged from prior inflammation may be palpable. In children up to 12 years of age, shotty cervical nodes up to 1 cm in diameter are almost always felt in the occipital region, the axillae, and the inguinal region. In adolescents and adults, palpable inguinal lymph nodes are very common and may be of little significance.

    b. Examination techniques including inspection and palpation. Compare sides, using middle three fingers for palpation. Use slow, gentle movements; fingers should oscillate up and down, back and forth, and in a rotary motion.

    c. Recording of findings. Include five characteristics:

        (1) Location

        (2) Size—diameter in centimeters. Include any descriptive terms, such as split-pea, bean, almond.

        (3) Tenderness

        (4) Degree of fixation (movable, matted, fixed)

        (5) Texture (hard, soft, firm)

2. Three regional groups of lymph nodes.

    a. Cervicofacial and supraclavicular nodes. Palpation must be light, or small nodes will escape notice. Look for asymmetry and lymphadenopathy.

        (1) Methods of palpation

            (a) Anterior approach (Fig. 4-1). In this approach, the hand not used for palpation controls the head.

            (b) Posterior approach (Fig. 4-2). Flex patient's neck to obtain proper relaxation of muscles, and palpate both sides simultaneously.

        (2) Examination procedure. Begin above and posteriorly (Fig.4-3), and proceed downward as follows:

            (a) Occipital and postauricular

            (b) Submaxillary and submental

            (c) Anterior triangle (upper end of deep cervical chain)

            (d) Downward along the sternocleidomastoid muscle (superficial cervical nodes)

            (e) Posterior triangle (lower end of deep cervical chain)

            (f) Supraclavicular

    b. Axillary and epitrochlear nodes

        (1) Axillary nodes. Patient may be sitting or supine. Support the patient's arm (Fig. 4-4), but do not abduct the arm too far. Cup hand slightly and reach as high into the apex of the axilla as possible. Pull down, exerting gentle pressure against the thorax with finger-

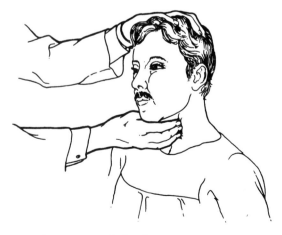

Fig. 4-1. Palpation of anterior cervical nodes.

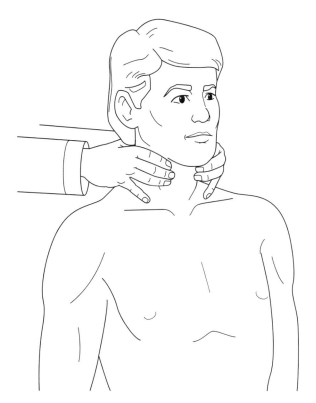

Fig. 4-2. Technique of exmaination of cervicofacial lymph nodes, posterior approach.

tips. Repeat several times, checking the following in this order: lateral group (posterior), central group, pectoral group.

(2) Epitrochlear nodes. Palpate as shown in Figure 4-5.

c. Inguinal and femoral nodes. Palpate using the rotary motion described above. The nodes in the inguinal region are commonly enlarged; this is a poor site for biopsy. Femoral node enlargement is more commonly of pathologic significance.

B. Spleen. Patient lies supine, arms at sides, knees flexed slightly.

1. Percussion. Begin by outlining the area of splenic dullness; this will delineate the size of the spleen and loosen the abdomen.

2. Palpation. Normally, the spleen is not palpable in the adult. It must be two or three times normal size before it becomes palpable. If the spleen is greatly enlarged, direct initial palpation to the left lower portion of abdomen. The keys to proper splenic palpation are proper instructions to the patient about breathing and gentleness by the examiner.

a. Place left hand under patient's left flank, and lightly press the tips of the index and middle fingers of the right hand to a point just beneath the costal margin (Fig.4-6A). Ask the patient to turn his or her head away from you and take a long, deep breath through the mouth. Do not move your hand as the patient inhales. The edge of an enlarged spleen (splenomegaly) will brush against your fingers, lifting them slightly upward. As patient exhales, probe more deeply, moving the fingertips in

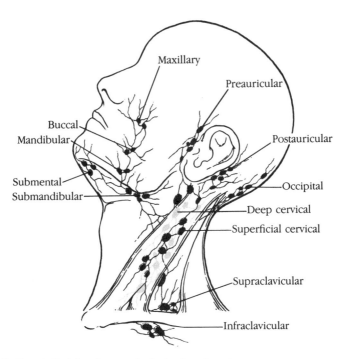

Fig. 4-3. Cervicofacial and supraclavicular lymph nodes.

a slightly rotary motion. If nothing is felt, drop hand about 1 cm and re-peat. Do not dig; this will cause muscle spasm.

b. Special maneuver no. 1. Have patient slip left forearm under the small of the back (see Fig.4-6B). This will tend to thrust the spleen upward.

c. Special maneuver no. 2. Roll patient on right side, with right leg straight and left knee flexed (see Fig.4-6C). The left shoulder is sup-ported by the flexed left arm, and it rotates posteriorly to the left; this thrusts the spleen forward and medially. Place the tips of your fingers 1 or 2 cm below the costal margin.

C. Liver. The technique for examining the liver is described in Chapter 9.

III. Cardinal Symptoms and Abnormal Findings

  A. Common clinical disorders

   1. Anemia. Important general symptoms are pallor, ease of fatigue, weak-ness, headache, lassitude, shortness of breath on exertion, faintness, and vertigo. These are due to increased circulatory effort, caused by deficient oxygenation of the tissues, especially the brain. In an otherwise healthy person, a gradual fall in hemoglobin level may not become conspicuous until hemoglobin is lowered to half its normal value, unless there is a fall in blood volume. Aerobic activity will exacerbate an anemia, causing symptomatology earlier than will sedentary activity.

   2. Leukemias and lymphomas commonly give rise to anemia, leukopenia, and thrombocytopenia.

    a. General symptoms: epistaxis, gum bleeding, petechiae, purpura, frank hemorrhage anywhere in body.

    b. Systemic symptoms: weight loss, fatigue, heat intolerance, night sweats, fever, pruritus.

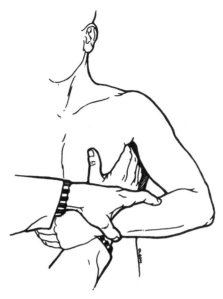

Fig. 4-4. Palpation of axillary nodes.

    c. Lymph nodes. Rapidly enlarging lymph nodes with acute distention of the capsule may be sore to exquisitely tender. Slowly enlarging nodes produce no symptoms until mechanical difficulties occur.
       (1) Enlarged mediastinal and hilar lymph nodes can compress the trachea, causing respiratory embarrassment with a dry, brassy cough, progressive dyspnea, orthopnea, and cyanosis. Swelling of face and neck (superior mediastinal syndrome) may be caused by obstruction to lymphatic and venous return.
       (2) Enlarged retroperitoneal, periaortic, and perifemoral nodes can cause ascites and edema of lower extremities.
       (3) Enlarged spleen. Early satiety, constipation, or diarrhea may occur if the spleen encroaches on the stomach and intestine.
  3. Polycythemia vera and secondary polycythemia. Total blood volume and blood viscosity are increased, commonly causing congestive heart failure, headache, flushing, hemorrhage, and thromboembolic phenomena.
B. Lymph nodes. It is often not possible to determine whether a node is normal or abnormal simply by its texture. Any node may show changes on microscopic examination.
  1. Localized lymphadenopathy is usually due to inflammation or neoplasm.
    a. Acute lymphadenitis. Inflammation causes enlarged, tender, rather soft nodes, sometimes associated with induration and the red streaks of lymphangitis. The primary site of infection is usually obvious.
    b. Metastatic lymphadenopathy. Nodes are usually stony hard, nontender, and somewhat fixed to underlying structures. To estimate the most likely site of a primary lesion, knowledge of the various patterns of lymphatic drainage is necessary.
    c. Other causes of localized lymphadenopathy are Hodgkin's disease or chronic granulomatous processes such as tuberculosis.

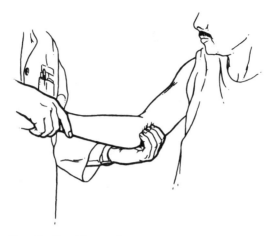

Fig. 4-5. Palpation of epitrochlear nodes.

2. Generalized lymphadenopathy is usually due to inflammation or neo-plasm. Many disorders not listed here are associated at times with generalized lymphadenopathy.

  a. Inflammation. Acute generalized lymphadenopathy is commonly caused by secondary syphilis, viral infections (infectious mononucleosis, measles), and hypersensitivity reactions (serum sickness). Such nodes are soft, movable, and slightly tender. Chronic systemic infections may produce generalized lymphadenopathy.

  b. Neoplasm

   (1) Lymphomas initially may cause painless, progressive, discrete enlargement of the nodes—often localized. Later, the enlargement often becomes generalized with firm, matted, and fixed nodes.

   (2) Acute leukemia rarely produces generalized lymphadenopathy. In monocytic leukemia with oropharyngeal infection, lymphadenopathy is most conspicuous in the cervicosubmandibular areas. Chronic lymphocytic leukemia often results in generalized lymphadenopathy, with nodes 1 to 3 cm in diameter, nontender, elastic (rubbery), and freely movable. Other varieties of leukemia produce variable degrees of lymph node enlargement.

C. Spleen. If greatly enlarged, the spleen may be missed on palpation. Careful inspection, preliminary percussion, and repeated palpation at ever lower levels of the abdomen can prevent this pitfall. If the splenic capsule has been acutely distended (as in infectious mononucleosis, splenic infarction, intrasplenic hemorrhage), use great caution to avoid splenic rupture. If the area is tender, listen for a splenic friction rub—a common finding with splenic infarction.

  1. Splenic hyperplasia occurs as a response to many systemic bacterial, parasitic, viral, or mycotic infections.

   a. Acute enlargement occurs with hematogenous dissemination of infectious organisms, such as in bacterial endocarditis, septicemia, and miliary tuberculosis.

   b. Chronic enlargement occurs with malaria, rheumatoid arthritis, other relapsing or progressive inflammatory diseases, chronic anemias, and polycythemia vera.

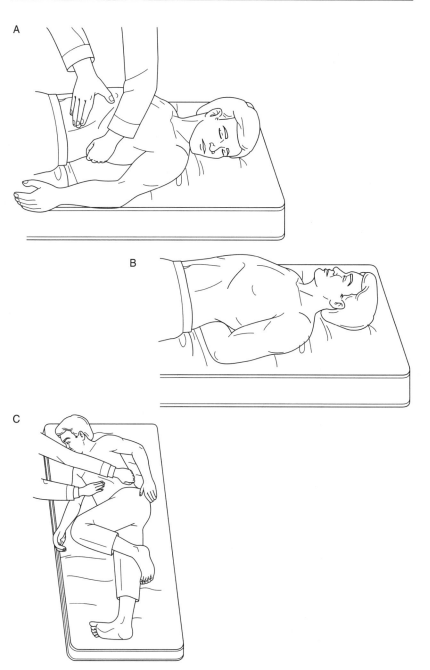

Fig. 4-6. Palpation of the spleen. **(A)** Positioning of examiner's hands. **(B)** Placement of patient's left forearm to elevate his left flank. **(C)** Examination of patient positioned on his right side to bring spleen forward.

Table 4-1. Classification of Splenomegaly[a]

Slight Enlargement (1–4 cm)	Moderate Enlargement (4–8 cm)	Great Enlargement (>8 cm)
Subacute bacterial endocarditis	Cirrhosis of the liver	Chronic granulocytic leukemia
Miliary tuberculosis	Acute leukemia	Chronic malaria
Septicemia	Chronic lymphocytic leukemia	Congenital syphilis in infant
Rheumatoid arthritis	Lymphoblastoma	Amyloidosis
Syphilis	Infectious mononucleosis	Agnogenic myeloid metaplasia
Typhoid	Polycythemia vera	Rare diseases: Gaucher's disease, Niemann-Pick disease, kala-azar, tropical eosinophilia
Brucellosis	Hemolytic anemia	
Congestive heart failure	Sarcoidosis	
Acute hepatitis	Rickets	
Acute malaria		
Pernicious anemia		

[a]Distance of splenic edge below the left costal margin on deep inspiration.

    2. Splenic congestion is due to portal hypertension and may be secondary to chronic hepatic disease, congestive heart failure, or occlusion of splenic or portal veins. Cirrhosis of the liver is the most common cause.

    3. Splenic infiltration. Splenic pulp may be replaced by neoplasm (leukemias, lymphomas), amyloid, myeloid elements (extramedullary hematopoiesis), or lipid-filled reticuloendothelial cells (Gaucher's disease).

D. Skin. Many hematologic disorders have cutaneous manifestations.

    1. Pallor and coldness may occur in chronic anemia. Check nail beds and conjunctiva.

    2. Rubor, particularly of the face and neck, may occur with polycythemia vera and is often associated with dilatation of superficial veins and venules and with bloodshot eyes.

    3. Cyanosis may be associated with secondary polycythemia.

    4. Icterus (jaundice) may be a sign of rapid hemolysis.

    5. Purpura may occur with a number of deficiencies of the hemostatic mechanism.

        a. Petechiae: superficial, cutaneous, or mucosal hemorrhages less than 5 mm in size

        b. Ecchymoses: purplish lesions with irregular borders, greater than 5 mm in size

    6. Pruritus may be intense with certain lymphomas, resulting in extensive excoriation of the skin. Primary invasion of the skin and almost any type of secondary dermatitis can occur in lymphoma or leukemia (see Chapter 2).

E. Mucosa

    1. Glossitis and stomatitis are common with deficiency anemias. With long-standing anemia, atrophy of glossal papillae occurs, making the tongue pale and smooth. Gums may bleed whenever a blood disorder causes a hemorrhagic tendency.

    2. Gingival and mucosal ulcerations of mouth and pharynx occur with leukemia, particularly acute forms. A characteristic plum-colored swelling of the gingivae may be the most prominent physical finding in monocytic leukemia. Necrotic mucosal ulcers and pharyngitis are important signs of agranulocytosis.

F. Bone. Bone tenderness and pain commonly accompany disorders of the blood-forming organs.

1. Sternum. Exquisite tenderness may develop owing to increased intramedullary proliferation of blood cells, as in leukemias and regenerative anemias.

2. Localized bone tenderness may be due to invasion of bone by leukemia or other hematopoietic malignancies (e.g., multiple myeloma, Hodgkin's disease).

G. Ocular fundi. Many hematologic disorders produce fundoscopic signs (retinal edema, hemorrhages, exudates, venous dilatation, and tortuosity) due to hypoxemia, thrombocytopenia, stasis, capillary injury, or metabolic deficiencies (see Chapter 5).

IV. Available Technology

A. Examination of peripheral blood. A complete blood count should be performed on all patients.

B. Examination of bone marrow. Aspiration and needle biopsy of bone marrow and interpretation of bone marrow films can detect infiltrative processes and determine the effectiveness of hematopoiesis.

C. Lymph node biopsy. Excisional biopsy of a peripheral node (cervical, supraclavicular, axillary preferred) is a simple way to establish a tissue diagnosis.

D. Positive-pressure test for capillary fragility (Rumpel-Leede phenomenon). Place blood pressure cuff around upper arm; determine systolic and diastolic pressures. Inflate cuff to midway between these levels, but not higher than 100 mmHg. Observe for 5 minutes for petechiae. Normally, not more than one petechia forms. Grade 0 to 4+, depending on speed and number of petechiae formed. If petechiae begin to form promptly, discontinue the test immediately to avoid severe purpuric skin damage.

E. X-ray. Chest x-rays, including lateral views, are essential in evaluating intrathoracic lymphadenopathy.

F. Lymphangiography (serial filming of the trunk after the injection of a radiopaque medium into peripheral lymphatics) can determine the size, contour, and texture of deep femoral, iliac, and periaortic nodes. The mesenteric nodes are not visualized.

G. Nuclear medicine imaging

1. Gallium scan. Most lymphomas are gallium-avid tumors, especially Hodgkin's disease tumors. The most useful application is in determining whether residual adenopathy contains viable tumor following Hodgkin's therapy. Gallium scans are most useful when evaluating disease above the diaphragm and should be done before and after the completion of therapy.

2. Liver-spleen scan. The most useful application is in determining the presence of an accessory spleen after splenectomy in patients with immune thrombocytopenic purpura. It has limited usefulness in determining the size of liver or spleen or in determining whether space-occupying lesions are present, because better imaging studies are available.

3. Positron emission tomography. This technique identifies areas of metabolic activity and is therefore useful in distinguishing scar tissue from persistent malignancy.

4. Bone scan. This test highlights areas of osteoblastic activity but is not useful in multiple myeloma because lesions tend to have little osteoblastic activity. It can be useful in detecting areas of involvement by lymphoma that has demonstrated a predilection for the bone.

H. Imaging studies

1. Computed tomography (CT). CT remains the mainstay in evaluating activity of lymphoma and is the most effective test for assessing growth of lymphoma or its response to therapy.

2. Skeletal survey. The most useful test for evaluating the activity of myelomatous bone lesions, skeletal surveys should be done periodically on all patients with multiple myeloma to assess the efficacy of therapy and to prevent pathologic fractures.

3. Lymphangiogram. Useful in detecting occult disease below the diaphragm in patients with Hodgkin's disease above the diaphragm, it can detect space-occupying lesions in normal-sized lymph nodes up to the level of L1. The clinical usefulness is in deciding whether radiation therapy should be the primary treatment modality or in determining whether a staging laparotomy is indicated.

4. Magnetic resonance imaging (MRI). MRI is the most useful test in evaluating bone lymphoma. It is also the most sensitive test for lymphomatous involvement in the brain and in evaluating liver lesions.

I. The cost figures cited in this table are **basic direct costs**. The figures are difficult to obtain and change quickly. They include **only** the cost of the test itself (technician, equipment, time, and materials). No professional costs (interpretation) are included. Costs vary from region to region based on differences in some components such as labor. However, the relative cost ranking should remain similar.

Procedure	Code
Complete blood count	$
Examination of bone marrow	$$$
Lymph node biopsy	$$
Positive-pressure test for capillary fragility (Rumpel-Leede phenomenon)	*
Chest x-rays, including lateral views	$
Lymphangiography	$$$$
Nuclear studies	
Gallium scan	$$$$
Liver-spleen scan	$$$$
Positron emission tomography (PET)	$$$$$$
Bone scan	$$$$
Imaging studies	
Computed tomography (CT)	$$$
Skeletal survey	$
Lymphangiography	$$$$
Magnetic resonance imaging (MRI)	$$$$

$ = $0–$50; $$ = $50–$100; $$$ = $100–$200; $$$$ = $200–$500; $$$$$$ =>$1000; * = highly variable or not available.

V. Bibliography

Barkun AN, Camus M, Green L, et al. The bedside assessment of splenic enlargement. *Am J Med* 1991;91(5):512–518.

Burns CP, Armitage JO, Frey AL, et al. Analysis of the presenting features of adult acute leukemia: the French-American-British classification. *Cancer* 1981; 47(10):2460–2469.

Even-Sapir E, Bar-Shalom R, Israel O, et al. Single-photon emission computed tomography quantitation of gallium citrate uptake for the differentiation of lymphoma from benign hilar uptake. *J Clin Oncol* 1995;13(4):942–946.

Grover SA, Barkun AN, Sackett DL. Does this patient have splenomegaly? *JAMA* 1993;270(18):2218–2221.

Hoane BR, Shields AF, Porter BA, Borrow JW. Comparison of initial lymphoma staging using computed tomography (CT) and magnetic resonance (MR) imaging. *Am J Hematol* 1994;47(2):100–105.

Howard MR, Taylor PR, Lucraft HH, et al. Bone marrow examination in newly diagnosed Hodgkin's disease: current practice in the United Kingdom. *Br J Cancer* 1995;71(1):210–212.

Kyle RA. Multiple myeloma: review of 869 cases. *Mayo Clin Proc* 1975;50(1): 29–40.

Newman JS, Francis IR, Kaminski MS, Wahl RL. Imaging of lymphoma with PET with 2-[F-18]-fluoro-2-deoxy-D-glucose: correlation with CT. *Radiology* 1994; 190(1):111–116.

Pangalis GA, Vassilakopoulos TP, Boussiotis VA, Fessas P. Clinical approach to lymphadenopathy. *Semin Oncol* 1993;20(6):570–582.

Sandrasegaran K, Robinson PJ, Selby P. Staging of lymphoma in adults. *Clin Radiol* 1994;49(3):149–161.

Tamayo SG, Rickman LS, Mathews WC, et al. Examiner dependence on physical diagnostic tests for the detection of splenomegaly: a prospective study with multiple observers. *J Gen Intern Med* 1993;8(2):69–75.

VI. Key Search Words

The following key words reflect the content of this chapter. They are provided to assist with an on-line search of computer databases, such as MEDLINE, if you wish to pursue the topic of this chapter further.

Hepatomegaly
Leukemia
Lymphoma
Magnetic resonance imaging
Multiple myeloma
Physical examination
Positron-emission tomography
Splenomegaly
Tomography, x-ray computed

5. VISUAL SYSTEM

Terry J. Bergstrom

I. Glossary

Accommodation: increase in optical power (focus) by the eye to maintain a clear image as objects are moved closer (occurring through ciliary muscle contraction).

Amblyopia: decreased vision of an eye without detectable anatomic damage.

Anisocoria: inequality in size of the pupils.

Anterior segment: anterior third of the eye, from the anterior surface of the vitreous forward.

Anterior synechiae: adhesions between iris and cornea.

Arcus senilis: a white ring around the limbus of the cornea occurring in patients usually older than 60 years (also called *corneal arcus*).

Asthenopia: discomfort related to use of the eyes.

A-V nicking: the indentation of a retinal vein by a retinal arteriole in arteriolosclerosis/hypertension.

Cataract: opacity in the crystalline lens of the eye.

Conjunctivitis: inflammation of the conjunctiva.

Cycloplegia: paralysis of the ciliary muscles resulting in paralysis of accommodation.

Diplopia: double vision.

Ectropion: eversion of the lid border.

Entropion: inversion of the lid border.

Epiphora: the overflow of tears down the cheek.

Exophthalmos: abnormal protrusion of the eyeball, usually associated with thyroid abnormalities.

Funduscopy: examination of the interior of the eyeball using an ophthalmoscope (preferred term *ophthalmoscopy*).

Glaucoma: disease characterized by elevation of intraocular pressure resulting in damage to optic nerve and retinal nerve fibers.

Hyphema: presence of blood in the anterior chamber of the eye.

Hypopyon: presence of pus in the anterior chamber, often with a horizontal fluid level.

Intraocular pressure: fluid pressure inside the eye.

Iritis: inflammation of the iris.

Miosis: constriction of the pupil; a drug that constricts the pupil is called a *miotic.*

Mydriasis: dilation of the pupil; a drug that dilates the pupil is called a *mydriatic.*

Nystagmus: involuntary rhythmic movement of the eyes.

O.D.: abbreviation for the right eye *(oculus dexter).*

O.S.: abbreviation for the left eye *(oculus sinister).*

O.U.: abbreviation for both eyes *(oculus uterque).*

Optic atrophy: optic nerve degeneration characterized by paleness of the optic nerve and an irreversible loss of vision.

Papilledema: swelling of the optic nerve head associated with elevated intracranial pressure.

Phoria: latent tendency to deviation of the visual axes, which is held in check by the fusion mechanism.

Photophobia: sensitivity to and discomfort from light, which is usually associated with corneal or iris inflammation.

Posterior synechiae: adhesions between the iris and the lens.

Presbyopia: diminished power of accommodation of the eye because of aging of the crystalline lens.

Proptosis: abnormal protrusion or forward displacement of the eyeball.

Ptosis: drooping of the upper lid (blepharoptosis).

Tropia: constant deviation of the visual axes from parallelism that is not overcome by the fusion reflex.

Visual field: extent of space visible to an eye when the eye is directed straight ahead.

Yoke muscles: muscle pairs, one on each eye, which lead in a specific diagnostic position; for example, the right lateral rectus and the left medial rectus in gaze to the right side.

II. Techniques of Examination and Normal Findings

A. Components of the examination. A complete ocular examination includes:

1. Measurement of visual acuity.
2. Assessment of visual fields
3. External evaluation
4. Testing of the pupillary reactions
5. Evaluation of the extraocular muscles
6. Assessment of the ocular fundus
7. Measurement of the intraocular pressure

B. Procedure. To perform the examination in an orderly manner, begin from the outside of the eye and proceed toward the inside. Visual acuity measurement is always the first part of the examination, since it must be accomplished before palpation of the external structures or before the use of light to check pupils, and so on; these procedures will affect the visual acuity.

C. Requirements

1. Eye chart or reading card
2. Penlight type of flashlight
3. Ophthalmoscope
4. Mydriatic drops for pupillary dilation
5. Tonometer for measurement of intraocular pressure
6. Sufficiently darkened examining room

D. Visual acuity measurement. An accurate estimate of vision should be accomplished in all patients; it is mandatory in cases of head trauma or injury of face or eyes. If the patient customarily uses corrective lenses, measurement of visual acuity should be accomplished with the patient wearing those glasses or contact lenses.

1. Distance vision, measured by Snellen's chart

    a. Seat the patient 20 feet from the chart, test one eye at a time while completely covering the other eye; ask the patient to read the letters starting from the top of the chart proceeding downward.

    b. Snellen's chart is constructed to determine the distance at which a patient can read letters of a size that subtends an angle of 5 minutes of arc at the eye (Fig. 5-1). Each row of the chart represents a distance at which the normal eye can see the letters in 5 minutes of arc. The top is designated 20/200, which means that, when seated 20 feet from the chart, the patient is reading a letter that would ordinarily be read at 200 feet by someone with normal vision (in other words, that letter subtends a 5-minute arc 200 feet away). The numbers are not fractions: 20/200 does not equal 1/10th.

    c. Recording the results. Record which eye has been tested, the last row in which the patient is able to read the majority of the letters, and whether glasses or contact lenses are worn to correct the refractive error. Record in the following manner:

    OD 20/30−2 (meaning: missed two letters on the 20/30 row)
    OS 20/40+2 (meaning: 20/40 row read completely plus two letters on the 20/30 row)
    Add "with correction" or "without correction" as appropriate.

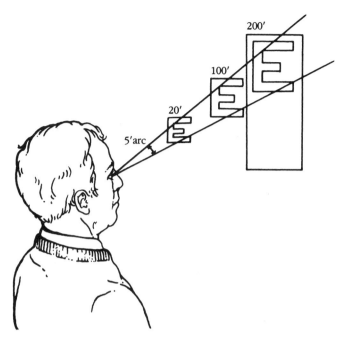

Fig. 5-1. Principle of testing visual acuity with Snellen's chart.

      d. Normal findings. Vision of 20/30 or better in each eye is acceptable, even though 20/20 vision is considered normal. There is usually no more than a one-line difference between the vision of the two eyes.
2. Near vision. Graded reading cards are available to measure near vision, but ordinary newsprint will suffice in a general examination. Persons over age 40 begin to have near-vision problems due to presbyopia and will require reading correction to appropriately measure the near vision. Have the patient hold the reading material at his or her usual reading distance (usually about 14 inches from the eyes). Test one eye at a time while completely covering the other, and note the reading distance the patient uses if markedly different from 14 inches.
3. Low vision
      a. Snellen's chart. Move the patient closer to the chart until he or she can read the large letter at the top. Record the distance at which the letter can be seen (e.g., 5/200 means the patient is seated 5 feet from the chart and reads the 200-size letter). If a person still cannot identify a letter on the chart, continue below.
      b. Finger/hand motions. Hold up your fingers and ask the patient to count them, recording the distance at which this occurs (e.g., "counts fingers at 2 feet"). If the patient is unable to do this, move your hand and record "hand movement" and the distance at which this occurs. If a person still does not respond to hand movement, continue below.
      c. Direction of light. If the patient can determine the direction from which a flashlight beam is shining, record "light projection." If light is perceived without recognition of direction, record "light perception." If no light is perceived, record "no light perception."

E. Visual field assessment with the confrontation method (if indicated by history)

   1. Assume position directly in front of the patient about 2 feet away so that your face is level with the patient's face.

   2. Instruct the patient to completely cover one eye (with an opaque occluder or palm of the hand—not the fingers) and to look at your open eye that is directly opposite that of the patient's noncovered eye. Close your corresponding (opposite) eye so that your visual field is roughly superimposed on that of the patient.

   3. Place your hand equidistant between yourself and the patient.

   4. Sequentially display one, two, or five fingers in one quadrant of the visual field, and ask the patient to identify how many fingers are displayed (don't let the patient look directly at the fingers, but direct him or her to continue to look at your open eye).

   5. Compare the patient's field of vision against your own.

   6. Test each of the four quadrants—upper left, upper right, lower left, and lower right.

   7. Have the patient occlude the other eye and repeat the above testing sequence.

F. External examination. Observe the face, orbits, eyelids, and eyes, and their general physical characteristics. Clues to general disease may be evident in facial and ocular expression. Compare one side of the face to the other with particular attention to the orbits and eyes regarding position of the orbits, eyebrows, and eyelids, size and shape of the orbital structures and eyes, alignment of the eyes, and prominence (bulging) or retraction of the eyes.

   1. Eyebrows. Note position and configuration and the presence of exudates and deposits and scaliness of the underlying skin.

   2. Eyelids. Inspect and palpate the eyelids, noting the position of the lids in relation to the globe, the condition and position of the eyelashes, the completeness of opening and closing of the lids, and any unusual color (e.g., redness, darkening), edema (swelling), or lesions. Many structural variations fall within the normal range. A slight difference in the palpebral fissures (distance between the lids when the eyes are open) is not usually significant unless associated with pupillary inequality. Differences in depth of the upper lid fold between patients are normal; racial differences can also be expected.

   3. Lacrimal apparatus (Fig. 5-2). Inspect and palpate the lacrimal gland area in the upper temporal orbit and the lacrimal drainage system nasally. Abnormalities include a palpable, tender lacrimal gland, excessive tearing, and swelling and tenderness over the area of the lacrimal sac between the eye and the nose.

   4. Conjunctiva and sclera. The conjunctiva covers the anterior eyeball (the white sclera not including the cornea) and is reflected back onto the posterior lid surfaces.

   a. Examination technique

   (1) Lower lid: With patient looking up, place your index finger firmly over the midpoint of the lid just above the bone of the lower orbital rim and pull the lid downward. This everts the lower lid allowing examination of the lower fornix with a penlight.

   (2) Upper lid: With patient looking down, elevate the upper lid and expose the sclera and conjunctiva. Do not apply pressure to the eyeball itself when pulling open the lid. Hold the lid against the rim of the bony orbit. To inspect the conjunctiva on the posterior surface of the lid, have the patient look down, then grasp the upper lashes gently with the thumb and forefinger of one hand while using the side of a tongue blade or the tip of a cotton-tipped applicator to form a fulcrum on the upper border of the tarsal plate (the firm cartilaginous structure forming the inferior-most portion of the upper lid). Push down on the tongue blade or cotton tipped ap-

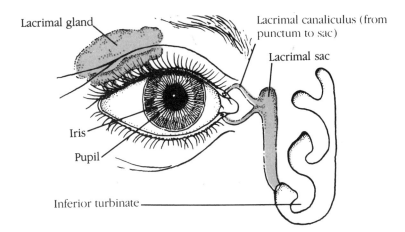

Lacrimal gland

Lacrimal canaliculus (from punctum to sac)

Lacrimal sac

Iris

Pupil

Inferior turbinate

Fig. 5-2. External eye and lacrimal apparatus.

plicator and pull upward on the lashes; this will evert the upper lid (Fig. 5-3). After inspection with a penlight, ask the patient to look up, and the lid will return to its normal position.

b. Variation in findings. Variations in vascularity are normal. Edema (swelling) or pallor should be noted. Pigmentation in darker-skinned races is usually normal but not normal in lighter-skinned races.

5. Cornea. Use a penlight with oblique and direct lighting to illuminate the cornea, which should appear continuous, shiny, and bright. Corneal scarring, vascularization, or ulceration will dull the light reflex. Photophobia (light sensitivity) may be a clue to corneal disease or intraocular inflammation.

6. Iris. Inspect the size, shape, markings, definition, and color of the iris. Check for equality of the pupils, although the size of the two pupils may vary slightly in a normal patient (anisocoria). Also, note the depth of the anterior chamber (distance between the iris and the cornea).

7. Lens. The lens, which is located behind the iris, is usually transparent and the pupil is usually black. Opacities in the lens make it visible through the pupil on examination with the penlight.

G. Pupillary testing

1. Test in dim light.

2. Instruct the patient not to focus on your penlight, but to look into the distance.

3. Position the penlight slightly below the patient's eyes to avoid fixation on the light and illuminate both eyes with the least amount of light possible to discern the pupil size and shape in dim illumination.

4. Shine the bright light on each pupil (in turn, not simultaneously) from a point slightly lateral to the patient's line of vision, and inspect for pupillary constriction in the eye that the light is shined into (direct response).

5. Perform the swinging flashlight test (changing the light rapidly from one pupil to the other and back again) to check for equal pupillary constriction.

6. Ask the patient to look into the distance and then at your finger (or a test object—not a light) held about 4 inches from the bridge of the patient's nose, and look for pupillary constriction in each eye when changing from distant focus to near focus (reaction to accommodation).

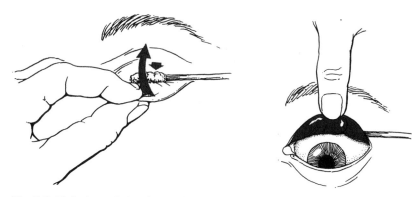

Fig. 5-3. Technique of visualizing the superior fornix and conjunctiva of the upper lid.

7. The rapidity of pupillary reflexes varies considerably in normal patients (it is sufficient if the response occurs and is equal in the two eyes).
H. Extraocular muscle examination (ocular motility)
   1. Technique. Assume a position directly in front of the patient so that your face is level with the patient's face.
      a. Corneal light reflex. Hold your flashlight in the midline between yourself and the patient. Ask the patient to look directly at the light. Note the position of the reflection of the light on each cornea with respect to the location of the pupils. Normally, the eyes have symmetrically located corneal light reflexes.
      b. Cardinal positions of gaze (Fig. 5-4). Cardinal positions are used to evaluate the possible weaknesses of the 12 individual extraocular muscles (six muscles on each eye; see Fig. 5-4A). Two primary muscles can be evaluated in each of the six positions (see Fig. 5-4B).
        (1) Staring straight ahead, direct the patient to follow your light to each of these positions: up to the right, directly to the right, down to the right, down to the left, directly to the left, and up to the left.
        (2) Pause during each gaze position to detect any possible nystagmus (oscillations of the eyes).
        (3) Ask the patient about the presence of diplopia (double vision). If the patient sees two lights in any position, this indicates the need for further analysis of that muscle pair.
      c. Convergence test
        (1) Ask the patient to follow your light as you slowly move it from a distance of approximately 2 feet toward the bridge of the patient's nose, and note the convergence of each eye.
        (2) Note the distance from the bridge of the nose at which the two eyes can no longer maintain convergence. The patient should be able to converge closer than his or her normal reading distance (about 14 inches).
      d. Cover/uncover test for muscle imbalances. Ask the patient to fixate on a distant target (over 10 feet away, if possible). Cover one eye while the patient is looking at the target, and notice whether the uncovered eye moves to regain fixation on the target. Then uncover both eyes and cover the previously uncovered eye to notice whether the now-uncovered eye moves to regain fixation on the target. A horizontal movement indicates weakness of one of the horizontal rectus muscles; a

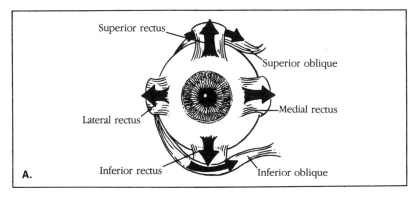

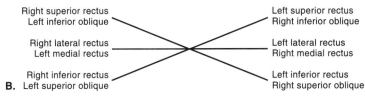

Fig. 5-4. Yoke muscles in diagnostic positions of gaze. **(A)** Extraocular muscles. **(B)** Primary extraocular muscles evaluated in cardinal positions of gaze. (Note: Vertical recti are evaluated in out-turned eye, obliques in in-turned eye.)

vertical movement indicates weakness of one of the vertical muscles (elevator or depressor).

    e. Alternate cover test for muscle imbalance. With both eyes uncovered and fixating on a distant target, cover one eye, then shift the cover from that eye to the other eye and note the movement that the uncovered eye makes to regain fixation. Then move the cover back to the first eye, and note the movement that the uncovered eye makes to regain fixation.

    f. If a patient complains of difficulty with near vision or reading, the cover/uncover test and the alternate cover test should be repeated with the patient fixating on a target (letter on a reading card, finger, or pencil) at 14 inches.

  2. Normal findings. Normally, the fusion reflex maintains the eyes in a parallel position, thus permitting binocular vision. The cover/uncover test checks for a *tropia,* which is a constant deviation of one of the eyes such that when both eyes are asked to fixate on a target, only one eye actually looks at the target and the other eye does not. The alternate cover test checks for a *phoria,* a deviation of direction that recovers when both eyes are allowed to fixate on a target at the same time.

I. Ophthalmoscopic examination. The examination of the fundus (interior surface of the eye) not only aids in the evaluation of the eye but also in the general physical evaluation of the patient.

  1. Technique

    a. Complete examination of the ocular fundus is best done with a dilated pupil.

      (1) Instill 1 drop of a mydriatic drug into each eye and allow at least 20 minutes for dilation to occur (some patients may need an additional drop of mydriatic, particularly if they have dark irises). Infrequently, mydriatic drugs can cause an elevation of intraocular pressure in patients with a type of glaucoma called angle-closure glaucoma. It is very difficult to determine whether a patient has this predisposing condition before actual dilation of the pupil occurs. However, some patients can tell you that they have had difficulty with dilating drops in the past, and these patients should not have a dilated eye examination.

(2) If the patient has significant discomfort after dilation has occurred, check the intraocular pressure at the end of the examination before the patient leaves the examination area.

(3) Do not dilate the eyes of patients with acute neurologic disease, head trauma, or similar conditions, when the observation of serial changes in the pupils is crucial in patient management.

b. Darken the examining area, have the patient be seated, and ask the patient to look straight ahead at a specific target in the distance and try not to move the eyes. Begin by standing on the right side of the patient examining the right eye with the ophthalmoscope in the right hand and using your right eye (Fig. 5-5). If you have a visually compromised eye, ask the patient to lie down for the examination, stand at the patient's head, and look at each eye with your "good" eye.

c. To assess the ocular media, set the ophthalmoscope to +6 to 8 diopters (the black or green numbers on the dial) and observe the pupil from a distance of 8 to 12 inches. This illuminates the retina, showing any opacity or obstruction as a dark spot or shadow against the red background of the fundus.

d. Procedure.

(1) Move in toward the patient's eye at an angle of 15 degrees to the side, and move closer to the patient until the hand holding the ophthalmoscope touches the patient's cheek or the head of the ophthalmoscope touches your thumb, which is resting on the upper lid/brow of the patient. You may need to hold the upper lid open with the thumb of your free hand.

(2) Adjust the ophthalmoscope lenses toward the setting of "0" on the ophthalmoscope, and note the lighter color of the optic disk.

(3) Refocus and align the ophthalmoscope until the details of the optic disk (nerve head) are clearly seen. Note the size, shape, color,

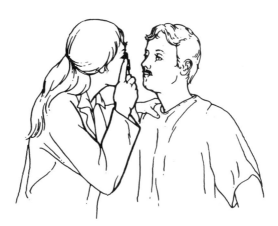

Fig. 5-5. The initial position for examination of the ocular media. The examiner then moves as close as possible to visualize the retina.

margins, central physiologic depression, and blood vessels of the optic nerve head.

(4) Measure any elevation of the optic nerve head by focusing on the highest part of the disk, then by focusing on the retina adjacent to the optic nerve head.

(5) Note the number of clicks as the focusing wheel turns, and read the difference directly from the instrument dial.

e. Assessment of the retina (Fig. 5-6). Always follow a definite order when evaluating the retina and retinal vessels, reserving the central or macular area until last to avoid dazzling the patient with your bright ophthalmoscope light. Four main pairs of blood vessels emerge from and enter the optic nerve head.

(1) Examine the superior nasal vessels and retina first, following them out as far as possible.

(2) Then examine the inferior nasal blood vessels and retina from peripherally toward the optic nerve head.

(3) To evaluate peripherally, have the patient move the eye up and nasally, then down and nasally during this part of the funduscopic examination.

(4) Proceed from the optic nerve head, examining the inferior temporal vessels and the adjacent retina as far peripherally as possible.

(5) From the periphery of the superior temporal vessels proceed toward the optic nerve head, evaluating the vessels and the adjacent retina.

(6) To evaluate peripherally, have the patient move the eye down and temporally, then up and temporally. Next, have the patient look straight ahead, and move the ophthalmoscope light from the optic nerve head temporally to the macula (center of the retina), asking the patient to look directly at the light, if necessary. The foveal pit (center of the macula) is seen as a small bright dot produced by the light reflection from the indentation of the fovea in the center of the macula.

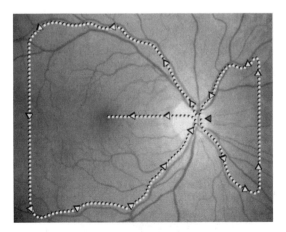

Fig. 5-6. Diagrammatic representation of retina, showing order in which areas are examined. Start at the optic nerve head (dark arrow head). Note that macular area is examined last.

      f. In a similar manner, examine the retina and retinal vessels for the left eye, standing on the left side of the patient, holding the ophthalmoscope in your left hand, and using your left eye.

  2. Normal findings. It is impossible to enumerate the myriad normal variations encountered in the ophthalmoscopic examination, since the pattern of the retinal vessels, the shape of the optic nerve, and so on, is unique for each patient. Considerable variation in the size and shape of the optic nerve head and the central physiologic depression may occur. If the optic nerve head is small, the nasal border may be blurred. If the eye is myopic (nearsighted), there may be an arc of retinal pallor or pigmentation along the temporal side of the optic nerve head. The position of the vessels on the nerve head may vary. The retinal vessels are usually gently sinuous in their courses, making approximate right angles at branching points. The retinal arterioles and venules usually cross each other without noticeable indentation. The veins are somewhat darker than the arterioles and about one third wider. The background color of the fundus may be darker in brunettes and very light in blonds, and the deeper, larger blood vessels of the choroid (vascular layer of the fundus) may become more prominent.

J. Measurement of intraocular pressure. Intraocular pressure should be recorded in every complete physical examination.

  1. The Schiötz tonometer measures the indentation of the cornea caused by a central plunger fitted into a curved foot plate with variable weights on the plunger (Fig. 5-7). The reading is translated into millimeters of mercury (mmHg), and the range of normal is from 8 to 21 mmHg. The patient is made comfortable in a reclining position, and 1 drop of a topical anesthetic such as 0.5% proparacaine hydrochloride or 0.5% tetracaine hydrochloride is instilled into each eye. After a few seconds, the eyes are anesthetized and the patient is directed to look straight toward the ceil-

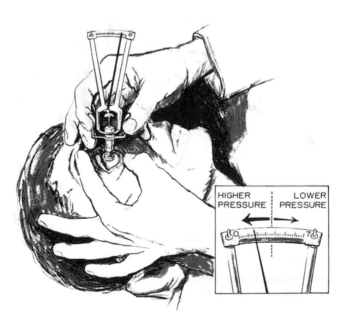

Fig. 5-7. Measurement of intraocular pressure by Schiötz tonometry.

ing, fixating either his or her finger at arm's length or a target on the ceiling. Hold the instrument lightly in one hand, and separate the lids gently with the fingers of the other hand. The foot plate is rested on the cornea, and the reading taken from the dial. A small rhythmic oscillation in the pointer should be observed (the transmitted pulse pressure) to ensure a proper end point. Care must be taken not to exert pressure on the lids, and the instrument must be kept meticulously clean. The reading from the dial is converted to mmHg by using the conversion chart that accompanies each tonometer. The Schiötz tonometer is only a screening instrument and if more exact intraocular pressure measurements are required, applanation tonometers (in every ophthalmologist's office) are more accurate.

2. A very rough estimate of the intraocular pressure can be obtained using the tactile method (Fig. 5-8). Ask the patient to look downward, and place the tips of both index fingers on the upper lid above the position of the down-turned cornea. While one index finger rests firmly on the globe, the other is pressed inward to indent the eyeball. This indentation is then alternated to the other index finger and repeated several times with a reciprocal piston-like movement, pressing directly toward the center of the globe. Only abnormally low intraocular pressures (a very soft eye) or a marked elevation of intraocular pressure (a very hard eye) can be determined in this way, and this method is no substitute for tonometry.

K. Screening examination. When a complete ophthalmologic examination is not required, a screening examination can be substituted:

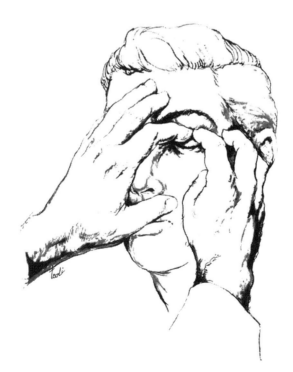

Fig. 5-8. Tactile test for intraocular pressure.

SCREENING OPHTHALMOLOGY EXAMINATION CHECKLIST

☐ *Visual acuity testing (check each eye with the fellow eye occluded)*
   1. Distance. Wear corrective lenses.
   2. Near. Be aware of presbyopic patient.
☐ *Visual fields (confrontation—compare patient's visual field with yours)*
   1. Position yourself so that your face is level with patient's face and about 2 feet away.
   2. Test one eye at a time by displaying one or two fingers in one quadrant and asking patient to identify how many fingers are displayed.
   3. Test all four quadrants.
☐ *External examination*
   1. Inspection and palpation
      a. Orbits, prominence, or retraction of eyes
      b. Eyebrows, eyelids, lacrimal apparatus
   2. Inspection (with penlight)
      a. Conjunctiva
         (1) Bulbar (on eyeball)
         (2) Palpebral (on lids)
         (3) *Cul-de-sacs* (fornices)—upper and lower
      b. Cornea, iris
☐ *Pupillary examination (test with room lights dimmed)*
   1. Size and shape
   2. Reaction to direct light (each eye)
   3. Swinging flashlight test (for afferent pupillary defect)
☐ *Motility examination*
   1. Cardinal positions of gaze (6)
      a. Presence of nystagmus or diplopia
   2. Convergence
   3. Tropias—distance and near
      a. Cover/uncover test (do for each eye)
   4. Phorias (optional)—distance and near
      a. Alternate cover test
☐ *Ophthalmoscopic examination (test with room lights dimmed)*
   1. Ocular media (at 12 inches)
   2. Fundus examination (close to eye)
      a. Optic nerve
      b. Retinal vessels
      c. Retinal periphery
      d. Macula
☐ *Intraocular pressure*

III. Cardinal Symptoms and Abnormal Findings
   A. Symptoms
      1. Pain. The complaint of pain in or about the eyes must be evaluated as to location, duration, type, and mode of onset. It may be related to a specific incident, as in the case of an injury to the eye with a foreign body sensation due either to a surface abrasion of the cornea or to an actual foreign particle on the cornea or the back of the eyelids.
         a. In acute iritis, the pain is throbbing, and injection (vascular dilation/congestion) occurs around the periphery of the cornea (circumcorneal injection). In addition, there may be a small pupil and photophobia (light sensitivity).
         b. Acute glaucoma also presents with a dull, throbbing pain but with more diffuse redness, a cloudy (edematous) cornea, high pressure, and a mid-dilated pupil.
         c. Very severe localized pain in one eye usually suggests surface disease such as a corneal abrasion, corneal infection, or corneal ulcer.
         d. Deep pain in the orbit may not be associated with local signs, but may indicate contiguous processes such as sinus disease or intracranial

sensory nerve involvement. Irritation of the meninges or increased intracranial pressure may also produce orbital pain.

2. Discomfort in the eye referred to the forehead may be the result of uncorrected refractive error or ocular muscle imbalance, in which case it will often follow prolonged use of the eyes as with reading or computer work (asthenopia). Almost all patients with headaches will ask whether the eyes are involved but few headaches will be secondary to eye disease; a typical unilateral migraine headache, for example, will often include severe ocular pain on that side but the headache is not caused by an eye problem.

3. Visual loss. This may range from blurring of vision to complete blindness in one or both eyes.

   a. Double vision. The earliest signs may be recognized by the patient only as a visual blur related to the overlapping images.

   b. Visual acuity. A reduction in visual acuity can reflect systemic disease, such as early diabetes in which a shift to myopia (nearsightedness) may occur. The early symptoms of cataract may include visual blurring, especially for distance.

   c. Secondary to either local or general disease. Reduced vision can be result from local or systemic disease, especially when the loss has been sudden or when recently prescribed glasses no longer improve the vision. *Any case of reduced vision, either unilateral or bilateral, demands an explanation.*

   (1) Causes can range from local ocular pathology, such as cataracts, macular degeneration, retinal detachment, and vitreous or retinal hemorrhage, to optic nerve or visual pathway involvement as a part of neurologic disease processes. Sudden changes may suggest circulatory insufficiencies of various types, such as cerebral hemorrhage, major carotid occlusions, central retinal artery occlusion, and the like.

   (2) Poor vision in one eye may be noted in many patients who had strabismus in childhood, resulting in suppression of central vision in one eye (amblyopia).

   (3) Visual field defects resulting from intracranial disease may be associated with complaints of visual loss, but the central acuity may be normal and a visual field examination is therefore necessary.

   d. Sudden loss of vision usually signals retinal or optic nerve disease and may be related either to inflammation or to vascular abnormalities. Central visual loss must be distinguished from that of peripheral visual field loss; the patient is usually much more aware of loss of central (reading) acuity than of peripheral involvement of the visual field.

4. Double vision. Double vision (diplopia) characteristically causes visual confusion, and the patient often closes or covers one eye for relief. In certain cases of incomplete paralysis of an eye muscle, the patient may assume an unusual head position to maintain single vision; for example, turning the head to the left with the eyes directed to the right in the case of a partial paralysis of the left lateral rectus muscle. Diplopia usually signifies either muscular or neurologic disease, but may indicate thyroid abnormalities. A lack of parallelism of the eyes may not be associated with double vision when it is the result of a "lazy" or amblyopic eye dating from a muscle imbalance in childhood.

5. Photophobia. Sensitivity to light varies considerably among normal individuals, and patients with light-colored irises may have more complaints than those with dark-colored irises. With more significant photophobia, there is usually disease of the cornea or of the anterior segment of the eye. In acute cases, corneal foreign body, corneal ulcer, corneal inflammation, or an iritis should be suspected. Old corneal scarring and vascularization, as well as cataracts, may also produce a sensitivity to light.

6. Discharge. Material coming from the eyelids that is either a watery or more viscous discharge usually suggests either conjunctival disease or abnormalities in the lacrimal drainage system.
   a. In acute infections, the discharge can be more purulent and may collect on the lid margins.
   b. When the lacrimal drainage system is occluded, an overflow of tears may occur and mucous may collect in the tear sac so that pressure over this structure between the eye and the nose causes regurgitation back into the eye.
   c. In allergic conjunctival disease, the consistency of the discharge is stringy and tenacious, and the patient will complain of itching.
   d. Abnormalities in the tear film may also cause a watery discharge and may cause some light sensitivity.
7. Redness. Conjunctival vascular dilation and congestion results in redness (hyperemia) of the eyes and must be evaluated in terms of other findings. In certain "florid" persons, it may not be significant unless other findings support the diagnosis of disease.
   a. If redness is greater toward the fornices of the conjunctiva, there is usually associated discharge and conjunctivitis.
   b. If redness is greater on the margin of the cornea, there may be associated corneal or anterior segment diseases such as keratitis or iritis.
   c. It may be generalized and related to surface irritation or sensitivity.
B. Abnormal findings
   1. External examination
      a. General appearance
         (1) Staring expression, retraction of upper lids, prominence of eyeballs: hyperthyroidism
         (2) Unilateral prominence *(proptosis)* of eyes indicates space-occupying lesion in the orbit. Bilateral prominence may indicate hyperthyroidism or disease of the blood-forming organs.
         (3) Drooping upper lids *(ptosis)* may be indication of extreme debility or neuromuscular disease. Partial ptosis may be part of Horner's syndrome. More marked ptosis of one lid associated with decreased pupillary light reflex may be an early indication of oculomotor paralysis.
         (4) Edema around the eyelids may be an early indication of systemic edema. Dermatologic conditions, local or generalized, may be present. In-turning of lid border *(entropion)* causes lashes to irritate the cornea and may be due to lid spasm or scar tissue. Eversion
            of lid border *(ectropion)* is associated with overflow of tears *(epiphora)* and may be due to scar tissue or senile laxity.
      b. Conjunctiva
         (1) Injection of the vessels and discharge *(conjunctivitis)* occur in almost all diseases affecting the conjunctiva. If infectious, the injection increases in the fornices and secretions are present. When more severe, small hemorrhages beneath the conjunctiva may occur.
         (2) Edema may be a sign of systemic fluid retention or a manifestation of endocrine exophthalmos, local inflammation, or vascular stasis.
         (3) Yellow color of sclera visible through conjunctiva may be an early indication of jaundice.
      c. Cornea
         (1) Severe pain and photophobia are usually present in acute corneal disease.
         (2) Increased redness of the globe around the corneal limbus occurs in abrasions or ulcers.
         (3) Loss of bright surface reflection, and a shadow on underlying iris are signs of surface lesions.

(4) Enlargement of cornea is commonest finding of infantile glaucoma, usually associated with clouding and photophobia.

(5) Edema of the cornea may be part of local disease or of acute glaucoma.

(6) Vascularization or visible white scarring is indicative of disease.

(7) White arcus around limbus in younger persons may indicate lipid metabolism abnormality.

(8) Brown ring of pigment around limbus (Kayser-Fleischer ring) occurs in hepatolenticular degeneration (Wilson's disease).

d. Anterior chamber. Any material visible is abnormal.

(1) Blood may be present after injury *(hyphema)* or after vitreal hemorrhage.

(2) Pus may level out in the lower chamber in corneal infection *(hypopyon)*.

(3) The chamber may be lost in a perforating wound with aqueous leakage.

e. Iris and pupils. The findings are often associated.

(1) Iritis is a nonspecific inflammation of the iris. Symptoms and signs may include throbbing pain, visual blurring, circumcorneal injection with a small pupil, decreased intraocular pressure, and an irregular pupil caused by posterior synechiae.

(2) Irregular pupil may be due to adhesions of the iris to the lens as a result of prior iritis.

(3) Multiple or displaced pupils may be congenital or due to tears of the iris base from prior trauma *(iridodialysis)*.

(4) Localized elevation of the iris is immediately suspect of tumor, especially if darkly pigmented.

f. Lacrimal ducts

(1) Overflow of tears *(epiphora)* is commonly seen with disease of lacrimal ducts.

(2) Secretions from tear sac regurgitating into eye indicates obstructed nasolacrimal duct. Associated redness and tenderness indicate secondary tear sac infection.

2. Pupillary reflexes. Loss of the pupillary light reflex is always important.

a. Pupils

(1) Unilateral loss of light reflex due to blindness. Neither direct nor consensual reflex will occur when blind eye is tested.

(2) Bilateral loss of light reflex in the presence of sight is usually caused by neurologic disease.

(3) Unilaterally fixed dilated pupil is a serious sign in a patient with recent head injury, indicating beginning involvement of the oculomotor nerve. This also may be caused by local trauma.

(4) Miotic pupil associated with drooping upper lid may indicate disease of the cervical sympathetic on that side and is a part of Horner's syndrome.

b. Lens. Visible clouding seen through pupil is an indication of cataract formation; this may also be seen as a dark shadow against the light of the fundus in the ophthalmoscopic examination. If the lens is removed or dislocated, the unsupported iris will flutter with quick movements of the eye *(iridodonesis)*.

3. Ocular motility. Any vertical shift, lack of parallelism in the diagnostic positions of gaze, or tropia is abnormal.

a. Paralysis of specific nerve supply to extraocular muscles produces characteristic findings.

(1) Oculomotor: eye turned down and out, ptosis of upper lid, no diplopia.

(2) Abducens: eye turned in toward nose (because of unopposed action of normal medial rectus), esotropia greater when looking in the direction of normal action of the affected muscle.

      (3) Trochlear: difficulty with vision in lower field, and if binocular vision is maintained, the head will be tilted toward the shoulder opposite the side of the paralysis. Both the trochlear and oculomotor nerves are involved in some conditions.

  b. Ocular muscle involvement may occur with certain neuromuscular diseases, may follow orbital or facial fractures, or may be a finding of the endocrine exophthalmos of thyroid disease.

  c. Nystagmus (irregular jerking movements of the eyes) may be a congenital abnormality or indicative of vestibular or central nervous system disease.

4. Ophthalmoscopic examination

  a. Media of the eye (cornea, lens, vitreous). Cataract, scarring, or localized opacities may be evident. Haziness of the vitreous may be present in intraocular inflammation.

  b. Optic nerve

      (1) Optic atrophy. Color of disk is paler than normal and may be chalky white. Superficial scar tissue and loss of substance may be present, with resultant decrease in vision.

      (2) Cupping of disk in glaucoma consists of exaggeration of the physiologic depression on the temporal side, extending to the border. Cup may be deep, is bluish-white, and retinal vessels may disappear behind the shelf at the edge of the cup and emerge at the base. A C/D ratio (ratio of cup diameter to horizontal disk diameter) of greater than 0.5 or asymmetry between eyes should cause suspicion.

      (3) Swelling of nerve head *(papilledema)* may be unilateral (localized optic nerve disease) or bilateral (increased intracranial pressure). Early signs of papilledema include filling in of physiologic depression, blurring of disk margins, fullness of retinal veins, and loss of spontaneous venous pulsations on disk. Superficial hemorrhages and exudates around disk occur in more advanced disease.

  c. Retinal vessels

      (1) Assessment of arteriosclerosis. Changes occur in the appearance of the retinal arteriole due to visibility of the vessel wall (shinier, copper-colored or silver reflection). Venous notching or nicking may occur where an involved arteriole crosses a retinal vein.

      (2) Assessment of hypertension. Localized or generalized narrowing of the arteriolar blood column can be identified by change in ratio of arteriolar to venule size. Leakage through vascular walls leads to hemorrhages and exudative deposits in retina; papilledema may ensue.

      (3) Hemorrhages and exudates in retina (e.g., in advanced hypertension, severe renal disease, collagen diseases, advanced diabetes, blood dyscrasias, severe retinal venous occlusions). Shape of hemorrhage indicates depth within retina.

         (a) Superficial hemorrhages lie in nerve fiber layer, are flame-shaped or splinter-like, and may occur with venous back pressure (occlusion of central retinal vein, papilledema); fuzzy white cotton wool patches (small ischemic infarcts) also lie in nerve fiber layer.

         (b) Deeper hemorrhages are round and blotchy, often associated with exudates (sharply defined yellow or white deposits representing incompletely absorbed residues of edema and blood).

         (c) Punctate or cluster-like venous microaneurysms in the macular and posterior pole area occur in early diabetic retinopathy.

      (4) Closure of central retinal artery results in ischemic edema of retina; if completely closed, the retina is pale and edematous with cherry red macular area.

      d. Retinal elevation. Any elevation is significant. A solid mass indicates tumor growth, usually in the choroid. If dark, consider melanoma; if lighter, think of metastatic malignancy. If the elevation is transparent and wrinkled, consider retinal detachment.

      e. Chorioretinal scarring

        (1) Sharply defined, irregular pigment deposits around a paler center indicate older scarring.

        (2) Fuzzy borders, hemorrhages along margin, or clouding in the vitreous indicate an active inflammatory process.

        (3) Irregular mottling of pigment and scar tissue change in macular area may be seen in the elderly with senile macular degeneration with an associated decrease in central vision.

  5. Intraocular pressure. Any increase is abnormal and should be investigated for the presence of glaucoma. Glaucoma is the greatest cause of blindness in people over 40, but glaucoma can be controlled and blindness prevented with early treatment. Measurement of intraocular pressure must be part of a complete physical examination in all persons over age 40.

      a. Chronic glaucoma may have no symptoms, or mild symptoms including variable visual blurring, minor headache, peripheral visual loss. Signs include moderately elevated intraocular pressure and early cupping of the optic nerve head.

      b. Acute glaucoma is rare and associated with decreased vision, pain in the eye, cloudy cornea, moderately dilated pupil, systemic symptoms such as severe headache, nausea, and vomiting.

C. Findings in the elderly (age >75)

  1. The visual acuity is usually worse than 20/20 secondary to opacities in the ocular media (cornea, lens, vitreous) and a decreased sensitivity of the retinal photoreceptors (rods and cones) occurring with age.

  2. There is mild to moderate atrophy of the orbital fat with some posterior movement of the eyeball into the orbit and deepening of the recess of the upper lids.

  3. The facial muscles may lose some of their tone resulting in mild to moderate sagging of the eyebrows over the orbital rims.

  4. The eyelids often become thinner with age, and there may be a slight lowering of the upper lids toward the pupillary margin.

  5. The conjunctiva, which has a bright reflex from the examining light in younger patients, may have a dullness of the light reflex in the elderly.

  6. A partial or complete white ring around the periphery of the cornea (corneal arcus) may occur in the elderly.

  7. The anterior chamber depth (space between cornea and iris) decreases with age.

  8. The color of the iris may change because of decreased pigmentation of the iris. Dark brown eyes become less brown and blue eyes tend to become somewhat more blue.

  9. The intraocular lens thickens with age and may develop opacities (cataracts).

  10. The pupil size decreases gradually with age and the pupils respond less briskly to stimulation by light.

  11. There is a mild to moderate bilateral restriction of both eyes in attempted upgaze and a mild to moderate decrease in the ability of the eyes to converge as targets are brought closer to the face.

  12. On ophthalmoscopic evaluation in the elderly, there may be the following findings:

      a. Some generalized narrowing of the retinal arterioles

      b. Mild indentation of the retinal veins at arteriolovenous crossings

      c. A decreased and, eventually, a loss of the sharp foveal reflex in the center of the macula

      d. Tiny drusen (small yellow-white deposits) underneath the central retina in the macular area

   e. Small, gray-black objects in various patterns occurring in the vitreous
   (the transparent colorless gel-like material that fills in the posterior
   two thirds of the interior of the eyeball between the lens and retina);
   solid aggregates of vitreous material that accumulate as a result of
   the aging process and result in a fairly common complaint of floaters
   in the elderly

IV. Available Technology

A. *Fluorescein staining* of the surface of the eye (conjunctiva and cornea) is useful in determining the integrity of the epithelium and is particularly valuable in cases of trauma and in epithelial diseases such as herpes simplex and
zoster. A strip of fluorescein is moistened and briefly applied to the inferior
conjunctival *cul-de-sac,* and the surface is evaluated with a cobalt blue light.
Fluorescein that collects in an epithelial defect will become very prominent.
Fluorescein in eye-drop form is also available and is combined with a topical
anesthetic.

B. Visual field defects occur in glaucoma, optic nerve diseases, and macular diseases. They may also occur in central nervous system disease as a result of a
process involving the optic nerve or the visual radiations in the brain. The visual field is grossly evaluated by the confrontation testing method (as men-
tioned before), but more accurate measurements are achieved by using special instruments called *perimeters* to record the extent of the peripheral field
as well as defects in any part of the visual field. A flat screen on which light
targets are positioned (tangent screen) can also be used to test the central visual field.

C. The refractive error (refraction) must be measured in every case of subnormal visual acuity: this can be accomplished with individual lenses placed in
a spectacle trial frame or with an instrument called a phoro-optometer
(such as a Phoropter) that is placed in front of the patient's eyes and contains a variety of correcting lenses in a rotating wheel. A new instrument,
called an autorefractor, can be used to determine an approximate refractive
error, but the findings must be confirmed using individual lenses, or a phoro-
optometer

D. A *biomicroscope* (slit lamp) is a special instrument used to visualize fine detail in the anterior segment, particularly the cornea, iris, and lens, and it can
also be used with special lenses to examine the angle of the anterior chamber, the vitreous, and the retina.

E. An *exophthalmometer* is an instrument is used to measure the degree of protrusion (exophthalmos) or retraction (enophthalmos) of the eyeball in patients with orbital disease, trauma, aging processes, or thyroid disease. The
instrument is placed on the bone of each of the lateral orbital rims and a mirror system allows the distance from the rim to the corneal apex to be measured in mm. Serial measurements are usually performed in order to follow
pathologic processes.

F. An *ophthalmodynamometer* is an instrument that measures the blood pressure in the central retinal artery and may be useful in patients with circulatory disease. The foot plate of the instrument is placed on the sclera in
the outer temporal area and pressure is applied while the observer watches
the central retinal artery. When pulsation of the central retinal artery begins, a diastolic reading is taken; with greater pressure, collapse of the
artery indicates the systolic pressure. A low diastolic and/or systolic level
or differences between the two eyes may be significant. Doppler and magnetic resonance angiography are now of more value in measuring blood
flow.

G. *Fluorescein angiography* is a photographic technique commonly used to show
the flow characteristics of the blood vessels in the retina and choroid. The fluorescein dye is given intravenously, and special photographic equipment is used
to record the flow in the retinal vessels and assess the functional integrity.
This is particularly valuable in evaluating patients for diabetic retinopathy
and retinal neovascularization in age-related macular degeneration.

H. *Imaging studies,* including computed tomography and magnetic resonance imaging are used to evaluate orbital disease, and to evaluate optic nerve or optic chiasm lesions as well as to evaluate intraocular or intraorbital trauma, particularly with foreign body penetrations and perforations.

I. *Ultrasonography* can be used to evaluate orbital disease or intraocular abnormalities concealed by opaque media. It is most commonly used to measure axial length (cornea to retina) to calculate the power for intraocular lens implantation after cataract extraction.

J. The cost figures cited in this table are **basic direct costs**. The figures are difficult to obtain and change quickly. They include **only** the cost of the test itself (technician, equipment, time, materials). No professional costs (interpretation) are included. Costs vary from region to region based on differences in some components such as labor. However, the relative cost ranking should remain similar

Procedure	Code
Fluorescein staining	*
Visual fields	$$
Refraction	$
Biomicroscope (slit-lamp)	*
Exophthalmometer	*
Ophthalmodynamometer	*
Doppler and magnetic resonance angiography	$$$$$$
Fluorescein angiography	$$$$$
Computed tomography (CT)	$$$
Magnetic resonance imaging (MRI)	$$$$
Ultrasonography	$$

$ = $0–$50; $$ = $50–$100; $$$ = $100–$200; $$$$ = $200–$500; $$$$$ = $500–$1000; $$$$$$ = >$1000; * = highly variable or not available.

V. Bibliography

Berson FG. *Basic Ophthalmology for Medical Students and Primary Care Residents,* 6th ed. San Francisco: American Academy of Ophthalmology; 1993.

Cassin B, Solomon S. *Dictionary of Ocular Terminology.* Gainesville, FL: Triad Publishing Company; 1984.

Judge RD, Zuidema GD, Fitzgerald FT. *Clinical Diagnosis,* 5th ed. Boston: Little, Brown; 1989.

Kwitko MI, Weinstock FJ. *Geriatric Ophthalmology.* Orlando: Grune & Stratton; 1985.

Newell FW. *Ophthalmology: Principles and Concepts,* 7th ed. St. Louis: CV Mosby; 1992.

Rosenbloom AA Jr, Morgan MW. *Vision and Aging.* New York: Professional Pressbooks, Fairchild Publications; 1986.

Trobe JD. *The Physician's Guide to Eye Care.* San Francisco: American Academy of Ophthalmology; 1993.

Vaughan DG, Asbury T, Riordan-Eva P. *General Ophthalmology*, 13th ed. Norwalk, CT: Appleton & Lange; 1992.

Weale RA. *The Senescence of Human Vision.* New York: Oxford University Press; 1992.

VI. Key Search Words

The following key words reflect the content of this chapter. They are provided to assist with an on-line search of computer databases, such as MEDLINE, if you wish to pursue the topic of this chapter further.

Blindness
Eye abnormalities
Eye diseases
Eye injuries
Eye movements
Eye, in old age
Headache
Intraocular pressure
Ocular motility disorders
Oculomotor paralysis
Optic disk
Optic nerve
Optic nerve diseases
Physical examination, eye
Pupil
Pupillary functions, abnormal
Reflex, pupillary
Refraction, ocular
Retina
Retinal diseases
Vision, subnormal
Visual acuity
Visual fields

6. UPPER RESPIRATORY AND AUDITORY SYSTEM

Carol R. Bradford

I. Glossary

Dysphagia: difficulty in swallowing.

Dysphonia: difficulty or pain in speaking.

Epiphora: tearing.

Epistaxis: nasal hemorrhage.

Laryngopharynx: lower pharynx extending from the lingual surface of the epiglottis to the trachea and esophagus.

Mucocele: intrasinus cyst arising from mucosal lining.

Nares: the openings into the nasal cavity.

Nasopharynx (epipharynx): upper pharynx extending from the choanae to the inferior border of the soft palate.

Odynophagia: painful swallowing.

Oropharynx: portion of pharynx directly behind the oral cavity extending from the inferior border of soft palate to the lingual surface of the epiglottis.

Otalgia: pain in the ear.

Otitis: infection of the ear.

Otorrhea: discharge from the ear.

Pyocele: infected mucocele.

Rhinorrhea: nasal discharge.

Stridor: noisy respiration.

Vallecula: space between the base of the tongue and the lingual surface of the epiglottis.

Vestibule: of the ear, the oval cavity in the middle of the bony labyrinth; of the nose, the area just inside the nares.

II. Techniques of Examination and Normal Findings

A. General considerations

    1. The patient should be seated for the examination.

    2. A light source (60- to 100-watt bulb) and head mirror are essential.

    3. Basic instruments are needed.

B. Nose

    1. Inspection

        a. External nose (look for any loss of structure or support)

        b. Internal nose

            (1) Use a nasal speculum to assess the nasal vestibule and determine the adequacy of the airways (Fig. 6-1). (Be careful not to overdilate the nasal orifice or touch the nasal septum with the speculum.) Look for a deviation of the nasal septum, check the color of the nasal mucosa, and determine whether the turbinates are normal, hypertrophic, or atrophic.

            (2) Spray the nose with 0.25% Neo-Synephrine (phenylephrine hydrochloride) or 1% ephedrine solution. After a few minutes, examine the posterior aspect of the nasal cavities and the superior nasopharynx, which can be visualized in most cases.

            (3) The rigid nasal endoscope can be used in the office setting to carefully examine the nasal cavities for drainage, polyps, or masses.

    2. Palpation

        a. External nose. Palpate for any loss of structure or support.

        b. Sinuses. Palpate the roof of the orbit, the ascending processes of the maxillae, and the canine fossae for tenderness or masses. If sinus dis-

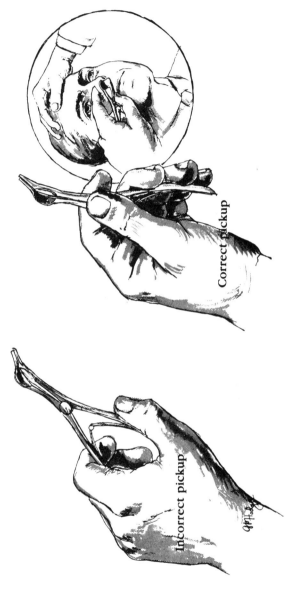

Fig. 6-1. Use of the nasal speculum.

ease is suspected, x-ray or computed tomography (CT) examination may be useful.

3. Normal findings (Fig. 6-2). The internal nose is the conditioner for inspired and expired air. There are two openings posteriorly, known as the *choanae,* which lead into the nasopharynx. Usually, the sinus orifices can be visualized only with nasal endoscopy.

C. Ear

1. External ear. Examine the lateral and medial surfaces of the auricle and the mastoid process. The main anatomic components of the auricle are the helix, antihelix, lobule, tragus, antitragus, and concha (Fig. 6-3).

2. Internal ear. Examine the ear canal and tympanic membrane with a head mirror and ear speculum or a pneumatic otoscope, which can also test the mobility of the tympanic membrane. Pull the auricle upward and backward (straight back in infants and small children) to obtain proper visualization.

3. Normal findings. The outer third of the canal contains hair follicles, sebaceous glands, and cerumen glands. At the junction of the middle and inner thirds of the canal is located a bony narrowing called the *isthmus.* Exostoses (benign bony projections usually associated with prolonged cold water swimming) are commonly found in the canal; however, these are rarely significant. The tympanic membrane is usually found on a slanted plane (Fig. 6-4). The anterior inferior quadrant is the farthest away from the examiner. This accounts for the triangle of light being re-

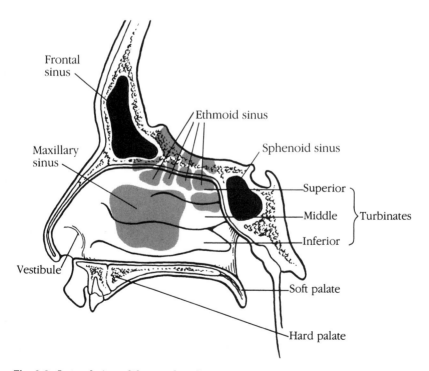

Fig. 6-2. Lateral view of the nasal cavity.

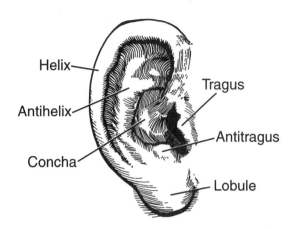

Fig. 6-3. External ear (auricle).

flected anteroinferiorly from the umbo. Note the relation of the various landmarks in Figure 4.
D. Nasopharynx (Fig. 6-5)
  1. Warm a size 0 to 3 mirror, or wipe with a thick soapy solution to prevent condensation. Sit directly in front of the patient, with heads at the same level. The patient's head is projected slightly forward. Encourage the patient to breathe normally through the nose during the examination. Using a tongue blade, depress the tongue into the floor of the mouth with your left hand (do not extend the tip of the blade posterior to the middle third of the tongue). Reflect light into the pharynx with a head mirror. Holding the mirror in the right hand like a pencil, slip the mirror behind and to one side of the uvula. Do not touch the base of the tongue. The gag reflex can be controlled, if needed, by spraying 2% tetracaine (do not exceed 80 mg) or 4% cocaine (do not exceed 20 mg) into the pharynx.

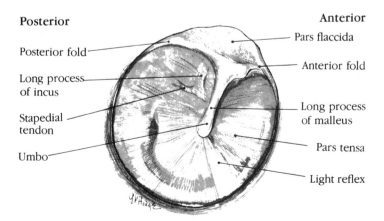

Fig. 6-4. Right tympanic membrane showing important landmarks.

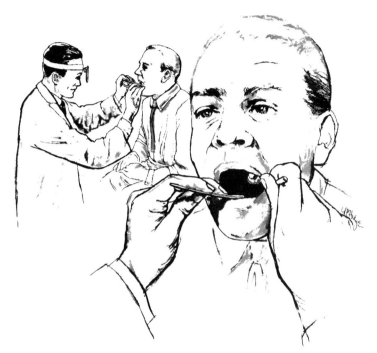

Fig. 6-5. Technique of examination of the nasopharynx.

2. Normal findings (Fig. 6-6). The nasopharynx extends from the choanae to the inferior border of the soft palate. Looking anteriorly from the nasopharynx into the nose, the posterior border of the nasal septum dividing the two choanae is seen. In each choana, the posterior tips of the middle and inferior turbinates can be visualized. Figure 6 shows the important landmarks.

Adenoid tissue is present on the posterior wall (usually absent by age 16 years). This mass of lymphoid tissue is also known as the *pharyngeal tonsil*. The adenoid is connected with the palatine and lingual tonsils by a band of lymphoid tissue extending down the lateral pharyngeal wall. This entire lymphoid complex is known as *Waldeyer's ring.*

E. Oral cavity and oropharynx (Fig. 6-7). Systemic diseases often have oral manifestations; reactive lesions to local injury are also common.

1. Palpation method. Ask patient to protrude the tongue and grasp it with folded gauze.

   a. Use index finger of opposite hand to palpate the soft, smooth tongue surfaces

   b. Release tongue and palpate the entire floor of the mouth, including the base of the tongue (small lesions can often be felt better than they can be seen). Palpate these sublingual structures with the opposite hand supporting the submental and submandibular tissues.

   c. Continue bimanual palpation between oral mucosa and facial skin in the cheek and lip regions.

   d. Conclude palpation with hard and soft palate area.

2. Oral mucous membranes

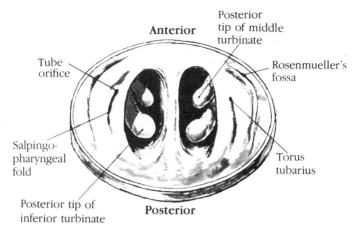

Fig. 6-6. Mirror view of the nasopharynx.

    a. Inspect and palpate all surfaces. Ask the patient to sequentially lift up his tongue and move the tongue right and left.
    b. Normal findings: normally pale coral pink, and moist. Oral mucous membranes are normally pigmented with generalized and local melanin on a racial basis. A horizontal white line extending from the commissure of the mouth to the retromolar pad may be seen, indicating the contact made by the occluding surfaces of the teeth. Hyperkeratotic reaction and shaggy superficial slough may occur if cheek biting is a habit.

  3. Lips

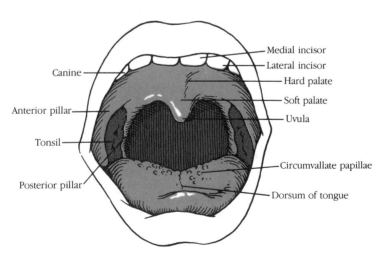

Fig. 6-7. Anatomy of the mouth.

a. Ask patient to purse lips; observe symmetry in form and function. Ask patient to remove dental appliances; then with patient's mouth slightly open, retract lips and cheek with the tongue blade and inspect the inner lip and cheek surfaces.

b. Normal findings. In the young, the vermilion surface has slight vertical linear markings and a smooth, pliable surface. With age, atrophic changes erase the strial pattern, and the sharp definition at the mucocutaneous border is lost.

4. Oral vestibule, buccal mucosa, gingivae

    a. Inspect all recesses of the gingivobuccal fornices and gums. A fine probe can be used to determine the level of gingival attachment and the presence of pocket lesions adjacent to the teeth.

    b. Normal findings. The posterior buccal mucosa may be prominent with large buccal fat pads. Small yellow macules or papules indicative of normal sebaceous gland deposition (Fordyce's spots) may be seen. The gingival tissues covering the alveolar process are normally pale coral pink and slightly stippled. The gingivae attach to the teeth, and gingival projections fill the interdental spaces as papillae.

5. Hard and soft palate

    a. Ask patient to open mouth wide and tilt head back. Depress dorsum of tongue with a blade, ask patient to say "ahh." Observe midline uvula elevation and coordinated pharynx constriction.

    b. Normal findings. A midline hard swelling or exostosis (torus palatinus) is a common variation (20% of adults) in hard palate structure; this is not significant unless ulceration occurs.

6. Tongue and floor of the mouth

    a. Ask patient to return head to original position and protrude the tongue. Note symmetry and muscle coordination of midline protrusion; note also the dorsal surface characteristics. Grasp the tongue with folded gauze, and retract it laterally to view its posterior surface. Ask patient to touch tip of tongue to the hard palate with mouth open; inspect the ventral surface of the tongue. Inspect the floor of the mouth as you inspect the lateral, posterior, and ventral surfaces of the tongue. Malignancy is common in this area.

    b. Normal findings—tongue. Many variations of the pattern of papillae are seen. Congenital variations may cause furrows or elevated areas. There is a V-shaped row of circumvallate papillae at the junction of the anterior two thirds and the posterior one third of the tongue.

    c. Salivary duct orifices (Figs. 6-8 and 6-9)

        (1) Submandibular duct (Wharton's duct). Ask patient to raise tip of the tongue; note the sublingual fold (frenulum, see Fig. 6-8). The elevation on either side is the sublingual papilla. The submandibular duct is one of at least 10 ducts that empty into the sublingual area. It can be expressed by massaging the submandibular gland. Note flow and secretion quality.

        (2) Parotid duct (Stensen's duct) enters the mouth through a small papilla in the lateral buccal mucosa opposite the lateral aspect of the second upper molar tooth (see Fig. 6-9).

    d. Salivary glands

        (1) Submandibular gland. With one index finger in the floor of the mouth between the lateral aspect of the tongue and the teeth, the other hand can palpate the submandibular gland externally, directly under the ramus of the mandible about halfway between the chin and the angle of the jaw. It has a firm, irregular consistency and normally becomes more prominent with advancing age.

        (2) Parotid gland. Located anterior to and below the auricle, the parotid gland normally extends from the sternomastoid muscle anteriorly to the masseter muscle.

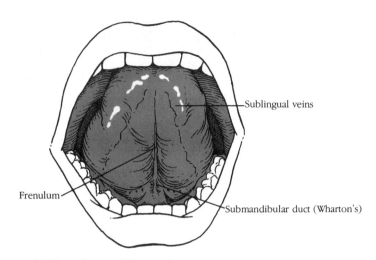

Fig. 6-8. Sublingual view of the mouth.

      (3) Sublingual glands. These numerous glands normally cannot be palpated with accuracy. They are located along the floor of the mouth around Wharton's duct.

  7. Tonsils. If present, note their size. If they are cryptic, note any debris (sebaceous material, pus, foreign bodies). Check for inflammation of the anterior or posterior pillars. Pull the tongue forward or use a laryngeal mirror to assess the status of the lingual tonsils.

  8. Teeth

    a. Examine for their form, function, and support in the jaws. Light percussion with a mirror handle may help to localize painful dental conditions.

    b. Normal findings. The teeth are firmly anchored in the alveolar process by the periodontal membrane, and the surface is smooth white enamel.

  9. Jaws

    a. Observe the excursions of the mandible and occlusion of the teeth.

    b. Temporomandibular joint. Palpate the condyles of this joint in motion by placing your fifth fingers in the external auditory canals during jaw excursions.

    c. Normal findings. Excursion of the jaws will admit the width of three contacting fingers of the patient's hand (3.5 to 4.5 cm). Excursions of the mandible are smooth and gliding.

 10. Regional lymph nodes. Evaluate for their relation to oral pathology.

F. Laryngopharynx. Hoarseness of more than 2 weeks' duration is the most common indication for careful laryngeal examination.

  1. Indirect laryngoscopy. (Gagging may be a problem with this examination. If necessary, spray the pharynx with 2% tetracaine, 4% cocaine, or Cetacaine spray, and resume the examination in 4 or 5 minutes.)

    a. Prepare a size 4 to 6 mirror. Ask patient to sit with head projected slightly forward. Grasp the tongue with folded gauze, with the thumb on top of tongue and second finger under tip of tongue; the index finger elevates the upper lip (Fig. 6-10). Insert the mirror in the oropharynx so that it elevates the uvula. (*Do not touch the lateral walls, tonsils, or back of tongue, because this will cause gagging.*)

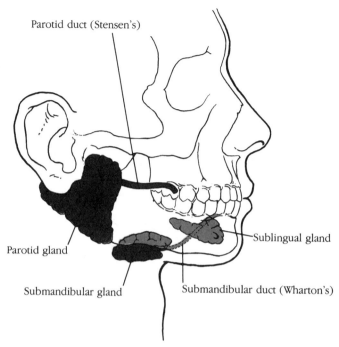

Fig. 6-9. Salivary system.

    b. Ask patient to breathe quietly, and reassure the patient that you will not obstruct the airway. Then ask the patient to say "eeeeeee." This will bring the epiglottis up and forward. Observe the following (Fig. 6-11):
      (1) Base of the tongue—lingual tonsils
      (2) Valleculae
      (3) Lingual surface and margins of the epiglottis
      (4) Arytenoid
      (5) Aryepiglottic folds
      (6) False and true vocal cords
      (7) Trachea
      (8) Walls of hypopharynx
      (9) Pyriform sinuses
     (10) Mouth of the esophagus
  2. Normal findings are normal movements of the vocal cords (tense, relax, abduct, adduct), and the sphincteric action of laryngopharynx during swallowing. Note three layers of sphincters: epiglottis and aryepiglottic folds, false cords, and true cords.
G. Consideration in geriatric patients (age >75).
  1. *Presbycusis.* Auditory dysfunction associated with the aging process includes several identifiable forms of degeneration of hearing. This common disorder may have a devastating effect on the older person by reducing the ability to communicate, jeopardizing autonomy, and limiting the opportunity to participate in society. Accurate estimates of the prevalence of presbycusis in particular and sensorineural hearing loss in general are not available. However, a recent survey demonstrated that 20.7 million Americans (8.8%) are hearing-impaired. The specific causes of

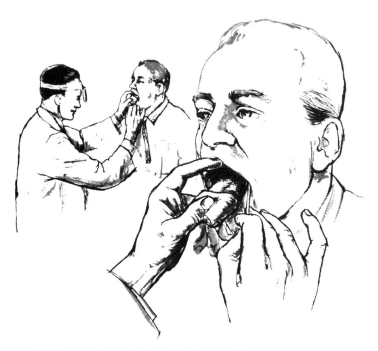

Fig. 6-10. Technique of examination of the laryngopharynx.

presbycusis are speculative, but likely represent a combination of effects of years of use and exposure to noise and chemicals, along with genetically programmed biologic degeneration.

2. *Presbystasis.* Presbystasis, the disequilibrium of aging, is a group of disorders affecting the mobility of a large number of elderly persons. As a result of degeneration of vestibular, proprioceptive, and visual senses, ability to walk and drive, as well as spatial orientation, can be reduced to the point of incapacitation. Estimates indicate that 12.5 million persons older than 65 years of age note that dizziness represents a serious impairment of their normal activities. The most significant complications of presbystasis are falls and hip fractures.

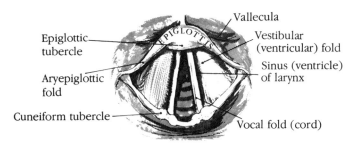

Fig. 6-11. Mirror view of the laryngopharynx.

3. *Presbylarynx.* Generally accepted characteristics of the senescent voice include weakness, hoarseness, tremulousness, and altered pitch. However, changes in voice and speech are more closely related to physiologic than chronologic age, and a change in vocal quality may herald significant local or systemic disease. Specific disease entities, such as cancer, neurologic illness, and endocrine dysfunction must be excluded before a diagnosis of senile dysphonia can be made. Atrophy of the vocal folds with bowing and prominence of the vocal processes of the arytenoid cartilages is the hallmark.

III. Cardinal Symptoms and Abnormal Findings
  A. Nose

1. Rhinitis (inflammation of the mucous membranes of the nose). Rhinitis is a common finding, usually caused by infection, allergy, or vasomotor changes.
   a. Watery rhinorrhea suggests a viral infection; thick, purulent discharge points to probable superimposed bacterial infection.
   b. Nasal allergy results in sneezing, watery rhinorrhea, stuffiness, and epiphora, with pale and boggy turbinates.
   c. Vasomotor rhinitis is similar to that caused by allergy, but with more reddened turbinates.

2. Sinusitis. Pain and tenderness over the involved sinus is common; generalized headache is rare. Orbital complications (proptosis, pain, diplopia, epiphora, swelling of lids, or tumor mass) often are first signs of sinusitis. In the nose, the turbinates are red and boggy, purulent nasal discharge is often present, and the nasal mucosa is red and edematous. Fever and prostration may occur.

3. Nasal obstruction
   a. Unilateral obstruction may be caused by a deviated septum, foreign bodies, or neoplasm.
   b. Bilateral obstruction is often the result of rhinitis or nasal polyps; an S-shaped deviated septum also can obstruct both airways. In children, adenoid hypertrophy is a common cause of obstruction.

4. Perforation of the nasal septum can result from trauma or infection.
   a. Anterior perforation occurs with tuberculosis; posterior perforation with syphilis and cocaine abuse.
   b. Epistaxis most frequently occurs in the anterior septum (Little's area), which is easily accessible. Epistaxis may also arise posteriorly from a branch of the sphenopalatine artery, or superiorly from an ethmoid vessel.

  B. Ear

1. Auricle. Frostbite, eczema, sebaceous cysts often affect the auricle.

2. External canals. Tenderness usually indicates furunculosis or external otitis. Obstruction may be due to cerumen or foreign bodies or certain tumors such as exostoses, cysts, and malignant neoplasms.

3. Tympanic membrane. Middle ear disease is mirrored in the tympanic membrane.
   a. Bulging. Landmarks become obscure; thickening and erythema indicate acute otitis media.
   b. Retraction. Landmarks are accentuated, usually indicating obstruction of the eustachian tube or scarring from past otitis.
   c. Color. Amber-colored membrane indicates serous otitis media; air bubbles or fluid level can sometimes be seen.
   d. Perforations. Usually old inflammatory disease is the cause of perforations. They vary in size, may be central (usually benign), anterior, or marginal.

4. Middle ear
   a. Discharges *(otorrhea)*. These are serous, mucoid, purulent, putrid, or sanguinous. Putrid, foul discharge usually indicates mastoid disease with bone destruction. Sanguinous discharge can occur with acute otitis, but neoplasm or injury must be ruled out.

    b. Cholesteatomas. Pearly white cystlike masses may occur in chronic otitis media. Retraction pockets in the tympanic membrane usually precede this condition.

  5. Hearing loss

    a. Conductive hearing loss. Any disturbance in the conduction of a sound impulse as it passes through the ear canal, tympanic membrane, middle ear, and ossicular chain to the footplate of the stapes is considered a conductive hearing loss. A person with this loss speaks softly, hears well on the telephone, hears best in a noisy environment.

    b. Sensorineural (perceptive) hearing loss. A disturbance anywhere from the cochlea, through the auditory nerve, to the hearing center in the cerebral cortex. A person with this loss speaks loudly, hears better in a quiet environment, does poorly in a crowd and on the telephone. He or she may hear but does not understand; sounds are garbled. This is indicative of poor discrimination.

    c. Mixed hearing loss is combined conductive and sensorineural.

C. Nasopharynx. Inflammatory, neoplastic, or congenital disease may occur.

  1. Thickened mucus secretions (postnasal drip), caused by nasal or environmental factors, which appear as white or yellow strands or webs in the nasopharynx

  2. Polyps and cysts (common)

  3. Obstruction may cause changes in voice quality, since normal voice resonance is produced by the nasopharynx. Inflammatory and neoplastic disease almost always produces obstruction of the eustachian tube orifice, resulting in hearing loss and otalgia, negative middle ear pressure, and transudation of serum into the middle ear space.

D. Oral cavity and oropharynx

  1. Oral mucous membranes

    a. Mucosal surfaces

      (1) Color. Bright red surfaces may indicate erythema and inflammation, pallor indicates localized ischemia or generalized anemia, cyanotic color changes may indicate local congestion or a systemic state that produces hypoxemia.

      (2) Deposits. Local deposits of brown pigment are seen in some metabolic conditions such as hypoadrenalism. Linear pigmentation of terminal capillary beds of the free gingival margin may indicate heavy metal absorption, which may correlate with toxic symptoms. Localized bluish pigmentation in the gingival areas may be due to accidental implantation of metal dental filling materials.

      (3) Ulcers, white patches. Ulceration is indicative of trauma or secondary lesions following initial vesicles of viral or other primary disease lesions. White, thickened patches are caused by increase in the layer of mucosal keratin. White plaques may be caused by monilial infection.

    b. Swelling. Oral mucosal and submucosal swelling are caused (in order of frequency) by inflammation, reactive hyperplasia, cysts, congenital deformities, or neoplasm. Careful palpation is necessary to detect many submucosal swellings. If bleeding occurs following palpation, great care is needed to locate the source of bleeding and the tissue characteristics of the bleeding source (inflammatory or neoplastic).

    c. Dry mouth (xerostomia). Atrophy of salivary glands is seen with senility, disease states, radiation, and many drugs that decrease salivary function.

    d. Excess saliva (ptyalism). Too much saliva may be caused by mucosal irritation, heavy metal toxicity, or pilocarpine-like drug action.

  2. Lips

    a. Ulcers: usually secondary to vesicular lesions of viral origin (such as herpes), and to trauma

    b. Numbness of lower lip: due to anesthesia or damage to the inferior alveolar nerve in the mandible

    c. Drooling: motor loss due to peripheral or central facial nerve paralysis

    d. Swelling: pronounced response to any inflammatory process; sometimes subtle as in angioneurotic edema and other allergic phenomena

    e. Surface keratosis, induration, ulceration: suggestive of squamous cell carcinoma and necessitates a biopsy

    f. Fissures at angle of mouth: seen in the aged with inflammation and loss of dental structures; also may be a feature of nutritional deficiency

    g. Mucocele of superficial accessory salivary glands: occasionally develop following injury

    h. Congenital anomalies: may result repair in parasagittal scars in the upper lip from congenital cleft

3. Oral vestibule, buccal mucosa, gingivae

    a. Submucosal hemorrhage. Small spots may be due to recent trauma of the buccal mucosa; similar lesions may be caused by blood dyscrasias with bleeding tendency.

    b. Gingival bleeding. This may be caused by local inflammation and infection or hemorrhagic disorders.

    c. Gingival recession. Recession of gingivae to low position on roots of teeth may be due to increased age, trauma from incorrect brushing, or chronic periodontitis.

    d. Gingival swelling. This is a common sign of odontogenic infection; sinus tracts draining dentoalveolar abscesses may also occur. Generalized enlargement of the gingivae may occur in chronic inflammation, pregnancy, endocrine disturbance, phenytoin medication, or blood dyscrasias, and may occur as a familial tendency to gingival fibromatosis.

    e. Gingivitis. A common inflammatory reaction due to irritation and infection, gingivitis is often caused by deposition of dental calculus around the necks of teeth, particularly the anterior mandibular teeth and the maxillary molar teeth near the salivary ducts.

    f. Chronic periodontitis. Epithelial attachment of the gingivae is lost, and pocket lesions form adjacent to teeth resulting in loss of supporting soft tissue and bone.

    g. Ulcerative gingival stomatitis (Vincent's infection). A combination of painful gums, bleeding from the free gingival margins and pseudomembrane, and loss of interdental papillae are manifestations of ulcerative gingival stomatitis. Anti-infective medication may attenuate the process, but comprehensive dental treatment is needed to eliminate the process.

    h. Pericoronitis. Common localized gum inflammation around a partially erupted third molar is seen in pericoronitis. Prompt removal of the molar is usually required.

4. Hard and soft palate

    a. Nodular papillomatosis may occur beneath a maxillary artificial denture because of irritation and altered function of the region.

    b. Congenital clefts involve both hard and soft palates and may extend through the alveolar ridge between canine and lateral incisor teeth. Evidence of the deformity or scar tissue from surgical repair may be noted. A submucosal cleft palate may include a bifid uvula with hypernasal speech.

    c. Nicotine stomatitis may produce general white mucosal hyperkeratosis and elevation of the accessory salivary glands with red dilated orifices.

    d. Neoplasm can occur in the posterior palatal vault; palpation may reveal submucosal nodular swelling as the only sign.

5. Tongue and floor of the mouth

a. Atrophy of the tongue produces a smooth-surfaced red appearance and suggests nutritional deficiency or pernicious anemia.

b. Hypertrophy and hyperkeratosis of the filiform papillae produces a furred, hairy, thick coat; this may be due to irritation and immobility caused by poor oral hygiene.

c. "Geographic tongue," with a striking pattern of arcuate variations in papillary distribution, is a transient, benign condition.

d. Macroglossia (large tongue) may be due to hypothyroidism or to several inflammatory, cystic, congenital, and neoplastic conditions. Asymmetric tongue enlargement may be caused by hemangioma, lymphangioma, or neurofibroma.

e. Burning tongue is chiefly a psychogenic disorder.

f. Abnormal tongue motility may be due to neuromuscular disorders such as stroke and myasthenia gravis and may cause speech disturbance; fixed, firm tongue may result from infiltration with malignant neoplasm, usually squamous cell carcinoma.

g. Retention cysts of the sublingual glands produce soft, translucent swellings on the floor of the mouth.

h. A localized, palpable stone in the course of the submaxillary duct may produce obstructive symptoms.

i. Exostosis of the mandible is manifested by a hard mass projecting toward the floor of the mouth from the region of bone supporting the premolar teeth (torus mandibularis).

j. Similar hard swelling may occur in the midline of the mandible at the genial tubercles, especially prominent when teeth are gone and alveolar process has atrophied.

6. Tonsils. Large tonsils may not be diseased, unless they interfere with respiration or swallowing. Acute tonsillitis is easily recognized. Malignant and benign tumors may also arise from the tonsils.

7. Teeth

a. Darkened teeth may be caused by surface stains and by devitalization of the pulp through trauma or disease.

b. Irregular, short, or broken teeth may be caused by congenital hypoplasia, attrition, or dental caries. Congenital syphilis causes hypoplasia of incisors resulting in notched and barrel-shaped Hutchinson's incisor.

c. Hypermobility of permanent teeth may be due to injury; more commonly this is due to advanced periodontal disease. Localized hypermobility may be an indication of alveolar bone destruction caused by primary or metastatic neoplastic disease.

8. Jaws

a. Restriction of the mandible may be caused by disturbances of the temporomandibular joint, extra-articular restriction by scar tissue, and trismus from spasm of the elevating muscles of mastication from any inflammatory cause.

b. Crepitus or pain may be caused by disturbances in the temporomandibular joint.

9. Tumors

a. Malignant tumors of the oral cavity/oropharynx are usually squamous cell carcinomas. The typical cause is tobacco and ethanol abuse. Symptoms may include odynophagia, dysphagia, altered speech, otalgia, loose teeth, altered fit of dentures, weight loss, and neck mass. Diagnosis is by visualization, palpation, and biopsy. Malignant tumors are typically indurated on palpation. The appearance may be ulcerated or friable.

E. Laryngopharynx. Hoarseness is the main symptom of laryngopharyngeal disease, although it may also result from congenital abnormalities.

1. Acute inflammation (laryngitis). Laryngeal mucosa is red and edematous; true vocal cords remain pale at first, later become fiery red; secretions may be seen on the cords; ecchymotic spots may develop due to coughing. Symptoms can include aphonia (loss of voice).

2. Chronic laryngitis. Repeated infections, voice abuse, smoking, gastroesophageal reflux, and poor nasal respiration may cause chronic laryngitis. Laryngeal mucosa is dull red; true vocal cords lose pearly white appearance and are boggy; engorged capillaries may be present on the cords; and thick stringy secretions are seen. In tuberculous laryngitis, additional signs include pallor and ulceration of the laryngeal mucosa.

3. Tumors
   a. Benign tumors. Occasionally these tumors cause hoarseness.
   b. Carcinoma of the larynx. Hoarseness is an extremely important symptom, and may be the only early symptom. Advanced signs include stridor, dysphagia, severe pain, otalgia, halitosis, widening of the thyroid cartilages, hemoptysis, and cervical adenopathy.

4. Paralysis of the vocal cords. Hoarseness may occur when paralysis is incomplete. Cord paralysis indicates interruption of the recurrent laryngeal nerve on the same side, which can result from many traumatic, operative, inflammatory, neoplastic, or vascular abnormalities, and occasionally from central nervous system disease.

IV. Available Technology

A. Weber test
   1. The Weber test is a test of lateralization.
   2. The tuning fork is set into motion, and its stem is placed on the midline of the patient's skull. The patient must state where the tone is louder: in the left ear, right ear, both ears, or the midline.
   3. Patients with normal hearing or equal amounts of hearing loss in both ears (conductive, sensorineural, or mixed loss) will experience a midline sensation.
   4. Patients with a unilateral sensorineural loss will hear the tone in their better ear.
   5. Patients with a unilateral conductive loss will hear the tone in their poorer ear.

B. Rinne test
   1. The Rinne test compares a patient's air and bone conduction hearing.
   2. The tuning fork is struck and its stem placed first on the mastoid process (as closely as possible to the posterosuperior edge of the canal without touching it), then approximately 2 inches lateral to the opening of the external ear canal. The patient reports whether the tone sounds louder with the fork behind or in front of the ear.
   3. Patients with normal hearing or sensorineural hearing loss will perceive the tone as louder in front of the ear (positive Rinne).
   4. Patients with conductive hearing loss will perceive the sound as louder behind the ear (negative Rinne).

C. Audiogram. The pure tone audiogram is the standard measure of hearing acuity. It is a test of an individual's sensitivity to air and bone conduction from 250 to 8000 Hz. Masking, the introduction of noise into the nontest ear, prevents it from listening when assessing the test ear. Routine speech audiometry measures speech reception threshold (SRT) and speech discrimination score (SDS). The SRT is the softest level at which a person can hear and correctly repeat words in 50% of presentations. The SDS assesses how clearly a person can hear speech.

D. Auditory brain-stem response audiometry (ABR). Surface electrodes are used to measure the potentials arising in the auditory nerve and brain-stem structures. The stimulus is a wide-band click. The three main clinical uses of brain-stem audiometry are threshold testing of infants, young children, and malingerers; diagnosis of acoustic neuromas; and diagnosis of brain-stem lesions and neuropathies.

E. Caloric test. This is a test of vestibular function. Each ear is stimulated by water that is warmer and cooler than body temperature (30° C and 40° C).

Water is placed in the external auditory canal, and the eyes are observed for onset, direction, and duration of nystagmus. The normal response is as follows:
1. Latent period of 15 to 30 seconds
2. Duration of nystagmus for 30 to 75 seconds
   a. Cool stimulus will produce nystagmus whose fast phase is away from the stimulated ear.
   b. Warm stimulus will produce nystagmus whose fast phase is toward the stimulated ear (*COWS*: cold opposite, warm same).

F. Sinus x-rays. Radiographic examination of the paranasal sinuses consists of four standard projections: Waters', lateral, submentovertex, and Caldwell's. Sinus x-rays are best for detection of acute sinusitis (air-fluid levels). Chronic sinusitis is better delineated on CT scans.

G. Computed tomography (CT) and magnetic resonance imaging (MRI). These diagnostic studies have revolutionized head and neck imaging. Their cross-sectional display of anatomy has added new dimensions in the diagnostic workup. CT is better in its evaluation of bony structures. MRI is a noninvasive, nonradiologic imaging technique with no known biologic hazards. One of the major advantages of MRI in head and neck imaging is its superior display of soft tissue detail in any plane, coronal, axial, or sagittal without moving the patient.

H. The cost figures cited in this table are **basic direct costs**. The figures are difficult to obtain and change quickly. They include **only** the cost of the test itself (technician, equipment, time, and materials). No professional costs (interpretation) are included. Costs vary from region to region based on differences in some components such as labor. However, the relative cost ranking should remain similar.

Procedure	Code
Weber test	$
Rinne test	$
Audiogram	$$
Auditory brainstem response audiometry (ABR)	$$
Caloric test	$$
Sinus x-rays	$
Computed tomography (CT)	$$$
Magnetic resonance imaging (MRI)—head	$$$$

$ = $0–$50; $$ = $50–$100; $$$ = $100–$200; $$$$ = $200–$500.

V. Bibliography

Ballenger JJ, ed. *Diseases of the Nose, Throat, Ear, Head & Neck*, 14th ed. Philadelphia: Lea & Febiger; 1991.

Cummings CW, Frederickson JM, Harker LA, et al. *Otolaryngology—Head and Neck Surgery,* 2nd ed. St. Louis: CV Mosby; 1993.

DeWeese DD, Saunders WH, Schuller DE, Schleuning AJ II. *Textbook of Otolaryngology,* 7th ed. St. Louis: CV Mosby; 1988.

Kerr DA, Ash MM Jr, Milard HD. *Oral Diagnosis*, 6th ed. St. Louis: CV Mosby; 1983.

Lee KJ, ed. *Essential Otolaryngology: Head and Neck Surgery,* 6th ed. Norwalk, CT: Appleton & Lange; 1995.

Lynch MA, Brightman VJ, Greenberg MS. *Burkett's Oral Medicine: Diagnosis and Treatment,* 9th ed. Philadelphia: JB Lippincott; 1994.

Robinson HBG, Miller AS. *Colby, Kerr and Robinson's Color Atlas of Oral Pathology,* 5th ed. Philadelphia: JB Lippincott; 1990.

Shafer WG, Hines MK, Levy BM. *A Textbook of Oral Pathology,* 4th ed. Philadelphia: WB Saunders; 1983.

VI. Key Search Words

The following key words reflect the content of this chapter. They are provided to assist with an on-line search of computer databases, such as MEDLINE, if you wish to pursue the topic of this chapter further.

Diagnosis, oral
Diagnostic imaging
Head and neck neoplasms
Hearing disorders
Hearing tests
Hypopharynx
Larynx
Nasopharynx
Oral health
Oropharynx
Neoplasms, squamous cell
Salivary glands
Salivary gland diseases
Salivary gland neoplasms
Sinusitis

7. RESPIRATORY SYSTEM

Cyril M. Grum

I. Glossary

Adventitious sounds: extra sounds not normally present, such as rales, rhonchi, wheezes, stridor, and rubs.

Asthma: a disease characterized by increased responsiveness and inflammation of the trachea and the bronchi to various stimuli manifested by widespread narrowing of the airways, characterized clinically as wheezing or cough; changes in severity can occur spontaneously or as a result of therapy.

Atelectasis: partial or complete airlessness with collapse of the affected segment, lobe, or entire lung; reduction in the volume; with or without locally obstructed bronchi; chronic or acute. Atelectasis also refers to diffuse small areas with loss of volume—microatelectasis.

Breath sounds: sounds due to the movement of air through the lungs and air passages appreciated by auscultation; *bronchial* (also called tubular), abnormal breath sounds, similar to tracheal sounds, heard over consolidated lung; *bronchovesicular,* sounds intermediate between vesicular and tracheal, heard over the major bronchi; *tracheal,* normal to-and-fro sounds heard over the trachea; *vesicular,* the normal breath sounds, predominantly inspiratory, heard over most of the lung.

Bronchiectasis: a disease characterized by chronic dilatation of bronchial walls associated with chronic production of mucopurulent phlegm; causes obstructive ventilatory defect.

Bronchitis: acute or chronic bronchial inflammation.

Chronic bronchitis: a clinical entity characterized by cough and sputum production on most days for at least 3 months in at least 2 successive years without a specific cause, usually associated with airways obstruction and a history of cigarette smoking.

Chronic obstructive pulmonary disease (COPD): a general term describing diseases characterized by diffuse airways obstruction, especially chronic bronchitis and emphysema.

Clubbing: deforming enlargement of the terminal phalanges, usually acquired, associated with certain cardiac and pulmonary diseases; characterized by loss of the normal angle between the skin and nail base due to proliferative soft tissue at the nail base.

Collapse: reduction in lung volume, acute or chronic, due to bronchial or parenchymal disease.

Compression: mechanical reduction of lung volume by pressure.

Consolidation: filling of pulmonary parenchyma; usually refers to the lung becoming firm as the air spaces are filled with exudate in pneumonia.

Crackle: adventitial lung sound, often used synonymously with rale.

Cyanosis: a blue color of the skin and mucous membranes due to severe arterial oxygen desaturation, caused by excessive levels of reduced hemoglobin.

Dyspnea: the subjective sensation of abnormal or inappropriate shortness of breath or difficulty in breathing.

Emphysema: a chronic obstructive lung disease characterized pathologically as destruction and dilatation of alveoli; usually associated with a history of cigarette smoking; characterized clinically by dyspnea, a minimally productive

This chapter builds on the foundation established by the previous authors of this section, Drs. Robert A. Green and John G. Weg. They are superb clinicians and educators and have been leaders of Michigan Pulmonology for a generation.

or nonproductive cough, persistent hyperinflation of the lung, and decreased breath sounds; *Compensatory emphysema*: secondary dilatation of air spaces adjacent to areas volume loss, or removal. *Subcutaneous emphysema*: air or other gas in subcutaneous tissues.

Empyema: pus in the pleural cavity; pyothorax. Empyema is classified as an exudative effusion.

Forced expiratory time (FET): the time required to empty the lungs completely with maximal effort from full inspiration to full expiration; normally less than 3 seconds, increased with obstructive lung diseases.

Forced vital capacity (FVC): the total volume of air exhaled from the lungs from a maximum inspiration to a maximum expiration, with expiration as rapid and forceful as possible.

Fremitus: a palpable vibration or thrill; *tactile* or *vocal fremitus*, vibration felt from voice sounds; often the words "ninety-nine" or "blue moon" are used to elicit.

Friction rub: grating sensation, heard or palpated, which arises from inflamed serous surfaces, such as pleural or pericardial.

Hemoptysis: expectoration of gross blood by coughing from the larynx or lower respiratory tract.

Kyphosis: increased convexity of the spine in the anteroposterior plane.

Müller's maneuver: production of increased negative intrapleural pressure by an attempt to inhale forcibly against a closed glottis.

Pleural effusion: fluid of any type in the pleural cavity; classified as transudate or exudate based on etiology. Thoracentesis is required for specific identification.

Pleurisy: any pleural inflammation; loosely, the pain associated with disease of the pleura.

Pneumoconiosis: condition resulting from inhalation and deposition of inorganic (mineral) or organic dusts and the inflammatory reaction of lung tissue to its presence; this parenchymal pulmonary disease is usually of environmental or occupational cause, including reactions to fumes, gases, and so on.

Pneumonia: clinical term that most commonly refers to pulmonary inflammation and consolidation due to infection.

Pneumonitis: any pulmonary inflammation.

Pneumothorax: air within pleural cavity; *tension pneumothorax,* a pneumothorax characterized by increased pressure such that vascular flow and normal ventilation is compromised.

Rale: (also crackle), discontinuous adventitial sound usually heard only in inspiration; crisp, discrete, short, crackling sound believed to be due to opening of collapsed peripheral airways and alveoli, or to gas flowing through secretions. *Fine, medium, coarse rale:* classifying terms referring to loudness, duration, and quality of rales; coarse rales are louder, longer, and lower in pitch than fine rales. *Dry, moist, crepitant, Velcro, cellophane, sibilant, sonorous rales:* descriptive terms that have not been shown to have diagnostic value.

Respiration, variations in. *Apnea*: the absence of breathing; *bradypnea*: breathing at a slow rate; *Cheyne-Stokes*: a cyclic breathing pattern in which there is increased depth and rate of respiration between periods of apnea; *hyperpnea*: increased depth and usually rate of respiration; *orthopnea*: inability to breathe comfortably while supine, relieved by sitting up; *tachypnea*: increased rate of respiration.

Rhonchi: continuous coarse sounds arising from the trachea or bronchi; longer in duration than rales, lower pitch than wheezes, caused by turbulence around mucus in airways; may be inspiratory or expiratory and often changes in character with cough.

Scoliosis: lateral deviation of the spine.

Stridor: difficult respiration due to upper airways obstruction, characterized by high-pitched crowing sounds in inspiration.

Valsalva's maneuver: production of decreased negative intrapleural pressure by an attempt, after deep inspiration, to expire forcibly against a closed glottis.

Voice sounds: the vibrations of the spoken voice transmitted through the lungs and appreciated by auscultation; also called vocal resonance and, rarely, vocal fremitus. Voice sounds are often altered when the lung has consolidation; three examples—*bronchophony*: increased intensity of voice sounds; *egophony*: a peculiar nasal quality of voice sounds in which a spoken long e ("eee") simulates a long a (ay); *whispered pectoriloquy*: distinct transmission of whispered words.

Wheeze: a high-pitched whistling sound associated with airflow through a partially obstructed, vibrating airway.

II. Techniques of Examination and Normal Findings
  A. Important factors and considerations
   1. Evaluation of the respiratory system requires thorough physical examination using four techniques (inspection, palpation, percussion, and auscultation) and careful correlation with diagnostic studies (e.g., roentgenograms, arterial blood gases, pulmonary function studies).
   2. Examination of the respiratory system consists primarily of examination of the chest. Develop a thorough, systematic routine that can be applied to all patients. Interpret findings first in terms of pathologic changes; after review of diagnostic studies, specific disease entities can be considered.
   3. Knowledge of the anatomy of the lungs is essential to a proper examination. Chest wall landmarks are shown in Figures 7-1 and 7-2. The sternal angle (angle of Louis) is a prominent landmark and the best guide to accurate numbering of the ribs. A series of imaginary lines are useful to document topographic location. Each bronchopulmonary segment should

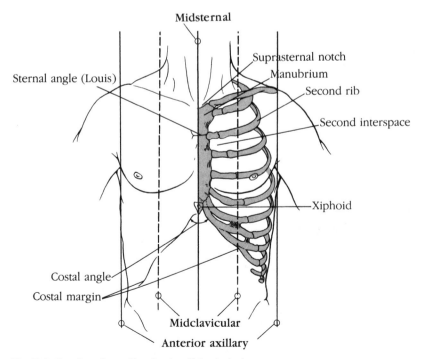

Fig. 7-1. Landmarks on the chest wall (anterior).

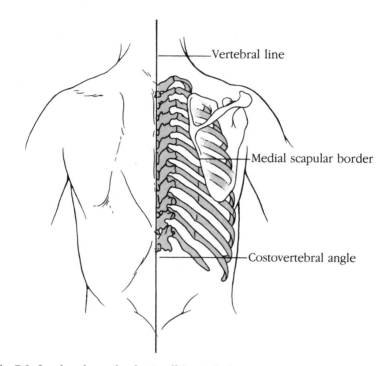

Fig. 7-2. Landmarks on the chest wall (posterior).

be checked in a thorough examination. Anatomic distribution of lung lobes and segments is shown in Figures 7-3 through 7-6.

4. Strengths and limitations of the physical examination must be appreciated. The physical examination allows excellent evaluation of ventilatory function but not efficacy of gas exchange. It allows estimation of the volume of exchanging gas and the rate and distribution of air flow. The physical examination does not allow evaluation of diffusion, perfusion, the relation of ventilation to perfusion (gas exchange), and other functions of the lung.

B. Examination techniques

1. Inspection. Major value: observation of symmetry, both of ventilation and structure, of the two sides of the thorax. Minor variations are common.

   a. Technique

   (1) A quiet, well-lit room is required.

   (2) Patient sits erect, exposed to the waist, and supported by an aide if necessary. Patient should be relaxed and comfortable.

   (3) While seated, inspect the front, back, and side of the chest. Stand behind the patient and look down over the patient's shoulders at the anterior chest.

   b. Respiratory rate. A normal examination should have the following features:

   (1) A resting rate between 12 to 16 breaths per minute (should be counted for at least 30 seconds)

   (2) A regular rhythm of respiration

   (3) Inspiration 1½ times as long as expiration

   (4) Quiet respiration; not noisy or audible

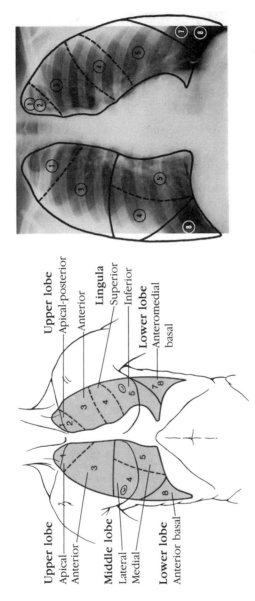

Fig. 7-3. Segmental pulmonary anatomy (anterior).

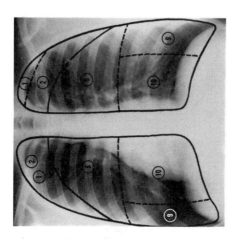

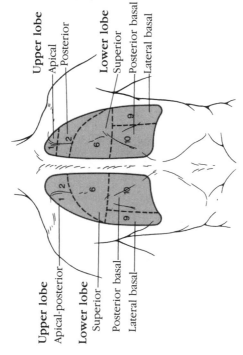

Upper lobe
Apical
Posterior

Lower lobe
Superior
Posterior basal
Lateral basal

Upper lobe
Apical-posterior

Lower lobe
Superior
Posterior basal
Lateral basal

Fig. 7-4. Segmental pulmonary anatomy (posterior).

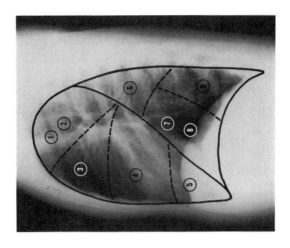

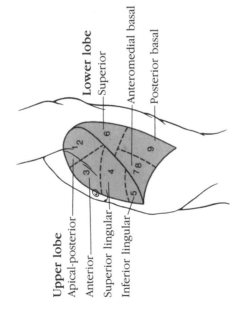

Upper lobe
Apical-posterior
Anterior
Superior lingular
Inferior lingular

Lower lobe
Superior
Anteromedial basal
Posterior basal

Fig. 7-5. Segmental pulmonary anatomy (left lateral).

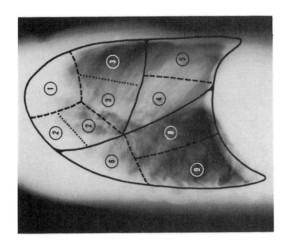

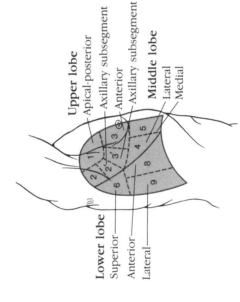

Upper lobe
Apical-posterior
Axillary subsegment
Anterior
Axillary subsegment

Middle lobe
Lateral
Medial

Lower lobe
Superior
Anterior
Lateral

Fig. 7-6. Segmental pulmonary anatomy (right lateral).

    (5) Diaphragmatic respirations with no accessory muscle use (e.g., bulging or retraction of intercostal muscle or use of sternocleidomastiod muscle)

    (6) Respiration not labored or painful

c. Chest. People usually breathe predominantly with their thoracic cage when erect. While supine, respiration is usually largely abdominal, with the abdomen moving out during inspiration.

    (1) Observe the following during quiet respiration:

        (a) Status of skin and breasts

        (b) Muscular development or loss

        (c) State of nutrition

        (d) Position of cardiac apex impulse

        (e) Size, shape, contour, and symmetry of chest

        (f) Angle of costal margins at the xyphoid (normally <90 degrees>; widens with inspiration); the angle the ribs make posteriorly with vertebrae (normally approximately 45 degrees); the slope of the ribs

    (2) Exclude the following abnormalities:

        (a) Asymmetry of chest wall motion (e.g., lag of a hemithorax)

        (b) Interspaces that retract or bulge during ventilation—general or limited

        (c) Flaring or lag of the chest wall

        (d) Scars, prior surgery, sinus tract openings

        (e) Thoracic deformities, bilateral or unilateral; minor variations shown in Figure 7-7: *pectus excavatum* (funnel-shaped depression of lower portion of sternum); *pectus carinatum* or pigeon breast (sternum projects beyond frontal plane of abdomen); *scoliosis* (lateral curvature of the spine); *kyphosis* (increased convexity of the spine, often associated with scoliosis)

        (f) Vascular pulsation or dilatation

d. Chest. Forced vital capacity (FVC) maneuver:

    (1) Patient takes in maximum breath and forces it out with mouth wide open until lungs are completely empty. It is helpful to demonstrate this to the patient first, then have patient perform it two or three times.

    (2) Listen with stethoscope over cervical trachea.

    (3) Measure and record, in seconds, the time to complete this maneuver—the forced expiratory time (FET). Normal: 3.5 seconds or less. Prolonged: 4 seconds or more, indicative of obstruction to airflow.

e. Inspect related anatomy. Exclude the following abnormalities:

    (1) Cyanosis

    (2) Digital clubbing

    (3) Jugular venous distention

    (4) Pedal edema

    (5) Facial plethora or flushing

2. Palpation. Major value is evaluation of degree and symmetry of thoracic expansion with respiration and appreciation of transmitted vibrations of the spoken voice. It is complementary to inspection in the evaluation of respiratory excursion.

a. Technique

    (1) Use both hands to palpate symmetric areas of the thorax simultaneously. Glide your hands over every square inch. Be sure your hands are warm.

    (2) Use fingertips, palms, or ulnar edges of the hands. Palpate from above down during normal and deep respiration and while patient phonates.

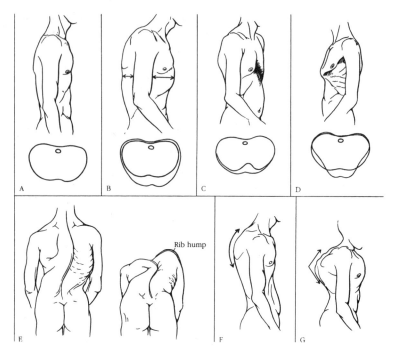

Fig. 7-7. Chest wall contours. **(A)** Normal. **(B)** Barrel chest (emphysema). **(C)** Pectus excavatum (funnel chest). **(D)** Pectus carinatum (pigeon breast). **(E)** Scoliosis. **(F)** Kyphosis. **(G)** Gibbus (extreme kyphosis).

b. Stand behind patient; place hands on lower chest with thumbs adjacent near the spine (Fig. 7-8). Tell patient to inhale deeply; compare the symmetry of onset and depth of inspiration. Normal costal expansion is 4 to 6 cm. Repeat with hands over lower lateral chest, and, still standing behind patient, with hands over the shoulders onto the anterior chest below the clavicles.

c. Palpate chest wall, noting general condition of skin, character of musculature, presence of any masses. Palpate each rib, noting any tenderness or vibrations that occur with respiration or heart beat.

d. Palpate the intrathoracic trachea (Fig. 7-9). Stand behind patient; let each index finger slide off the head of the clavicle deep into the sternal notch on either side. Note the position of the trachea (normally in the midline) and its distance from the posterior surface of the sternum.

e. Palpate supraclavicular areas for lymph nodes.

f. Check for scoliosis and deformities.

g. Evaluate tactile fremitus over all lung segments: palpate using the palmar aspect of fingers or ulnar aspect of hands as the patient speaks (Fig. 7-10). Have the patient repeat a standard phrase (e.g., "ninety-nine," "blue moon," "one, two, three"). Note the comparative increase, decrease, or absence of fremitus, which is most prominent over areas where the bronchi are relatively close to the chest wall. Fremitus increases as the intensity of the voice increases and as its pitch drops. It is normally symmetric except for a slightly greater intensity over the right upper lobe than over the left. Fremitus varies greatly

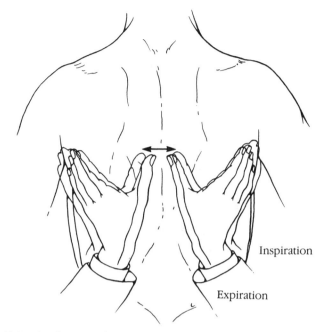

Inspiration

Expiration

Fig. 7-8. Palpation for expansion.

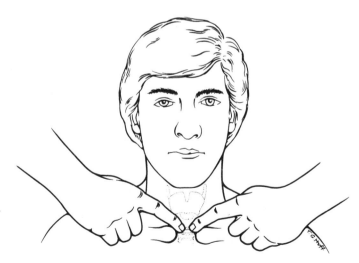

Fig. 7-9. Palpating the intrathoracic trachea. When the fingers slide down and are posterior to the clavicular head, the normal trachea can be felt in the midline.

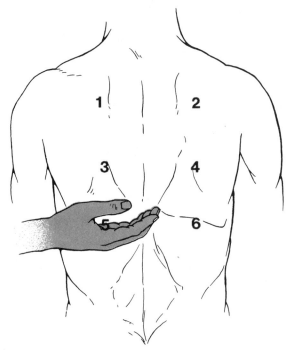

Fig. 7-10. Evaluation of tactile fremitus.

with chest wall thickness and pitch of voice (deep voice and thin chest are best for transmission of sound vibration).

   3. Percussion. Major value: determining the relative amount of air or solid material in the underlying lung; locating the boundaries of organs or portions of the lung that differ in structural density. Do not be discouraged if initial attempts are clumsy and unrewarding; skillful percussion requires much practice.
      a. Technique
         (1) Direct percussion (used very infrequently, as mediate percussion is standard practice). Tap the chest with the middle or ring finger. This is especially valuable over the clavicle.
         (2) Indirect or mediate percussion (Fig. 7-11):
            (a) Place distal two phalanges of middle finger of left hand firmly against chest wall in intercostal spaces parallel with ribs.
            (b) Strike the distal interphalangeal joint with the tip of the middle finger of right hand, one or two rapid sharp blows in succession. Hold forearm stationary, make striking motion with the wrist. Proper striking motion should attempt to induce resonance, as in striking a bass drum.
         (3) Percuss gently though firmly and with equal force at all points. The amount of force used depends on the thickness of the chest wall. Note the sound elicited, the sense of resistance, and the vibration under the finger.
      b. Percuss from side to side, comparing symmetric areas of the chest.
      c. Percuss the lower margins of the lungs, the width of the heart and upper mediastinum.

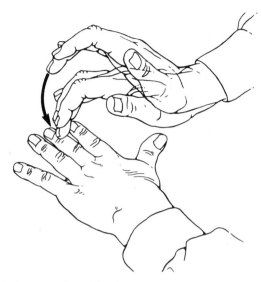

Fig. 7-11. Mediate percussion of the chest.

    d. Ascertain the extent and equality of diaphragmatic excursion (also well-evaluated by fluoroscopy) (Fig. 7-12).

        (1) Ask patient to inhale deeply and hold breath. Note line of change in percussion note between resonant lung and dull abdominal viscera posteriorly.

        (2) Ask patient to exhale completely and hold breath. Note the lower level of pulmonary resonance, which has moved upward.

        (3) The distance between these two points is the diaphragmatic excursion. Normal excursion is 3 cm in women and 5 to 6 cm in men.

        (4) Costal expansion is a complementary value. Measure with a flexible tape measure placed around the chest at nipple level.

    e. Evaluate percussion sounds. Normal percussion note is resonant over all of the lungs except over organs (heart, liver) where dullness is detected. The note varies with thickness of chest wall and force applied (Fig. 7-13).

        (1) *Resonance*: the clear, long, low-pitched sound elicited over the normal lung. When patients are examined while lying on the side, the dependent lung has less resonance.

        (2) *Dullness*: short, high-pitched, soft, thudding, without vibration. Dullness occurs when the air content of the underlying tissue is decreased and solidity increased. It is heard normally over the heart, accompanied by increased sense of resistance in the finger.

        (3) *Flatness*: absolute dullness; very short, feeble, high-pitched. It occurs when no air is present in underlying tissues; this sound may be demonstrated by percussion of arm or thigh muscles.

        (4) *Hyperresonance*: the vibrant, lower-pitched, louder, and longer sound heard normally over the lungs during full inspiration, or in the presence of a pneumothorax.

        (5) *Tympany*: high-pitched, clear, hollow, drumlike, moderately loud, fairly well-sustained, musical sound normally heard in left upper quadrant of the abdomen over the air-filled stomach or over any hollow viscus.

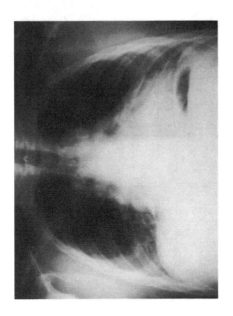

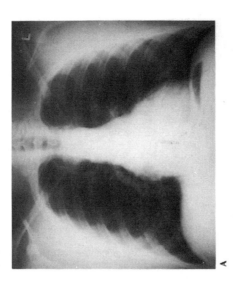

Fig. 7-12. Normal diaphragmatic excursion. **(A)** Full inspiration *(left)* and full expiration *(right)*. **(B)** Inspiration and expiration.

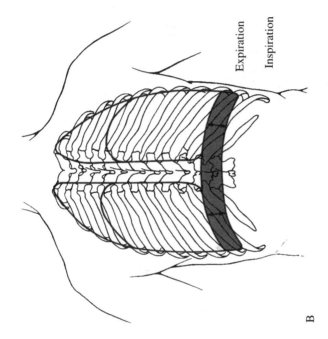

Expiration

Inspiration

B

Fig. 7-12. *Continued*

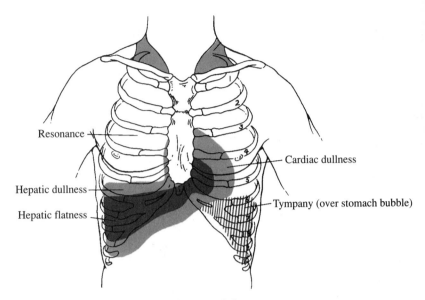

Fig. 7-13. Percussion notes over the normal chest.

4. Auscultation. Major value: appreciation of normal breath sounds and abnormal (adventitial) sounds arising from diseased areas; and comparison of the state of bronchial patency of various lung divisions. A quiet room is essential.
   a. Technique
      (1) Prior to auscultation with a stethoscope, listen to the patient breathing. It is quiet in health, but heard at a distance in obstructive lung diseases.
      (2) Use stethoscope fitted with both a diaphragm and a bell (a bell is helpful in very thin patients with deep intercostal spaces when the larger diaphragm does not make full contact).
      (3) Apply stethoscope firmly to the chest wall, avoiding factitious (artificial) sounds due to chest hair or rubbing against the stethoscope.
   b. Cover all portions of both lung fields systematically, from below to above—posteriorly, laterally, and anteriorly, comparing areas side to side. Be sure to cover each bronchopulmonary segment.
   c. Breath sounds. Instruct the patient to breathe a little deeper and faster than normal with mouth open; demonstrate this yourself to the patient. Note the character of the breath sounds and the presence of abnormal sounds, and note any changes that occur during more rapid and deep respiration (normally the breath sounds should increase in intensity, called *recruitment*). Direct the patient with instructions such as "a little deeper, please," "a little faster, please," "not quite so hard," until you are certain of what you hear. Factitious noise is often confusing (e.g., chest hair rubbing against the stethoscope).
      (1) *Vesicular* breathing is normal over most of the lungs. Vesicular breath sounds are breezy or swishy in character. The inspiratory

phase predominates; the pitch is high. Expiration is heard as a short, faint, lower-pitched puff less than 25% as long as inspiration. Vesicular sounds are more muffled than bronchial breath sounds. Think about air going into a sponge (the lung parenchyma).

(2) *Bronchial* breathing is heard normally over the trachea and the main bronchi. Inspiration is louder and higher-pitched. Expiration is increased in duration and is actually longer than inspiration; its pitch is high, intensity greater. Its quality is hollow or tubular and rather harsh. More hollow than vesicular breath sounds. Think about air going through a tube (the bronchi).

(3) *Bronchovesicular* breath sounds are an intermediate stage heard normally in the second interspaces anteriorly, the interscapular area posteriorly, and often at the medial right apex. Expiration is as loud, as long, and similar in pitch to inspiration. It is a transition between bronchial to vesicular sounds.

(4) *Exaggerated vesicular* breathing is heard normally in thin people and children, during exercise, and in loud and rapid respiration. Expiration is more prominent than in vesicular breathing, but not of bronchovesicular character.

d. Vocal resonance. Ask the patient to phonate, and note the character of the vocal resonance. Differences due to chest wall thickness and the area being auscultated will be heard. Voice sounds are heard best near the trachea and major bronchi; exaggerated voice sounds (*bronchophony*) are normally heard over the trachea and right upper lobe posteriorly. Speech is heard as indistinct noise. The whispered voice should not be heard over much of the lung parenchyma.

e. Adventitial sounds. Rhonchi, wheezing, and so on, are not heard in the normal chest. Rales are usually abnormal, but have been described at the lung bases in normal persons inspiring from residual volume to total lung capacity. Breath sounds are in general symmetric bilaterally, but much variation may exist. Therefore, when breath sounds are not symmetric, it may be impossible to determine whether pathology exists without the aid of a chest roentgenogram.

III. Cardinal Symptoms and Abnormal Findings

A. Cardinal symptoms. A single abnormal finding is rarely diagnostic; correlation with other physical abnormalities and with the chest roentgenogram is necessary before the status of the underlying lung can be deduced with confidence.

1. Cough. A cough is always abnormal; it helps clear the airways of extraneous material.

a. Due to inhaled irritant, aspirated material, focal anatomic lesions (pulmonary or upper airway), or diffuse airway or parenchymal abnormality. Isolated cough, especially in a young, healthy individual is most likely to be indicative of bronchospasm (e.g., asthma).

b. Productive or nonproductive of sputum, paroxysmal, brassy, loud and high-pitched, or whoop-like.

2. Sputum production. This is always abnormal and often accompanies cough when irritation or inflammation leads to transudation or exudation of fluids. The tracheobronchial tree's normal secretions of 60 to 90 mL/day are swallowed.

a. Record nature (color, odor, consistency) and quantity of sputum. Sputum volume may vary from 1 teaspoon daily to 1 pint or more. Patients are often unaware of sputum production if it has increased gradually. Ask about sputum production in several different ways (e.g., clearing throat, smoker's cough). Morning expectoration usually implies accumulation of secretions during the night. A extremely fetid odor often indicates anaerobic infection.

b. Specifically examine for the presence of blood. (Analysis of sputum is described in the section on Special Techniques.)

3. Hemoptysis. A substantive proportion of patients with hemoptysis have serious disease.
   a. It can result from a single anatomic lesion, proximal or distal, which inflames or destroys the lung or bronchus involved.
   b. It can occur with diffuse increase in pulmonary capillary pressure, as in cardiac disease.
   c. Acute respiratory tract infections followed by neoplasm are the two most common causes. Table 7-1 lists common causes of hemoptysis.
   d. Significant blood loss into lung can occur with minimal external evidence of bleeding. Blood streaking of sputum is commonly seen in diffuse or localized inflammatory diseases and can be brought on by coughing paroxysms.
   e. Hemoptysis can be confused with hematemesis, oral, or nasopharyngeal bleeding. Table 7-2 lists characteristics useful in distinguishing hemoptysis from hematemesis.

4. Chest pain
   a. The pulmonary parenchyma is relatively insensitive to pain; consequently, chest pain usually indicates pleural origin (very rich in nerve endings) or other organ system (e.g., cardiac, esophageal, musculoskeletal/chest wall).
   b. Constant, deep, aching pain can result from major bronchial and peribronchial disease. Sharp, intermittent pain that varies with respiration is caused by pleural disease. Pain similar to angina pectoris may be due to pulmonary hypertension. Chest wall pain is usually associated with localized tenderness. Table 7-3 lists some common sources of chest pain.

5. Dyspnea
   a. Dyspnea is a subjective finding, that is, the patient's perception of inappropriate shortness of breath. Careful questioning and precise documentation are required to ascertain its presence, character, and causes. The documentation of dyspnea needs to include relation to daily activity. Precise description of activities inducing dyspnea is essential. Duration of dyspnea in relation to activity, time to recovery, and progression over time should be recorded.
   b. Dyspnea is usually due to physiologic abnormalities, such as diffuse and extensive pulmonary disease or ventilation problems, although extensive lung disease, cardiac disease, and anxiety also can cause dyspnea. The respiratory rate is nearly always increased with dyspnea of an organic nature; a normal rate associated with sighing usually indicates an anxiety state.
   c. Common mechanisms of dyspnea include increased work of breathing (e.g., obstructed airways or decreased compliance) and inadequate ventilation with increased carbon dioxide tension and falling pH. Despite common belief, hypoxemia does not cause dyspnea. Hypoxemia can be a silent killer.

6. Other important findings
   a. Symptoms that may occur in chest diseases include the following:
      (1) Hoarseness; may be caused by damage to laryngeal nerve by tumor or inflammation, or may be secondary to vocal cord trauma with coughing (because the left recurrent laryngeal nerve passes under the pulmonary artery before reaching its destination, intrathoracic pathology may cause hoarseness)
      (2) Fever; may be indicative of inflammatory or neoplastic disease
      (3) Chills or rigors
      (4) Weight loss
      (5) Edema
      (6) Snoring; occurs commonly and is often merely irritating to others in the same or adjacent room; may indicate the presence of obstructive sleep apnea, which is often associated with frequent

Table 7-1. Some Causes of Hemoptysis

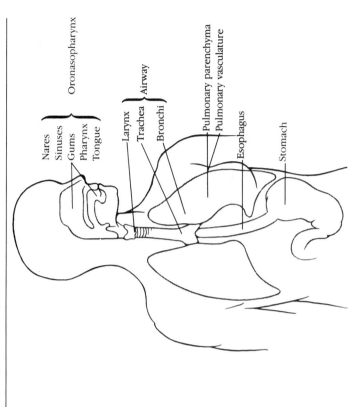

INFECTIONS
Acute bronchitis
Pneumonia
Bronchiectasis
Lung abscess
Tuberculosis
Fungal infections (histoplasmosis,
coccidioidomycosis, aspergillosis)
Parasites (e.g., paragonimiasis,
schistosomiasis, ascariasis,
amebiasis, echinococcosis,
strongyloidiasis)

NEOPLASTIC
Bronchogenic carcinoma
Bronchial adenoma
Metastatic neoplasms

TRAUMATIC
Lung contusion
Bronchial rupture
Postintubation

VASCULAR
Pulmonary infarction
Pulmonary vasculitis
Arteriovenous fistula
Anomalous vessels

CARDIOVASCULAR
Pulmonary edema
Mitral stenosis
Aortic aneurysm

Table 7-1. *Continued*

PARENCHYMAL
  Diffuse interstitial fibrosis
  Systemic diseases and vasculitis: Wegener's granulomatosis, rheumatoid
    arthritis, systemic lupus erythematosus, Goodpasture's syndrome, and others
  Sarcoidosis and hemosiderosis
  Other diffuse lung diseases

OTHER
  Cystic fibrosis
  Endometrial implants
  Broncholiths
  Coagulopathies (with generalized bleeding)
  Nonrespiratory tract (esophagus, stomach)
  Spurious

Table 7-2. Distinctive Characteristics of Hemoptysis and Hematemesis[a]

Hemoptysis	Hematemesis
1. Blood coughed up	1. Blood vomited up
2. Blood may be frothy	2. Blood not frothy
3. Blood mixed with sputum	3. Blood mixed with food
4. Bright red blood	4. Dark blood ("coffee grounds")
5. Stools may be tarry black (melena) if enough blood is swallowed	5. Stools often tarry black
6. History of chest disease	6. History of gastrointestinal disease
7. Patient says blood from lungs[b]	7. Patient says blood from stomach
8. Hemosiderin-laden macrophages in sputum	8. No hemosiderin-laden macrophages in sputum

[a]If the amount of blood is very large, patient will often swallow some blood, which may be vomited; likewise some blood may be aspirated with massive hematemisis and subsequently coughed up.
[b]Patients are sometimes remarkably perceptive in this regard and may even tell you the area of the lung the blood is coming from.

Table 7-3. Some Sources of Chest Pain

EXTRATHORACIC
  Migraine
  Cervical arthritis
  Subdiaphragmatic disease (e.g., appendicitis, hepatitis, splenic infarct, pancreatitis, ulcer, gallstones)

CHEST WALL
  Rib fracture, neoplasm
  Intercostal muscle spasm, inflammation (Bornholm disease)
  Herpes zoster
  Costochondritis
  Thoracic vertebral pain
  Thoracic nerve disease (radiculitis)

PLEURA
  Pleurisy (infectious, neoplastic, vasculitic, irritative)

LUNG PARENCHYMA
  Pneumonia
  Neoplasia } (pain uncommon with pure parenchymal lesions)

LUNG VASCULATURE
  Pulmonary infarction
  Pulmonary hypertension

MEDIASTINAL STRUCTURES
  Lymph nodes (pain with lymphoma, cancer)
  Esophagitis
  Aortic dissection
  Tracheobronchitis
  Pericarditis
  Myocardial pain (angina, infarct)

awakenings, mental confusion, daytime hypersomnolence, personality changes, pulmonary hypertension, and hypoxemia
- **b.** Past history often may be a guide to abnormalities:
    - **(1)** Pneumonia in childhood, recurrent pneumonia, or whooping cough may indicate a predisposition to respiratory tract infection. Chronic obstructive pulmonary disease (COPD) may be suspected with a history of bronchiectasis, congenital anomalies, or genetic defects (e.g., cystic fibrosis, hypogammaglobulinemia, IgA deficiency).
    - **(2)** Use of oily nose drops, poor oral hygiene, recent dental extraction, alcoholism, or unconsciousness may indicate aspiration pneumonia or lung abscess.
    - **(3)** Exposure to tuberculosis, occupational exposure to certain mineral or organic dusts, travel to an area with endemic disease, or inhalant allergies (e.g., hay fever) provides important clues in the diagnostic evaluation of pulmonary symptoms.
- **B.** Abnormal findings
    - **1.** Inspection. It is important to inspect beyond the thorax; many extrathoracic signs (e.g., clubbing, cyanosis, marked sweating, peripheral thrombophlebitis) are important indicators of intrathoracic disease.
        - **a.** Extrathoracic signs of lung disease
            - **(1)** Clubbing: soft tissue swelling at the ends of the fingers and toes (possible causes: diffuse interstitial fibrosis, cystic fibrosis, carcinoma of the lung with pulmonary osteoarthropathy).
            - **(2)** Cyanosis: a blue discoloration of the skin, nail beds, and mucous membranes, caused by elevated levels of reduced hemoglobin; that is, ≥ 5 g/dL (possible causes: decreased oxygenation as in COPD or congenital heart disease; decreased perfusion of tissue beds with increased oxygen extraction).
        - **b.** Asymmetry
            - **(1)** Skewness of chest wall (possible causes: scoliosis, kyphosis)
            - **(2)** Localized prominence of chest wall (possible causes: large tumors, large pleural effusions)
            - **(3)** Localized contraction of chest wall (possible causes: scarring of the lung and pleura, localized lung parenchymal volume loss)
            - **(4)** Barrel-shaped chest, that is, anterior-posterior dimension approximating same as the side-to-side dimension; the ribs are more horizontal, and the subcostal angle is greater than 90 degrees without variation during respiration (possible cause: COPD; barrel shape may be normal in older patients)
            - **(5)** Localized areas of diminished excursion (possible causes: local disease, effects of severe pain with splinting, phrenic nerve paralysis)
            - **(6)** Local inspiratory retraction of intercostal spaces (possible cause: local bronchial obstruction)
            - **(7)** Generalized retractions or bulging of intercostal spaces (possible causes: COPD, asthma, chronic bronchitis, emphysema)
            - **(8)** Dilated chest wall veins (possible causes: compression of venous flow within mediastinum, superior vena cava syndrome)
            - **(9)** Subcutaneous swellings (possible causes: metastatic tumor nodules, abscesses, pointing of empyema)
            - **(10)** Sinus tract openings, scars (possible causes: underlying infection)
        - **c.** Abnormal respiratory rate and rhythm
            - **(1)** Extremely slow respiration (possible causes: central nervous system respiratory depression due to disease or drugs)
            - **(2)** Periodic or Cheyne-Stokes respiration: rhythmic waxing and waning of depth of respiration with regular periods of apnea (possible cause: serious cardiopulmonary or cerebral disorders)

   (3) Biot's respiration: irregular periods of apnea alternating with periods of four to five breaths of identical depth (possible cause: increased intracranial pressure)
   (4) Extreme tachypnea (possible causes: chronic pulmonary or cardiac disease, or systemic disorders such as shock, severe pain, acidosis, anxiety).
   (5) Use of accessory muscle of respiration; that is, sternocleidomastiod, intercostal (possible causes: inadequacy of ventilation, inadequacy of diaphragmatic function, or both)
   (6) Paradoxical abdominal motion: an inward motion of the abdominal wall during inspiration (usually indicative of severe respiratory muscle weakness, or diaphragmatic paralysis)
   d. Abnormal preference for a particular position (cause)
   (1) Sitting (possible cause: cardiac disease, COPD)
   (2) Sitting, leaning forward (possible cause: pericardial disease)
   (3) Unable to lie flat comfortably, orthopnea (possible cause: cardiac disease, pulmonary edema, large amounts of sputum)
   (4) Preference for one side or the other (possible causes: local pathologic processes, lung abscess)
   e. Limited costal expansion (possible causes: diffuse obstruction, fibrosis, muscle weakness, ankylosing spondylitis)
2. Palpation
   a. Tenderness
   (1) Chest wall, ribs (possible causes: local trauma, tumor, underlying pleural inflammation)
   (2) Costal cartilage (possible cause: inflammation such as Tietze's syndrome)
   (3) Rib (possible cause: fracture can occur with even minor trauma or coughing)
   b. Anatomic position changes
   (1) Shift of trachea (possible cause: increased volume of one hemithorax causing shift of entire mediastinum to opposite side: large bulky tumor, pleural effusion, pneumothorax; decreased volume of one hemithorax causing drawing of mediastinum to same side: obstructing tumor, chronic inflammatory parenchymal and pleural disease)
   (2) Shift of cardiac apex beat (possible cause: cardiomegaly and causes listed for shift of trachea)
   (3) Increased distance from posterior sternum to trachea (patients with emphysema, anterior mediastinal tumor)
   (4) Limited costal expansion (possible causes: diffuse obstruction or fibrosis, muscle weakness, diaphragmatic paralysis, or ankylosing spinal disease)
   c. Subcutaneous emphysema: crackling sensation of air bubbles under the skin caused by air leaking from lung or other air-containing viscus. Subcutaneous emphysema is usually felt earliest in the supraclavicular area, but may spread into the face and eyelids, over the trunk, into the scrotum, and down to the toes (possible causes: by trauma, mediastinal emphysema, pneumothorax, asthma, or barotrauma in patients on mechanical ventilation.)
   d. Lymph nodes in supraclavicular area; these may be brought up to the examining finger by having the patient perform Valsalva's maneuver (possible causes: sarcoidosis, tumor metastases)
   e. Abnormal fremitus. The intensity of fremitus and the breath sounds are influenced in the same direction by the same physical factors—diminished fremitus with diminished breath sounds, increased fremitus with loud or bronchial breathing. If discrepancy exists, auscultatory findings are usually more reliable in the assessment of fremitus.

      (1) Rhonchal fremitus: coarse vibrations associated with noisy respiration, primarily inspiration, which may clear with coughing (possible cause: exudate in the trachea or larger bronchial tubes).

      (2) Pleural friction rub-grating vibration commonly associated with pain and involving both inspiration and expiration, unaffected by cough. It is localized, unilateral, sound heard close to ear, accentuated by pressure of hand or stethoscope (possible cause: any inflammatory lesion in the pleura, e.g., viral, bacterial, or tuberculous pleurisy, uremia, or tumors).

      (3) Tactile or vocal fremitus: symmetric increases or decreases are rarely significant.

        (a) Localized diminution of fremitus; implies that transmission of sound is blocked or discontinuous (possible cause: obstructed bronchus, air or fluid in pleural space, thickened or edematous chest wall)

        (b) Generalized diminution of fremitus (possible cause: diffuse bronchial obstruction)

        (c) Localized increased fremitus (possible cause: consolidation, e.g., denser lung with patent bronchus, compression above pleural effusion)

3. Percussion

  a. Generalized hyperresonance: more vibrant, lower-pitched, louder and longer than normal (possible cause: hyperinflation)

  b. Localized hyperresonance (possible cause: pneumothorax, solitary bulla)

  c. Impaired resonance (near areas of greater pathology, over partially consolidated lungs as in diffuse bronchopneumonia)

  d. Dullness: occurs when air content of underlying lung is decreased (possible cause: pulmonary infiltration, pleural thickening or filling)

  e. Flatness: absolute dullness, no air present, very short, feeble, and high-pitched sound (possible cause: pleural effusion).

  f. Tympany: musical quality tone similar to hyperresonance, but of a specific pitch, hollow, high-pitched, clear, drumlike, normally heard over stomach bubble (possible cause: large pneumothorax)

  g. Diaphragmatic excursion, symmetrically reduced (possible cause: hyperinflation, muscular weakness)

  h. Diaphragmatic excursion, unilateral reduction (possible cause: phrenic nerve paralysis)

4. Auscultation. Abnormal breath sounds have great significance. Determination is often difficult, especially for the novice, because what is normal in one area may be pathologic elsewhere. Considerable auscultatory experience is necessary with the wide range of normal breath sounds to distinguish abnormal sounds. Anatomic differences may make sound amplitudes vary widely. Auscultatory findings on one side must be compared with the other side and correlated with other examination techniques and roentgenograms. Visual representation and classification of lung sounds are shown in Table 7-4.

  a. Normal breath sounds in abnormal locations.

      (1) Bronchial breath sounds in areas where vesicular sounds are heard (possible cause: consolidated lung, shift in trachea or large bronchi)

      (2) Accelerated transition from bronchial to vesicular breath sounds (possible cause: partial consolidation, compression, fibrosis, atelectasis)

  b. Continuous adventitial sounds. Major distinction is on the basis of pitch. These sounds are generated when airway walls or intraluminal secretions are set in rapid oscillation.

      (1) Wheezing: high-pitched, musical, hissing, whistling sound of more than 250 msec in duration; frequency of 400 Hz or more.

Wheezing can be inspiratory, expiratory, or both (possible cause: luminal narrowing, or partial obstruction; e.g., asthma, bronchospasm, congestive heart failure, foreign body, vocal cord paralysis). The disappearance of wheezing may be an ominous sign indicating increasing or total obstruction with lack of airflow.

(2) Rhonchi: low-pitched, snoring, slurping sound of more than 250 msec in duration, frequency of 200 Hz or less. Rhonchi can be inspiratory, expiratory, or both; the sound may partially or totally clear with cough or position change (characteristic of secretions in the airways, such as acute or chronic bronchitis; partial endobronchial obstruction, such as tumor, foreign body, or granuloma).

(3) Transmitted laryngeal sounds: monophonic wheezing (i.e., sounds all of the same pitch) in both inspiration and expiration originating from the larynx. These may simulate diffuse airway obstruction, especially asthma. Wheezes are heard best over the larynx. Although the person may be appear ill, arterial blood gases are normal, and a chest x-ray does not show obstruction.

c. Discontinuous adventitial sounds, called crackles or rales: short, intermittent, explosive sounds, usually less than 20 msec. These sounds are believed to be generated by the sudden explosive opening of small airways, the intermittent passage of air through a closed airway, or the bubbling of air through secretions.

(1) Fine rales: high-pitched, described as the separation of cellophane or Velcro strips; simulated by rubbing of hair together. These sounds tend to recur at same point in inspiration and are not altered by cough. They are more frequent at bases or in dependent areas (possible cause: early pulmonary edema, atelectasis, or areas of decreased ventilation, diffuse interstitial fibrosis, or resolving pneumonia).

(2) Coarse rales: low-pitched, less frequent, and louder than fine rales (possible cause: chronic bronchitis, emphysema, bronchiectasis; bubbling of air through secretions).

d. Other adventitial sounds

(1) Pleural friction rub: low-pitched, coarse, grating, loud sound heard close to ear usually during both phases of respiration. It disappears when patient holds breath (possible cause: inflammation of the pleura; most commonly infectious or neoplastic).

(2) Mediastinal crunch, that is, Hamman's sign: extremely loud, knocking, crunching sound synchronous with heartbeat along left sternal border (possible cause: mediastinal emphysema, left pneumothorax), often accompanied by subcutaneous emphysema in neck.

(3) Stridor: a loud harsh, high-pitched, whooping, or crowing musical sound (laryngeal or upper airway obstruction), usually louder in inspiration.

e. Alterations in transmitted voice sounds—abnormal vocal resonance.

(1) Decreased intensity of the spoken voice (pleural disease, diffuse or local obstruction of ventilation)

(2) Bronchophony: increased intensity and clarity of the spoken voice (heard over areas of consolidation, e.g., lobar pneumonia); this finding is normal over the trachea.

(3) Egophony, also called bronchoegophony: a change in the quality of voice sounds such that a spoken long e ("eee") simulates a long a ("ay") (possible cause: dense consolidation, compressed area above a pleural effusion).

(4) Whispered pectoriloquy: distinct transmission of whispered words (possible cause: partial consolidation).

Table 7-4. Classification of Common Lung Sounds

	Acoustic Characteristics	American Thoracic Society Nomenclature	Common Synonyms
Normal	200–600 Hz Decreasing power with increase Hz	Normal	Vesicular Pulmonary
	75–1600 Hz Flat until sharp decrease in power (900 Hz)	Bronchial	Bronchial Tracheal
		Broncho-vesicular	Broncho-vesicular
Adventitious		Adventitous	Abnormal
	Discontinuous, interrupted explosive sounds (loud, low pitch), early inspiratory or expiratory	Coarse crackle	Coarse rale
	Discontinuous, interrupted explosive sounds (less loud than above and of shorter duration; higher in pitch than coarse crackles or rales), mid to late inspiratory	Fine crackle	Fine rale, crepitation
	Continuous sounds (>250 msec, high-pitched; dominant frequency of ≥400 Hz, a hissing sound)	Wheeze	Sibilant rhonchus
	Continuous sounds (>250 msec, low-pitched; dominant frequency ≤200 Hz, a snoring sound)	Rhonchus	Sonorous rhonchus

IV. Classic Physical Findings in Common Respiratory Disorders

A. Diffuse obstructive airway disease

1. Asthma (examination is usually normal between episodes of exacerbation)

   a. Inspection: patient complains of dyspnea; increased respiratory rate. Degree of respiratory distress depends on severity of attack; patient may have paroxysms of coughing. The use of accessory muscles of respiration and the presence of cyanosis indicate a life-threatening attack.

   b. Palpation—usually not helpful.

   c. Percussion note—goes from resonant (normal) to hyperresonant with increasing severity of air trapping.

   d. Auscultation: diffuse wheezing, with diminished breath sounds. Prolongation of forced expiratory time (FET) may be only evidence of airway obstruction in mild disease. As obstruction increases, the pitch of the wheeze becomes higher. In a dyspneic patient, the disappearance of wheezing (i.e., a silent chest) is an ominous sign, indicating lack of airflow.

2. Bronchitis

Table 7-4. (*continued*)

Representation of Sound at Chest Wall

Inspiration , Expiration

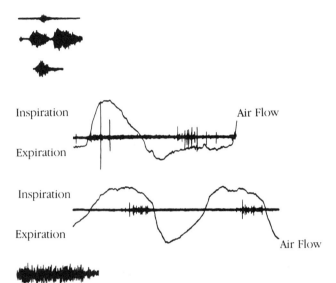

a. Inspection: patient may have no respiratory distress but will have increased respiratory rate; often a productive cough during the examination. Patient may have large barrel-shaped chest, wide interspaces that retract with inspiration, and have cyanosis.
   b. Palpation: fremitus decreased.
   c. Percussion note: resonant.
   d. Auscultation: breath sounds normal. Wheezes, rales, and rhonchi are often present. Adventitial sounds often change with cough; FET is prolonged.
3. Emphysema
   a. Inspection: patient may be in respiratory distress, may have increased respiratory rate, usually has large barrel-shaped chest, wide interspaces that retract with inspiration. Patient often uses accessory muscles of respiration and usually breathes with pursed lips.
   b. Palpation: fremitus decreased.
   c. Percussion note: hyperresonant.
   d. Auscultation: breath sounds diffusely diminished or almost inaudible; few or no rhonchi or rales with quiet breathing. Sounds may be elicited by deep breathing or the FVC maneuver, but breath sounds do

not increase. Patient's diaphragms are low and do not move well. FET is prolonged.

B. Bronchial obstruction

1. Local bronchial obstruction

a. Inspection: Ventilation may lag, the patient may have contracted thorax, and trachea and mediastinal contents may be shifted toward side of obstruction. Shift may increase further with inspiration and decrease with expiration.

b. Palpation: fremitus decreased.

c. Percussion note: dull.

d. Auscultation: breath sounds diminished or absent; no rales.

e. Causes: bronchogenic carcinoma, tumors, foreign bodies, inflammatory stenosing lesions of the bronchi.

C. Pleural disease

1. Pleural effusion

a. Inspection: Patient may or may not appear ill, depending on cause, accumulated volume, and duration. Affected side of hemithorax may bulge. Ventilation may lag and be diminished. Trachea and mediastinum may be shifted to opposite side.

b. Palpation: fremitus markedly decreased or absent.

c. Percussion note: flat.

d. Auscultation: breath sounds absent, no rales. (If moderate, breath sounds may be heard underlying the effusion, physical findings of compression noted above it.)

e. Causes: congestive heart failure, pneumonia, cancer, and so on.

2. Pleural inflammation without effusion

a. Inspection: normal or splinting on the affected side

b. Palpation: possible pleural friction rub heard

c. Percussion note: slight dullness

d. Auscultation: possible pleural friction rub sound

e. Causes: inflammation; e.g., viral pleurisy, uremic pleurisy

3. Pneumothorax. Symptoms depend on extent, acuteness, rapidity of progression, and adequacy of remainder of lung.

a. Inspection: affected side may bulge if pneumothorax large enough; inspiratory lag is seen on the affected side.

b. Palpation: fremitus absent.

c. Percussion note: hyperresonant.

d. Auscultation: breath sounds absent or markedly diminished.

e. Causes: spontaneous, iatrogenic (e.g., central line placement), trauma, secondary to lung disease (e.g., obstructive lung diseases).

D. Parenchymal lung diseases

1. Lung compression: an otherwise normal lung compressed above a pleural effusion

a. Inspection: usually normal

b. Palpation: fremitus increased

c. Percussion note: dull or tympanic

d. Auscultation: bronchovesicular or bronchial breath sounds; possible elicitation of egophony and whispered pectoriloquy

e. Causes: pleural effusion

2. Consolidation

a. Inspection: usually ill appearance, ventilation usually deep and rapid

b. Palpation: fremitus increased

c. Percussion note: dull

d. Auscultation: breath sounds loud and bronchovesicular or bronchial; fine and medium moist rales, consonating in quality; possible presence of bronchophony and pectoriloquy

e. Causes: pulmonary infections (e.g., pneumonia), large areas of pulmonary infarction

3. Pulmonary congestion or edema

    a. Inspection: If congestion is acute and severe, the patient is in extreme distress (i.e., pulmonary edema); if partial or chronic, minimal dyspnea may be present. Respiratory rate and use of accessory muscles reflect this.

    b. Palpation: fremitus normal or slightly decreased.

    c. Percussion note: possible signs of pleural effusion at the base.

    d. Auscultation: breath sounds of fair quality; resonance normal or slightly impaired; fine and medium rales that do not sound close to the ear. Rales and occasionally wheezes are more prevalent in dependent positions and shift after prolonged change of position. Bubbling coarse rales are heard with marked pulmonary edema; in patients with emphysema, breath sounds may increase in intensity toward normal.

    e. Causes: congestive heart failure.

  4. Diffuse interstitial fibrosis

    a. Inspection: usually normal, or decreased respiratory excursion; in extensive disease, shallow and rapid breaths

    b. Palpation: normal, decreased respiratory excursion with advanced disease

    c. Percussion note: normal

    d. Auscultation: fine late inspiratory crackles; initially at bases, spreading higher throughout chest with advanced disease

    e. Causes: idiopathic, drug reactions, connective tissue diseases, occupational and environmental exposures, hypersensitivity pneumonitis, and sarcoid

E. Mediastinal disease

  1. Mediastinal mass

    a. Inspection: Patient may be asymptomatic or quite ill and may be unable to lie on back. Veins are distended if great vessels within mediastinum are compressed (e.g., superior vena cava syndrome). Distance from sternum back toward trachea is increased if mass is in anterior mediastinum. Lungs may be normal.

    b. Palpation: usually normal.

    c. Percussion: possible increased width of dullness anteriorly extending laterally across the midline.

    d. Auscultation: often normal unless lung compressed or atelectatic.

    e. Causes: tumors, enlarged lymph nodes, esophageal disease, vascular disease (e.g., aneurysm, pulmonary hypertension).

F. Acute respiratory failure

  1. Acute respiratory failure

    a. Inspection: An increase in respiratory rate is the first, most sensitive, and quite specific sign of respiratory failure. A rate of 35 or greater is ominous. Observe for breathing through an open mouth, with pursed lips on expiration in obstructive diseases, flaring of nasal folds, sitting bent forward, sweating, anxiety, and tachycardia. Use of accessory muscles of respiration is common. Mental status changes or a reduction in respiratory rate indicate need for intubation and mechanical ventilation.

    b. Palpation: Patient often may have paradoxical respirations while supine. Palpate an inward movement of the abdomen with a decrease of intra-abdominal pressure.

    c. Percussion note: varied depending on cause.

    d. Auscultation: varied depending on cause.

    e. Causes: acute pulmonary edema, flare of asthma or COPD, fulminant pneumonia, septic shock, adult respiratory distress syndrome.

    f. Adjunctive studies: arterial blood gas analysis critical to determine severity; chest x-ray usually helpful. The decision to intubate and mechanically ventilate often precedes these studies in critical situations.

V. Available Technology

A. Roentgenogram. Reviewing the chest roentgenogram is usually an essential part of the examination. Be systematic when examining the roentgenogram. Check the soft tissues, bones of the shoulder, neck, spine, and ribs, visible abdomen, mediastinum, heart, diaphragm, and lungs. Give special attention to areas over which physical abnormalities were elicited. In turn, the roentgenogram can identify areas that require special attention on physical examination. It may be necessary to change the patient's position or perform additional physical studies to find the signs. Go back and forth between physical examination and roentgenogram, if necessary, until careful correlation leads to accurate diagnosis. If abnormalities are found, try to get previous roentgenograms for comparison.

B. Computed tomography (CT). A CT scan is often of enormous value in the diagnosis of abnormal pulmonary findings. It provides cross-sectional images that are helpful in delineating the anatomic structure and location of abnormal pulmonary findings. It is useful to see areas not well seen by the standard chest roentgenogram and hard to evaluate with the physical examination (e.g., the mediastinum, subpleural region, costophrenic sulci). CT may detect occult abnormalities and will provide three-dimensional size, shape, and location.

C. Arterial blood gasses are important to obtain in patients with respiratory distress, respiratory rate irregularities (e.g., dyspnea, tachypnea, bradypnea), or significant roentgenographic abnormalities because signs and symptoms of respiratory failure (hypoxemia or hypercarbia) and acid-base imbalance may be late and nonspecific. Four values are obtained: the partial pressure of oxygen (Pao_2), partial pressure of carbon dioxide ($Paco_2$), pH, and percent saturation of hemoglobin (Sao_2).

D. Pulmonary function studies are indicated to determine whether respiratory dysfunction exists, to characterize the type of dysfunction (i.e., obstructive or restrictive ventilatory defect), to objectively determine the amount of physiologic impairment, and to monitor the response to therapy. Spirometry refers to dynamic lung volumes and flow rates obtained from a forced exhalation from a maximum inspiratory effort, followed by a forced total inhalation. Full pulmonary function studies include spirometric data and add static lung volumes, residual volumes, total lung capacity, resistance, and diffusion (Table 7-5).

E. Cardiopulmonary exercise testing allows evaluation of both the heart and lungs under conditions that stress the body's functional reserves. Primary uses include differentiation between cardiac and respiratory exercise limi-

Table 7-5. Typical Pulmonary Function Values

	Men (height 6 ft)		Women (height 5 ft, 6 in)	
	Age 20 y	Age 70 y	Age 20 y	Age 70 y
FVC/L	5.92	4.67	4.88	3.63
FEV1/L	4.72	3.12	4.08	2.48
FEV1/FVC(%)	80	67	84	68
TLC/L	7.72	6.97	6.05	5.30
FRC/L	4.14	4.14	3.31	3.31
RV/L	1.83	2.68	1.35	2.20
RV/TLC(%)	24	41	24	41
D_LCO(mL/min/mm Hg)	38.43	26.98	35.50	24.05

FVC = forced vital capacity; FEV_1 = forced expiratory volume in 1 second; TLC = total lung capacity; FRC = functional residual capacity; RV = residual volume; D_LCO = diffusing capacity for carbon monoxide.

tation (especially in the evaluation of unexplained dyspnea), determination of work capacity (e.g., in the evaluation of disability), documentation of the need for supplementary oxygen and assessment of required level, and monitoring of disease progression or therapeutic improvement. Cardiopulmonary exercise testing is often an important part of a preoperative evaluation before thoracotomy, especially if functional lung parenchymal tissue are to be removed.

F. Sputum examination. Expectorated sputum may be sent for microbiologic and cytologic studies. The quality of expectorated sputum is determined by assessing the quantity of squamous epithelial cells (indicating oropharyngeal contamination) and the quantity of polymorphonuclear leukocytes, ciliated epithelial cells, and alveolar macrophages (indicating tracheobronchial origin). If an infective process is suspected, sputum should be sent for stain and culture. Gram's stain may reveal the category of bacteria that is present; fungal and acid-fast stains search for fungal and mycobacterial diseases, respectively. Special stains may be indicated for specific diseases (e.g., Gomori methenamine silver for *Pneumocystis*). Cultures for aerobic and anaerobic bacteria, fungi, acid-fast bacteria (AFB), and special organisms are ordered as appropriate. Cytologic examination looks primarily for neoplastic diseases.

G. Flexible bronchoscopy, performed under mild sedation, permits direct visualization of the trachea and proximal bronchial tree. Brushes and biopsy forceps may be passed through the bronchoscope, and the specimens obtained submitted for cytologic and histologic analysis. Peripheral lesions can be visualized with fluoroscopy, which permits the passage of brushes and biopsy forceps to those sites. A lung segment may be isolated by wedging the bronchoscope and lavaged for cytologic and microbiologic examination (BAL; bronchoalveolar lavage). Lymph nodes and other abnormalities identified on radiologic studies (usually CT scan) that are adjacent to airways may be aspirated by passing a needle through the airway wall (transbronchial Wang needle biopsy).

H. Radioisotope ventilation and perfusion lung scans are used principally to assist in the diagnosis of pulmonary emboli. Aerosolized radioisotopes assess ventilation, while injected radioisotopes assess perfusion. The classic appearance in pulmonary embolism shows absence of perfusion with normal ventilation. Ventilation and perfusion lung scans are also useful in the assessment of lung function before surgical removal in patients with marginal reserve (e.g., pneumonectomy for lung cancer).

I. Pulmonary arteriography is used to visualize the pulmonary vasculature. Its major use is in the diagnosis of pulmonary embolism for which it is considered to be the gold standard.

J. Percutaneous needle lung biopsy, under fluoroscopic or CT guidance, is an option to the evaluation of lung parenchymal abnormalities, especially very peripheral lung nodules. Cytologic and microbiologic specimens are usually processed. The most common complication of this procedure, pneumothorax, may occur in 5% to 50% of patients.

K. The cost figures cited in the table on page 122 are **basic direct costs**. The figures are difficult to obtain and change quickly. They include **only** the cost of the test itself (technician, equipment, time, and materials). No professional costs (interpretation) are included. Costs vary from region to region based on differences in some components such as labor. However, the relative cost ranking should remain similar.

VI. Bibliography

Baughman RP, Shipley RT, Loudon RG, Lower EE. Crackles in interstitial lung disease. Comparison of sarcoidosis and fibrosing alveolitis. *Chest* 1991; 100(1):96–101.

Epler GR, Carrington CB, Gaensler EA. Crackles (rales) in the interstitial pulmonary diseases. *Chest* 1978;73(3):333–339.

Forgacs P. The functional basis of pulmonary sounds. *Chest* 1978;73(3):399–405.

Procedure	Code
Chest x-ray	$
Computed tomography (CT)	$$$
Arterial blood gases	$$
Pulmonary function studies	$$$
Cardiopulmonary exercise testing	$$$
Sputum examination	$
Flexible bronchoscopy	$$$$
Radioisotope ventilation and perfusion lung scans	$$$$
Pulmonary arteriography	$$$$$
Percutaneous needle lung biopsy	$

$ = $0–$50; $$ = $50–$100; $$$ = $100–$200; $$$$ = $200–$500; $$$$$ = $500–$1000.

Jaakkola MS, Jaakkola JJ, Ernst P, Becklake MR. Respiratory symptoms in young adults should not be overlooked. *Am Rev Respir Dis* 1993;147(2):359–366.

Light RW, Macgregor MI, Luchsinger PC, Ball WC Jr. Pleural effusions: the diagnostic separation of transudates and exudates. *Ann Intern Med* 1972;77(4):507–513.

Loudon R, Murphy RL Jr. Lung sounds. *Am Rev Respir Dis* 1984;130(4):663–673.

Mahagnah M, Gavriely N. Repeatability of measurements of normal lung sounds. *Am J Respir Crit Care Med* 1994;149(2 Pt 1):477–481.

Ploy-Song-Sang Y, Martin RR, Ross WR, et al. Breath sounds and regional ventilation. *Am Rev Respir Dis* 1977;116(2):187–199.

Pulmonary Terms and Symbols. A report of the ACCP–ATS Joint Committee on Pulmonary Nomenclature. *Chest* 1975;67(5):583–593.

Wilkins RL, Dexter JR, Murphy RL Jr, DelBono EA. Lung sound nomenclature survey. *Chest* 1990;98(4):886–889.

Workum P, Holford SK, Delbono EA, Murphy RL. The prevalence and character of crackles (rales) in young women without significant lung disease. *Am Rev Respir Dis* 1982;126(5):921–923.

VII. Key Search Words

The following key words reflect the content of this chapter. They are provided to assist with an on-line search of computer databases, such as MEDLINE, if you wish to pursue the topic of this chapter further.

Top priority
  Auscultation, thorax
  Palpation, thorax
  Percussion, thorax
  Physical examination, respiratory system
  Respiratory sounds
Secondary priority
  Clubbed fingers
  Crackles
  Cyanosis
  Rales
  Respiration/abnormalities
  Respiratory function tests
  Respiratory system
Cardinal symptoms
  Chest pain
  Cough
  Dyspnea
  Hemoptysis
  Sputum

8. CIRCULATORY SYSTEM

Richard D. Judge
Michael J. Shea

I. Glossary

Adrenergic: activated by adrenaline or the sympathetic nervous system.

Afterload: the mean pressure against which the ventricle pumps.

Akinesia: complete loss of the power to move.

Aneurysm: saccular dilatation of an artery or cardiac chamber.

Angina pectoris: literally, "strangulation of the chest," a paroxysmal, constricting substernal discomfort often of cardiac origin and brief duration.

Angiography: x-ray examination of the circulation by injection of radiopaque substances.

Apex (cardiac): pointed, most lateral portion of the heart, usually located near the left fifth intercostal space.

Arrhythmia: any variation from the normal regular rhythm of the heart.

Asystole: complete loss of cardiac contractile function.

Atrial fibrillation: grossly irregular ventricular rhythm associated with rapid, uncoordinated movements of the atria.

Atrial flutter: cardiac arrhythmia characterized by rapid, regular, uniform atrial contractions (about 300 per minute) and a ventricular rate and rhythm that vary with the grade of A-V block.

Auscultation: listening to sound within the body (usually with a stethoscope).

A-V block: slowing or interruption of impulse conduction from atria to ventricles.

Base (cardiac): region of the aortic and pulmonic outflow tracts; the second and third intercostal spaces parasternally.

Bradycardia: slow heart beat (less than 50 beats per minute [bpm]).

Bruit: extracardiac blowing sound heard at times over peripheral vessels, usually arterial.

Cannon wave: a prominent jugular venous pulsation produced by contraction of the right atrium against a closed tricuspid valve.

Chordae tendinae: string-like tendons connecting the A-V valves (mitral and tricuspid) to the ventricular wall.

Cor: synonym for heart (Greek or Latin).

Cor pulmonale: heart disease secondary to pulmonary disease.

Coronary artery disease (CAD): heart disease resulting from narrowing or occlusion of one or more coronary arteries.

CPR: cardiopulmonary resuscitation.

Cyanosis: bluish discoloration of the skin produced by inadequate oxygenation of the blood.

Diastole: dilatation; period of relaxation during which ventricles fill with blood; technically ends with the onset of the first heart sound.

Dyskinesia: abnormal motion; usually referring to expansion of a ventricular segment when it should be contracting.

Dyspnea: difficult or labored breathing.

Edema: presence of abnormal amounts of interstitial fluid in soft tissue or lungs.

Embolism: sudden occlusion of a vessel by clot or other obstruction carried to its place by the current of blood.

End-diastole: the period of the cardiac cycle immediately preceding the first heart sound.

Endocarditis: inflammation of the lining of the heart and its valves.

Friction rub: characteristic grating adventitious sound, usually pericardial or pleural, simulating noise made by friction between two rough surfaces.

Gallop rhythm: characteristic cadence produced by three heart sounds (first and second heart sounds with one or more extra sounds) in conjunction with tachycardia.

Holo-: entire or wholly.

Hyper-: abnormally increased (e.g., hyperkinesia).

Infarction: ischemic necrosis of tissue resulting from interference with its circulation.

Ischemia: localized tissue anemia due to obstruction of the inflow of arterial blood.

Murmur: adventitious sound resulting from turbulent blood flow within the heart or great vessels.

Orthopnea: inability to breath comfortably when supine.

Palpitation: a sensation of forceful beating or throbbing.

Paroxysmal: sudden, unexpected.

Presystolic: immediately preceding the first sound; occurring in the latter third of diastole.

Preload: the mean ventricular filling pressure in end-diastole (immediately before the first sound).

Pulse: expansile wave felt over an artery; propagated at a speed approximately 10 times that of the actual flow of blood into the system.

Raynaud's phenomenon: paroxysmal pallor or cyanosis of a distal extremity, induced by chilling or emotion.

Shock: acute circulatory collapse, with pallor, hypotension, and coldness of the skin; also a term used to describe a palpable heart sound.

Supraventricular tachycardia: an arrhythmia arising in the atria or A-V junction, usually characterized by rapid, extremely regular beating of the entire heart.

Syncope: temporary unconsciousness due to cerebral ischemia.

Systole: contraction; period of contraction during which the atria or ventricles eject blood; *ventricular systole* includes the first and second sounds and the period between them; when the term *systole* or *diastole* is used alone, it is assumed to refer to the ventricles.

Tachycardia: rapid regular heart beat (over 100 bpm in adults).

Thrill: palpable vibrations (palpable murmur).

Varicose: dilated.

Ventricular tachycardia: arrhythmia originating in the ventricles, characterized by rapid relatively regular heartbeat.

II. General Considerations
  A. Approach
    1. Technology (echocardiography, Doppler, cardiac catheterization, magnetic resonance imaging [MRI]) is usually necessary for accurate diagnosis of cardiovascular disorders. The initial examination directs the selection and timing of costly confirmatory tests.
    2. The cardiovascular examination is especially challenging because of the following:
      a. Cardiovascular phenomena are passing by on an ever-moving time axis.
      b. The cardiovascular system continually adapts to the environment. Sitting, standing, breathing, and anxiety modify cardiovascular phenomena such as blood pressure, pulse rate, loudness of sounds, and amplitude of pulsations.
    3. It is often necessary to use two senses simultaneously to time your observations (e.g., palpating the carotid while observing the jugular pulse).
    4. The arteries and veins of the neck and extremities are as important a part of the system as the heart sounds. Look carefully, feel carefully, and then listen.

B. Surface anatomy. The cardiovascular system is assessed primarily from the surface of the chest, neck, and extremities. The three major cardiothoracic landmark areas are base, precordium, and apex (Fig. 8-1).

1. Right side landmarks (Fig. 8-2A and B)
   a. Jugular veins, superior vena cava, and right atrium form one functional unit with no effective valves above the tricuspid valve (see Fig. 8-2A).
   b. Right ventricle is anterior (see Fig. 8-2B); its movement is reflected in the left third and fourth interspace parasternally.
   c. Tricuspid valve is best observed (felt and heard) directly over its anatomic position (fourth left intercostal space next to sternum).
   d. Pulmonary valve is anterior (see Fig. 8-2B); best observed (felt and heard) close to its anatomic position (second left intercostal space next to sternum).

2. Left side landmarks (Fig. 8-3A and B)
   a. Carotid arteries are the closest "reachable" arteries for assessment.
   b. Left ventricle is behind right ventricle but wraps around anteriorly to form the left heart border and apex. The apex is normally left ventricular.
   c. Mitral valve is deep within chest (see Fig. 8-3B); best observed (felt and heard) inferolaterally from its anatomic position (note bottom arrow) at or near the apex. (The terms *mitral area* and *apex* may be used synonymously.)
   d. Aortic valve is deep within chest (see Fig. 8-3B); best observed *not* over its anatomic position, but in the second right interspace (note top arrows).

C. Physiology
1. Electrophysiology. Each mechanical contraction of the heart is preceded by electrical activation (Fig. 8-4).

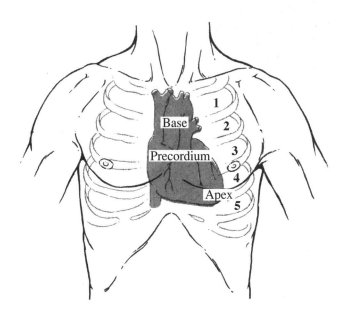

Fig. 8-1. Major cardiothoracic reference areas.

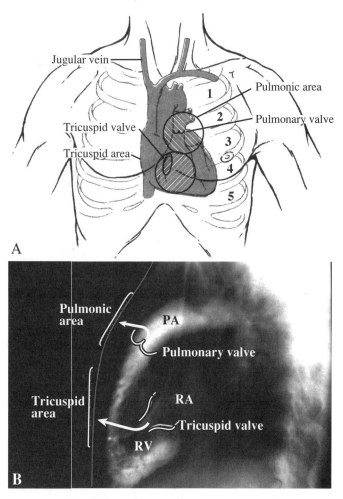

Fig. 8-2. Right-sided reference areas. Note that the tricuspid and pulmonic areas *(A)* are directly over their respective valves as shown in the angiogram *(B)*.

    a. The P wave represents atrial activation.
    b. The QRS complex represents ventricular activation.
    c. Contraction immediately follows activation; therefore, the atria normally contract about 160 msec before the ventricles do. This precise mechanical asynchrony is very important for normal function (Starling's principle) and is set electrically.
    d. Electrocardiography is the standard means for monitoring heart rate and rhythm, although arrhythmias often can be correctly diagnosed clinically.
  2. Intravascular pressures (Fig. 8-5)
    a. Two very different systems are part of mammalian circulation.
      (1) Pulmonary circulation. Low pressure, low resistance.
      (2) Systemic circulation. High pressure, high resistance.

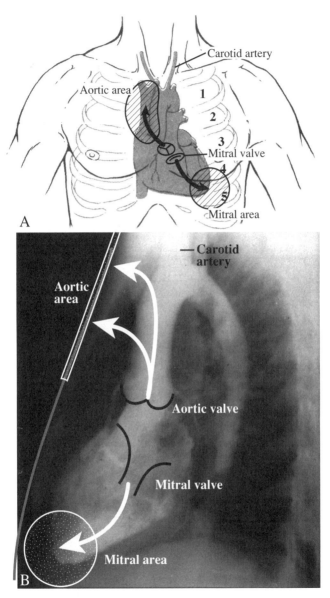

Fig. 8-3. Left-sided reference areas. Note that the mitral and aortic areas *(A)* are remote from their respective valves *(B)*. They are referred in the direction of blood flow. (The loudness of heart sounds diminishes as one moves farther from the valve.)

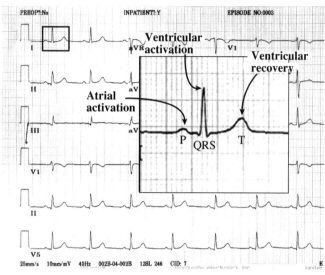

Fig. 8-4. The normal electrocardiogram.

   b. Direct measurements require cardiac catheterization, but much can be estimated at bedside. Three basic pressure contours:
     (1) Arterial (single peak)
     (2) Ventricular (single peak)
     (3) Atrial (double peak)
  3. Surface expressions of pressures. Pressure changes and intravascular flow are the basis of bedside examination—what is heard, seen, and felt (see Fig. 8-5).
   a. Systemic arterial pressure. This is measured with a sphygmomanometer; evaluated by palpating carotid artery (what you feel shown in bold black).
   b. Left ventricular pressure. This is evaluated by palpating the apex impulse; normal apical movement is generated by isovolumic contraction (shown in bold black).
   c. Left atrial pressure. This pressure is not normally accessible. However, left atrial contraction (shown in bold black) is palpable at the apex in a host of cardiac diseases (movement felt just before first heart sound).
   d. Pulmonary artery and right ventricular pressures. These are not normally accessible. Elevations are expressed as visible and palpable pulsations of the parasternal area and base.
   e. Right atrial pressure. Variations are seen as pulsations of jugular veins; atrial contraction and passive filling (shown in bold black) are normally visible but not palpable.
   f. Pressure changes open and close the cardiac valves (Fig. 8-6). Valve closure generates the first and second heart sounds; divides the cardiac cycle into systole and diastole. Cardiac sequence (also applies to right heart) is as follows:
     (1) Atrial activation—P wave.
     (2) Atrial contraction (silent)—A wave.
     (3) Ventricular activation—QRS.
     (4) Ventricular contraction.

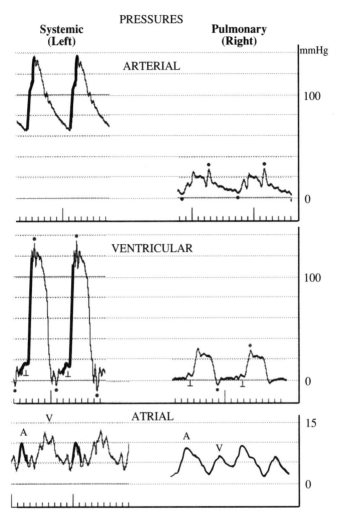

PRESSURES

Fig. 8-5. Surface expressions of intravascular pressures (see text).

    (5) When ventricular pressure exceeds atrial pressure, A-V valves (mitral/tricuspid) close, causing S_1.
    (6) When ventricular pressure falls below arterial pressure, semilunar valves (aortic/pulmonic) close, causing S_2.
    (7) The interval from S_1 to S_2 is systole. The interval from S_2 to S_1 is diastole.
  4. Intravascular flow
    a. Technology. Variations in motion and blood flow velocity are well demonstrated with echocardiography and Doppler technology.
      (1) Echocardiography demonstrates valve motion and ventricular wall motion, which underlie many normal and abnormal physical findings.

PRESSURE COMPOSITE

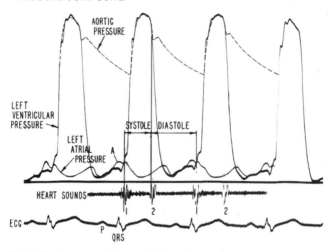

Fig. 8-6. Left-sided pressure changes during the cardiac cycle (see text).

  (2) Doppler technology demonstrates velocity, duration, direction of blood flow. Doppler flow velocities are expressed in meters per second. Low velocities are inaudible (e.g., 0.5 m/sec), but as velocities increase (e.g., 2.5 m/sec) they produce audible sound because of turbulence.
 b. Cardiac sequence. Figure 8-7 shows the relation between flow measurements by Doppler echocardiography and the sequence of cardiovascular sound generation. What is shown for the left heart is equally applicable to the right heart.
  (1) Mitral valve closure (along with tricuspid valve closure) generates S_1.
  (2) Left ventricular ejection. Doppler recording is from the aorta of a normal young subject, which shows the outflow of blood during systole after the aortic valve opens.
   (a) Velocity rises to a peak, then falls off.
   (b) Duration (ejection time) is 270 msec; peak velocity is 1.2 m/sec. This is inaudible; when velocities exceed 2.0 m/sec, a murmur often can be heard.
  (3) Aortic valve closure (along with pulmonary valve closure) generates S_2.
  (4) Early, passive left ventricular filling (see Fig. 8-7). Doppler tracing at mitral valve just inside the left ventricle is from normal young subject. Note the biphasic pattern of flow velocity reminiscent of atrial pressure. The first peak, E, is caused by the first rush of blood immediately following mitral valve opening. When the E velocity goes above 1.2 m/sec, an audible sound (S_3) is often present at the apex. This phase is the period of early passive filling and explains the S_3 in patients with heart failure.
  (5) Left atrial contraction (see Fig. 8-7). The second peak, A, of the Doppler tracing shows the effect of atrial contraction, and occurs just before mitral closure. The A velocity is normally inaudible, but an increased A velocity (>1.2 m/sec) often produces a low-pitched sound at the apex (S_4). This occurs in people with non-

FLOW COMPOSITE

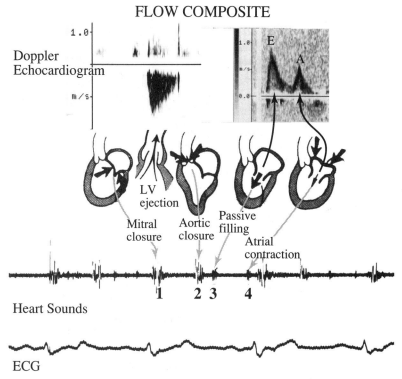

Fig. 8-7. The relation between flow measurements by Doppler echocardiography and the sequence of cardiovascular sound generation.

compliant left ventricles due to hypertension, coronary disease, or aortic valve disease.

5. Cardiovascular sound (Fig. 8-8)
   a. Audible cardiac sounds range between 25 and 600 cycles per second (cps). Most people can hear much higher frequencies (10,000 cps), but maximum sensitivity is usually 1000 to 2000 cps. Much cardiac sound is too soft to be heard; it falls below threshold (see Fig. 8-8).
   b. Loudness is subjective; what you hear with your stethoscope depends on the following:
      (1) Intensity of the sound at its origin
      (2) How well it is transmitted through the body
      (3) How good the stethoscope is
      (4) How good your hearing is (excellent hearing is less important when using a high-quality electronic stethoscope)
   c. To hear cardiac vibrations with a frequency of 50 cps (see Fig. 8-8):
      (1) The sound must have a higher intensity than sounds of 200 cps to be heard.

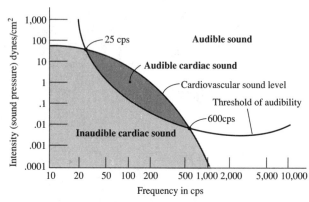

Fig. 8-8. Comparison of auditory threshold with average intensity of cardiac sound at various frequencies. Note that only sounds of 24 to 600 cps are in the audible range.

      (2) The bell of the stethoscope must be used. The bell is designed for low-pitched sounds; the diaphragm will completely filter out 50 cps sounds.

  d. Stethoscopes. Consider investing in a new electronic stethoscope (Fig. 8-9D), particularly if you are going into internal medicine, family practice, or pediatrics. The electronic devices are far superior to the standard variety. In selecting a stethoscope, consider the following:

      (1) Earpieces. A snug fit is important; if too small or too tight, the earpiece may partially or completely occlude against the anterior wall of the auditory canal rather than sitting comfortably in a position parallel with the long axis of your external auditory canal (see Fig. 8-9A). Try several types, and tailor the earpieces if necessary to achieve the proper fit.

      (2) Tubing. Tubing should be at least 1/8 inch inside diameter (smaller tubing will attenuate high frequencies), thick-walled to reject outside noise (plastic is better than thin, flexible rubber), double from the earpiece to the endpiece (rather than the Y configuration), and no longer than 15 inches in length (so that the overall distance from ear to chest is not greater than 21 inches).

      (3) Endpieces. The two standard types—bell and diaphragm—are available in many sizes. The 1-inch bell and the 1- to 1 1/2-inch diaphragm are most often used for examining adults (see Fig. 8-9B).

        (a) Diaphragm. The rigid diaphragm has a natural frequency of about 300 cps; it is best used to hear high-pitched sounds such as the second heart sound, high-pitched murmurs, some breath sounds. It acts as a band-pass filter, eliminating low-pitched sounds.

        (b) Bell. With the bell, the skin becomes the diaphragm and the natural frequency varies with the amount of pressure exerted, from 40 cps with light pressure to 200 cps with firm pressure. The bell is best used to hear low-pitched sounds and murmurs; therefore, it must be applied as lightly as possible (see Fig. 8-9C).

III. Techniques of Examination and Normal Findings

  A. Observation. Observe carefully during history-taking; especially watch body language while the patient is speaking.

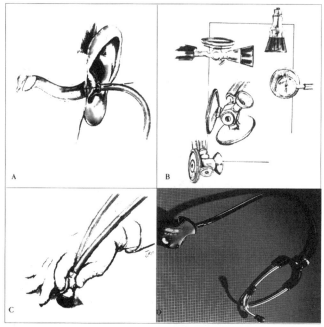

Fig. 8-9. The stethoscope. **(A)** Correct fit in auditory meatus. **(B)** Common types of stethoscope endpieces. **(C)** A method for holding the stethoscope endpiece. **(D)** An electronic stethoscope that offers electronic amplification of sound.

   B. Sequence of examination. Five basic positions are used for the cardiovascular examination (Fig. 8-10). (The details of several of the examinations are covered elsewhere.)
      1. Sitting
      2. Recumbent, head elevated to 45 degrees
      3. Left decubitus
      4. Sitting (for special listening)
      5. Standing, special maneuvers (e.g., squatting, Valsalva's position, and so on)
   C. Sitting
      1. Begin by facing the patient. Inspect the following:
         a. General appearance
         b. Respiratory pattern
         c. Face
         d. Eyes and fundi
         e. Lips and mouth
         f. Neck (quick look)
      2. Move behind the patient and examine the following:
         a. Posterior chest
         b. Thyroid
      3. Take the blood pressure (Fig. 8-11).
         a. Apply cuff 1 inch above elbow.
         b. Take systolic pressure by palpation (see Fig. 8-11A).
         c. Use auscultatory method (see Fig. 8-11B).

Sequence of the Directed Cardiovascular Examination

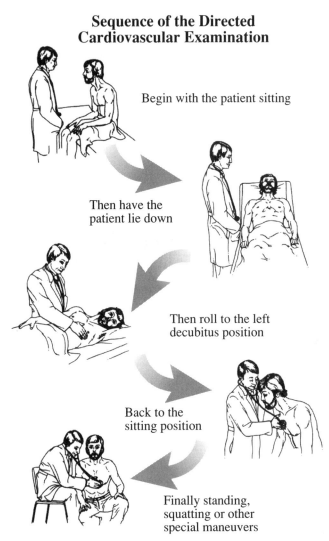

Begin with the patient sitting

Then have the patient lie down

Then roll to the left decubitus position

Back to the sitting position

Finally standing, squatting or other special maneuvers

Fig. 8-10. The five basic positions used for the cardiovascular examination.

    (1) Phase I: onset of Korotkoff's sounds indicates the systolic pressure level.
    (2) Phase II: bruit replaces sound; no significance.
    (3) Phase III: sudden intensification of sound (bruit disappears).
    (4) Phase IV: sudden dampening of sound (not diastolic pressure level).
    (5) Silence: indicates diastolic pressure level.
  d. When sounds are heard all the way to 0 pressure:
    (1) Point of muffling (phase IV) is recorded as the diastolic pressure
    (2) Record: 140/60–0

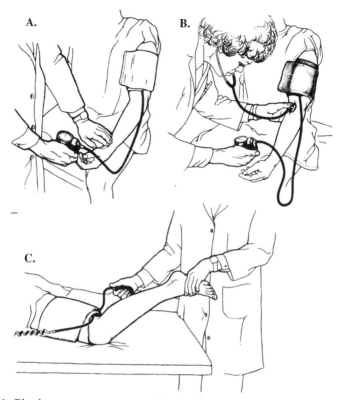

Fig. 8-11. Blood pressure measurement (see text).

e. Very faint sounds may cause uncertainty of the blood pressure values. To hear the sounds better, raise the patient's arm to drain the venous system, inflate the cuff with the arm raised, then lower the arm to listen. Sounds will be louder.
f. Leg pressures (see Fig. 8-11C). Apply an oversized cuff to the calf or thigh. The systolic pressure is usually sufficient; take by palpating the posterior tibial or dorsalis pedis artery.
g. Recording blood pressure. Always note the site and body position (e.g., 120/80 left arm sitting; 130/70 right arm standing).
h. Range of normal
   (1) Normal is 90 to 140/60 to 90.
   (2) Pulse pressure = systolic pressure − diastolic pressure.
   (3) Mean pressure = diastolic pressure + 1/3 pulse pressure.
   (4) Difference of 5 to 10 mmHg between arms is common.
   (5) Systolic pressure in leg is usually ±10 mmHg higher than in arm.
   (6) Standing normally causes a small and variable effect on arm blood pressure, such as a slight drop in systolic pressure (±10 mmHg) and a slight rise in diastolic pressure (±5 mmHg).
i. Common sources of error

(1) Undersized cuff: in an obese person, false elevation of pressure may be read. It may be necessary to settle for palpatory systolic pressure only, with cuff applied to the forearm.

(2) Oversized cuff: in an emaciated person, false depression may be read.

(3) Loose cuff: false elevation may be read.

(4) Feeble Korotkoff's sounds: systolic pressure can be determined by palpation, if Doppler imaging is not available.

D. Recumbent. With the patient recumbent and head elevated 45 degrees, examine the extremities, neck, and precordium.

1. Extremities. Examine upper extremities first, then the lower. Observe six things in the following order:

   a. Nails.

   b. Skin color and temperature. Note temperature and color gradation in lower extremities.

   c. Hair distribution.

   d. Venous pattern.

   e. Swelling or atrophy.

   f. Peripheral arterial pulsations. Use two fingers (index and middle) to palpate the pulses. Occlude the vessel and gradually release. For each pulse, note the following in order: rate, rhythm, amplitude, and elasticity of vessel wall. Check the following pulses (Fig. 8-12):

      (1) Radial
      (2) Brachial
      (3) Dorsalis pedis
      (4) Posterior tibial
      (5) Femoral

   g. Range of normal vascular tone.

      (1) Vasoconstriction may be caused by smoking, apprehension or chilling; it results in pallor, coldness, cyanosis, collapsed superficial veins.

      (2) Vasodilation may be caused by heat, exercise, and alcohol; it results in rubor, warmth, throbbing, distention of superficial veins.

   h. Range of normal arterial pulse.

      (1) Normal pulse rate: 50 to 100 bpm

      (2) Sinus arrhythmia common, especially in children and adolescents; transient *in*crease in rate with *in*spiration

      (3) Occasional premature beats common

      (4) Amplitude

         (a) Highly subjective
         (b) Function of pulse pressure
         (c) Increased by exercise, excitement, heat, alcohol, and slowing of rate
         (d) Recording of findings:
            (i) 2+ = normal
            (ii) 0 = absent
            (iii) 1+ = diminished
            (iv) 2+ = normal
            (v) 3+ = increased

      (5) Quality or contour

         (a) Use only carotid to assess quality.
         (b) The upstroke is all that is normally felt (Fig. 8-13B); it is less than 0.1 seconds in duration.
         (c) Brachial and femoral upstrokes are usually synchronous.

2. Neck. Observe three things in the following order:

   a. Carotid pulse (Table 8-1). Use two-finger method or thumb (see Fig. 8-13A). Palpate each artery just below the angle of the jaw, medial to the sternocleidomastoid muscle. (Many prefer to examine the carotid with the patient sitting.)

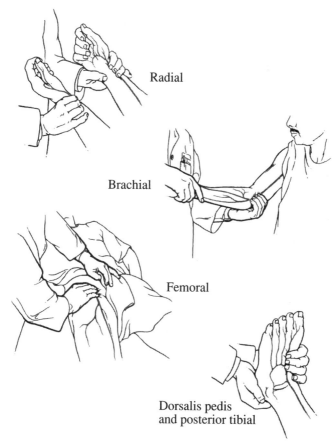

Radial

Brachial

Femoral

Dorsalis pedis
and posterior tibial

Fig. 8-12. Pulse examination (see text).

(1) Note amplitude and quality of the upstroke (quick versus slow). Normally, the upstroke is swift and is the main thing that is felt. If stroke volume increases (as with excitement, exercise, or slowing of the heart rate), the pulse pressure widens, giving a forceful, throbbing quality on palpation. In older persons with stiff arteries, the carotid pulse is often very forceful.

Table 8-1. Differentiation of Jugular Pulsation From Carotid Pulsation

Jugular Pulsation	Carotid Pulsation
Nonpalpable	Palpable
Undulating, diffuse	Brisk
Usually double	Single
Disappears with pressure over the jugular bulb	Not affected by pressure
Disappears in sitting position	Persists in sitting position
Varies with respiration	No variation

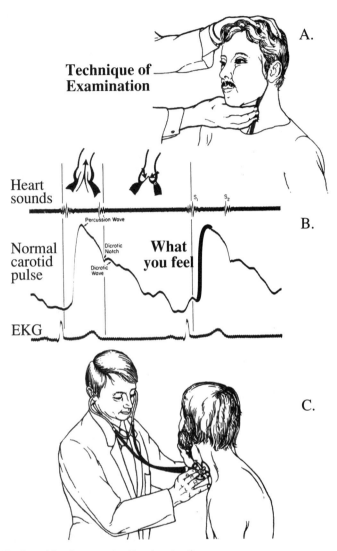

Fig. 8-13. Carotid pulse examination (see text).

> (2) Listen for bruits (see Fig. 8-13C).
> b. Jugular venous pulse. Patient is still at 45 degrees (Fig. 8-14).
>> (1) Step back and observe.
>> (2) Right internal jugular is usually best.
>> (3) Use penlight to illuminate neck.
>> (4) View neck border against white pillow background.
>> (5) Time motion by left carotid upstroke.
>> (6) The first peak of the waveform (see Fig. 8-14A) is due to right atrial contraction, the second to passive right atrial filling during ventric-

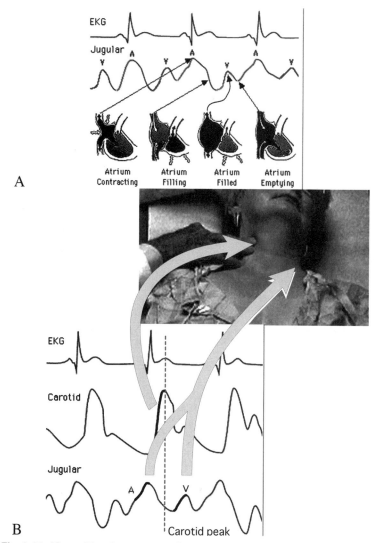

A

EKG

Jugular

Atrium
Contracting   Atrium
Filling   Atrium
Filled   Atrium
Emptying

EKG

Carotid

Jugular

B   Carotid peak

Fig. 8-14. Normal jugular venous pulse (see text).

ular systole. Palpate the carotid while you observe (see Fig. 8-14B): *the A wave occurs just before the carotid upstroke*; the V wave occurs just after the carotid upstroke. Note this relationship in Figure 14B.

c. Jugular venous pressure. Estimate the jugular venous pressure in the internal jugular from the location of the peak of the A wave (or V wave, if dominant). The sternal angle is the universal reference point (Fig. 8-15). Normal: up to 3 cm above the angle. If needed, precise

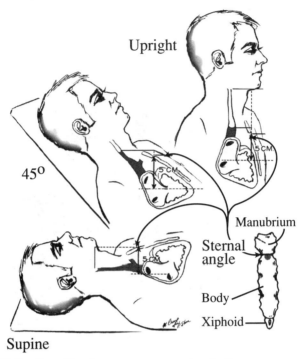

Fig. 8-15. Estimation of jugular venous pressure (see text).

measurement is possible with the patient at 45-degree angle. Add
5 cm to the height above the angle; normal is 7 to 8 cm.

3. Precordium. Inspection, percussion, and palpation are done in sequence,
   but often very rapidly. Findings are affected by position, respiration,
   chest configuration, amount of muscle and fat, and breast size (female).

   a. Inspection. Step back to inspect. Amplify any pulsation or movement
   by using a tongue blade or by asking the patient to expire and laying a
   tongue blade across the precordium. Time movements against the
   carotid pulse. Normally, no significant movement is present, although
   a visible apex impulse or gentle lift along the left sternal border may
   be seen in thin-chested adults.

   b. Percussion. Despite prevailing opinion, percussion is a useful and reliable method of assessing heart size.

   (1) Sensitivity is 94% when correlated with chest x-ray (see Heckerling et al and Schneiderman).

   (2) Mediate and direct method (Fig. 8-16) are equally accurate.

   (3) Direct allows left hand to hold away female breast.

   (4) Upper limit is 10.0 cm from midsternal line.

   (5) Record heart size in terms of cardiac enlargement (CE) (e.g., no
   CE, mild CE, and so on).

   c. Palpation.

   (1) Use middle three fingers; press lightly.

   (2) Begin at apex, then move to tricuspid, pulmonic and aortic areas.

   (3) Locate the apex impulse, if possible, and time it against the
   carotid upstroke. The normal apex impulse is a short outward
   tap that clearly precedes the carotid upstroke (Fig. 8-17). It can

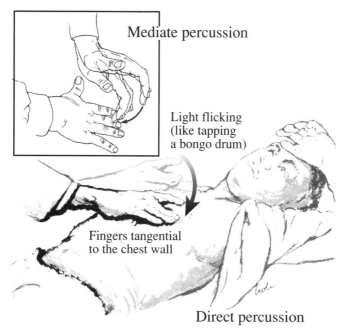

Fig. 8-16. Percussion for the estimation of heart size (see text).

be felt in about 30% of patients supine and about 60% of patients in the left decubitus position.

(4) Except for the apex impulse, the remaining precordium is normally quiet, although midprecordial movement can at times be present in healthy asthenic young people, and occasionally the heart sounds are felt in normal young adults (called "shocks").

(5) Always repeat palpation in the left decubitus position. Many normal and abnormal movements are identifiable only in this position (Fig. 8-18). A tongue blade can be used to amplify the apical movement.

d. Auscultation (mechanics).

(1) Assume a comfortable position in a place free of noise.

(2) Press bell lightly and diaphragm firmly.

(3) Follow same moves as palpation (apex, move medially, then upward to second left interspace, then across to second right interspace, and on up to the neck).

(4) Sequence (repeat with each move of the stethoscope).

(a) Observe and time the rate (fast or slow?) and rhythm (irregularities?).

(b) Identify the first and second sounds; listen to them separately (normal? accentuated? diminished?). Compare the first and second sounds in the various valve areas.

(c) Listen for extra sounds (not murmurs). Listen first in systole, then diastole.

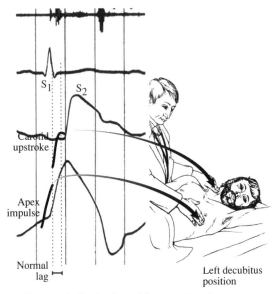

Two-handed palpation of the apex impulse

Fig. 8-17. Two-handed (simultaneous) method of palpating the apex impulse using the carotid upstroke as a timer (see text).

     (d) Listen for murmurs, first in systole, then diastole. Scan all major areas. Notice the point of maximum intensity and the transmission of murmurs.

  (5) If systole and diastole are difficult to identify, the following techniques may help:

     (a) Correlate the heart sounds with the carotid pulse, which is systolic in timing. The first sound should just precede the upstroke. (Peripheral arteries are not suitable for timing heart sounds.)

     (b) Locate the second sound at the base, which is always the loudest, then inch the stethoscope down toward the apex, keeping the sound "in your ear."

e. Auscultation (range of normal). Eight basic heart sound patterns can normally be heard: four basic auscultatory areas (apex, tricuspid, pulmonic, aortic), the physiologic third heart sound, the innocent murmur, the innocent arterial bruit, and the venous hum.

  (1) Apex. S_1 is usually louder and lower in pitch than S_2; both sounds range in frequency from 60 to 200 CPS. S_2 at the apex is due entirely to aortic closure. Splitting of S_1 is occasionally present, but S_1 at the apex is usually single and due primarily to mitral closure.

  (2) Tricuspid area. S_1 is almost always split with mitral closure occurring 0.02-0.03 seconds before tricuspid closure (rather like a grace note in music). S_2 is usually single and slightly softer than S_1.

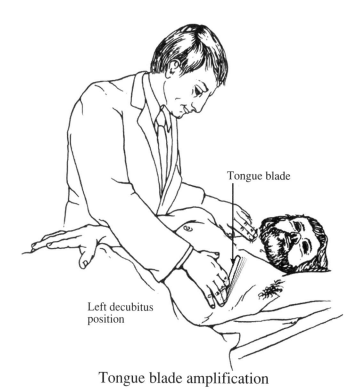

Tongue blade amplification

Fig. 8-18. Palpation in the left lateral decubitus position (see text).

    (3) Pulmonic area.
        (a) Physiologic splitting of S₂ occurs in most normal people.

        (b) Expiration: right and left ventricular systole are equal in duration; pulmonary and aortic valves close simultaneously.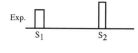

        (c) Inspiration:
            (i) Draws venous blood as well as air into the thorax
            (ii) Increased venous return to the right ventricle prolongs systole and delays pulmonary valve closure
            (iii) At the same time:
                (a) Expands lung volume with inspiration
                (b) Increases pulmonary vascular capacity
                (c) Reduces left ventricular venous return
                (d) Shortens left ventricular systole
                (e) Causes aortic valve to close earlier

            (iv) Results in transient splitting of S₂ that lasts for only three or four beats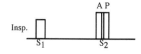

(a) Respiration must be normal and quiet, not forced or held.
(b) Physiologic splitting is at times well heard below the pulmonic area or medial (toward the aortic area).
(c) Physiologic splitting often disappears after age 60.

(4) Aortic area (2nd right interspace). S_1 is probably entirely due to mitral closure. S_2 is usually single and due to aortic closure, and is usually well heard over the right carotid. Physiologic splitting can sometimes be heard in normal people with unusually loud heart sounds.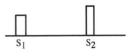

(5) Physiologic third heart sound (apex). This faint, inconstant, low-pitched (around 40 CPS) sound is best heard at the apex with the bell applied lightly to the skin, and with the patient in a left decubitus position. It often disappears in a sitting position. It varies in intensity with respiration, usually becoming louder with expiration. It is extremely common in children, young adults, and young pregnant women, but is seldom heard in normal persons over age 25 except in conditioned athletes, both male and female.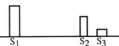

(6) Innocent systolic murmur
  (a) Common in children, adolescents, pregnant women, and conditioned athletes.
  (b) It is best heard in supine position.
  (c) Sound is short, low-pitched; it often disappears if person sits up, stands, or performs Valsalva's maneuver.
  (d) Two types
    (i) Vibratory or Still's murmur
      (a) First described in young children; often encountered during first two decades of life
      (b) Heard just medial to apex
      (c) Probably arises from left ventricle; has "twanging" quality
    (ii) Flow murmur
      (a) Older children and young adults
      (b) Best heard at or near pulmonic area
      (c) Medium-pitched, short, ejection
      (d) Probably arises from the pulmonary artery
      (e) No associated cardiac abnormality; they stand alone

(7) Innocent arterial bruit. Bruits are not uncommon in normal young people (particularly athletes), and they also stand alone. They are heard in the supraclavicular (carotid) area or abdomen. Because bruits are also signs of pathologic narrowing of arteries, it may be difficult to ascertain their innocence.

(8) Venous hum. This phasic roaring, heard in about 25% of normal young adults at the lower border of the right sternocleidomastoid muscle *in the sitting position*, is accentuated in diastole, and may be transmitted to the upper precordium. Hums are of no consequence and can be interrupted by compression over the jugular

vein, Valsalva's maneuver, and recumbency—unlike pathologic heart murmurs with which they can be confused.

E. Left decubitus position (see Figs. 8-17 and 8-18). Always repeat palpation and auscultation in this position. Several important findings often are identified only in this position:

   1. Apex impulse, normal or pathologic

   2. S_3, physiologic or pathologic

   3. S_4, palpable or audible or both

   4. Many pathologic systolic and diastolic murmurs and thrills

F. Sitting. Repeat palpation and auscultation (precordium and neck). Palpate over the aortic, pulmonic, and left parasternal areas; listen with patient leaning forward in full expiration (Fig. 8-19). Aortic diastolic murmurs are often heard only in this position; many murmurs are best heard sitting.

G. Standing and special maneuvers (Fig. 8-20). Perform any special maneuvers appropriate to your earlier findings (squatting, Valsalva's, isometric, amyl nitrite). These will be described later in the chapter.

IV. Cardinal Symptoms. Only major symptoms are considered here.

  A. Symptoms that indicate functional status (how bad?)

    1. Dyspnea

      a. Caused by decreased pulmonary compliance due to elevated pulmonary venous pressure plus a reduced cardiac output

      b. Onset

        (1) Abrupt: chordal rupture, pulmonary embolus

        (2) Rapid: paroxysmal nocturnal due to acute left ventricular failure

        (3) Gradual: congestive heart failure, valvular disease, cardiomyopathy

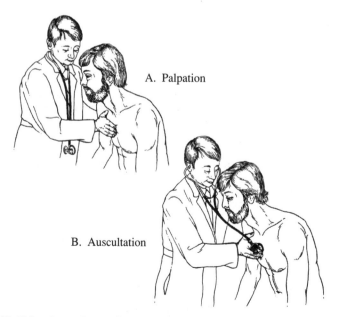

A. Palpation

B. Auscultation

Fig. 8-19. Palpation and auscultation in the sitting position (see text).

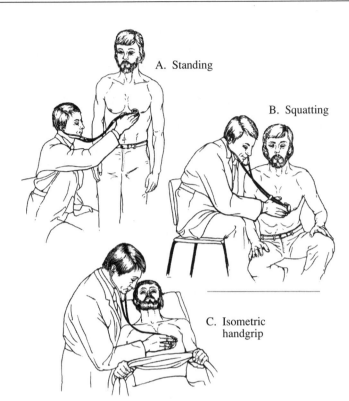

A. Standing

B. Squatting

C. Isometric handgrip

Fig. 8-20. Some special maneuvers for evaluation of heart murmurs.

   c. Severity (New York Heart Association classification)
      (1) Class I: only with strenuous exercise (athletic)
      (2) Class II: with above-average activity (three flights of stairs)
      (3) Class III: with average activity (walking on level/one flight of stairs)
      (4) Class IV: with no activity (at rest)
   2. Orthopnea
      a. Dyspnea with the recumbent position
      b. Graded by pillows (two pillow, three pillow, and so on)
      c. Usually with advanced disease
      d. Often improves with treatment
   3. Fatigue
      a. Many noncardiac causes
      b. Difficult to assess and quantify
      c. Common to many forms of advanced heart disease
B. Symptoms with special diagnostic significance (what's wrong?)
   1. Chest pain
      a. Instantaneous onset
         (1) Aortic dissection
         (2) Massive pulmonary embolus (pleuritic)
      b. Rapid onset
         (1) Coronary occlusion, often with diaphoresis, weakness, anxiety

          (2) Pericarditis; pleuritic, varies with position (improved by sitting forward)

  c. Gradual onset

      (1) Angina pectoris; comes on like a flush, builds to a peak, then subsides slowly

          (a) Angina pectoris (literally, strangulation of the chest) comes from the Latin *angere*, to strangle. It is often a more squeezing feeling than a painful one.

          (b) Induced by factors that increase cardiac work, such as exercise, excitement, cold, and meals.

          (c) Often radiates to throat, jaws, shoulders, and arms.

      (2) Unstable angina; occurs spontaneously without any unusual stress (rest angina)

      (3) Pulmonary hypertension; causes pain that is much like angina in character

  d. Mostly diffuse and anterior and spreads from the sternal area

2. Syncope

  a. Simple vasovagal faint (bradycardia and hypotension)

      (1) Prodrome of nausea, weakness, and diaphoresis

      (2) Short duration but total loss of consciousness

      (3) Usually benign

  b. Cardiac syncope due to arrhythmia

      (1) Very abrupt

      (2) Patient often incontinent

      (3) Arrhythmia usually not perceived

      (4) Caused by the following:

          (a) Excessive bradycardia with pulse rate <35 (e.g., complete A-V block)

          (b) Excessive tachycardia (particularly ventricular) with pulse rate >180

      (5) Rapid return of mental status without awareness of postictal state; no neurologic sequelae

  c. Orthostasis

      (1) Posturally related (standing up)

      (2) Often drug-related (vasodilators, diuretics)

3. Palpitation (sense of pounding in chest or neck). Simulate rhythms by tapping your chest when evaluating this symptom.

  a. Rare skips (premature beats)

  b. Rapid and regular

      (1) Sinus tachycardia

      (2) Supraventricular tachycardia, atrial flutter

      (3) Ventricular tachycardia (less common)

  c. Rapid and irregular (atrial fibrillation and atrial flutter)

  d. Slow, regular, and forceful (often benign)

V. Abnormal Findings

  A. Blood pressure

  1. Hypertension: persistent elevation (>140/90 mmHg in adults, 160/90 in elderly) of the systemic blood pressure. Labile elevations are common and not true hypertension.

  2. Widened pulse pressure: greater than usual difference between the diastolic and systolic pressures.

    a. This is common to all conditions producing an increased stroke volume, such as simple bradycardia, fever, anemia, hypermetabolic states (e.g., 150/70).

    b. Incompetence of the aortic valve lowers the diastolic pressure (e.g., 150/30).

    c. Diminished elasticity of the great arteries, as with aging, increases the systolic pressure (e.g., 165/80); this is sometimes called *isolated systolic hypertension.*

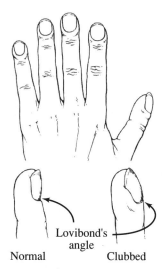

Normal   Clubbed

Lovibond's angle

Fig. 8-21. Clubbing of the digits (see text).

    3. Hypotension: systemic blood pressure below 90/60.
        a. Many children and some adults normally have systolic blood pressures of about 90 mmHg.
        b. Shock is not present unless there is evidence of decreased regional blood flow, such as syncope, sweating, oliguria, and obtundation.
        c. Systemic hypotension or shock may result from inadequate cardiac output, decreased peripheral resistance, or inadequate blood volume and is usually associated with dizziness, visual blurring, seating, or sometimes syncope.
  B. Inspection and palpation
    1. Extremities
        a. *Clubbing* of the digits: proliferative change in soft tissues (Fig. 8-21).

Table 8-2. Some Causes of Symmetric Clubbing

Cardiovascular Disease	Pulmonary Disease	Extrathoracic Disease
Congenital, cyanotic	Inflammatory	Gastrointestinal
Subacute infective endocarditis	Abscess	Hepatic cirrhosis
	Bronchiectasis	Chronic ulcerative colitis
	Empyema	Regional enteritis
	Neoplasm	(Crohn's disease)
	Primary lung cancer	Chronic diarrhea and
	Metastatic lung cancer	malabsorption
	Mesothelioma	syndromes
	Pulmonary fibrosis	Familial
	Cystic fibrosis	Pachydermoperiostosis
	Pulmonary arteriovenous	Primary
	malformations	Secondary (hypertrophic osteoarthropathy)

(1) Early clubbing shows loss of normal angle at base of nail (Lovibond's angle); Later, an increase in longitudinal curvature of the nail occurs.

(2) Etiology is uncertain, but is probably related to increased blood flow through multiple arteriovenous shunts in the distal phalanges (see classification in Table 8-2).

b. *Cyanosis:* a bluish skin color caused by a relative decrease in oxygen saturation of cutaneous capillary blood.

  (1) May be central or peripheral.

  (2) Manifests when arterial saturation falls below 85% (normal is about 95%; venous saturation about 70%), provided the patient is not severely anemic (Table 8-3).

c. *Edema:* excessive fluid in the tissues.

  (1) Has many causes.

  (2) Cardiac edema usually dependent (feet, ankles) and a common sign of congestive heart failure.

  (3) Graded (1+ to 4+) on the basis of pitting produced by sustained light pressure with the thumb over the medial malleolus or pretibial area.

  (4) Occurs unilaterally after occlusion of a major vein; peripheral arterial occlusion may cause mild "brawny" (nonpitting) edema.

2. Peripheral venous circulation

a. Varicose veins: dilatation of the superficial leg veins, with diminished blood flow and increased intraluminal pressure

  (1) Primary varicose veins. These varicosities are caused by inherent weakness of the vessel wall or incompetent venous valves.

  (2) Secondary varicose veins. These are due to proximal obstruction in the vena cava, pelvic veins, or iliofemoral veins. Both greater and lesser saphenous systems may be involved. Both greater and lesser saphenous veins communicate with the deep femoral venous system; when the valves in the perforating veins are incompetent, the superficial saphenous varicosities may fill from the deep venous system.

  (3) Diagnosis.

    (a) Inspection and tourniquet tests of the dependent limbs are sufficient in 80% to 90% of patients.

    (b) If severe, pigmentation, edema, or ulceration of the skin in the region of the medial malleolus point to significant venostasis.

    (c) Two facts must be determined: the competency of the valves in the veins communicating between the superficial and deep systems and the patency of the deep veins.

b. Venous thrombosis: may be acute (thrombophlebitis) or silent

Table 8-3. Some Causes of Cyanosis

Central Cyanosis	Peripheral Cyanosis[a]
Decreased oxygenation of blood	Congestive heart failure
Pulmonary disease	Hyperviscosity
Arteriovenous pulmonary shunts	Hypotension
Right-to-left intracardiac shunts	Distal vasoconstriction
Increased desaturated hemoglobin (>5 g/100 mL)	Drugs
Erythrocytosis	Cold
Methemoglobinemia	Raynaud's phenomenon

[a]Due to increased tissue oxygen extraction with slow flow.

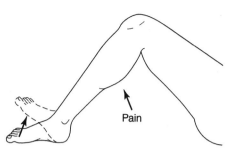

Fig. 8-22. Homan's sign.

(1) Superficial: produces redness, induration, tenderness adjacent to the involved venous segment, which is thickened and cord-like. This may be associated with deep thrombosis.

(2) Deep venous: involves the deep femoral and pelvic veins and may be entirely asymptomatic—fatal pulmonary embolism may occur without warning, especially in bedridden or postsurgical patients. Prophylaxis is very effective; watch for minor signs, including the following:

(a) Tenderness in popliteal space and calf

(b) Mild swelling detectable only by measuring the circumference of both thighs and calves at several levels

(c) Unexplained low-grade fever or tachycardia

(d) Calf pain on sharp dorsiflexion of the foot with the knee slightly flexed (Homans' sign) (Fig. 8-22).

(i) Distinguish from Achilles tendon pain, which is sometimes seen in women who wear high heels and people in flat slippers.

(ii) More than 50% of all deep vein thromboses are clinically silent; screening with ultrasound scanning, impedance plethysmography, or venography is needed for diagnosis (Fig. 8-23).

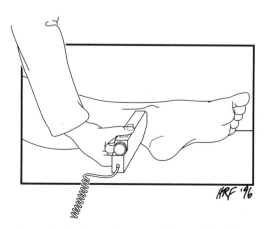

Fig. 8-23. A Doppler evaluation is a routine part of the peripheral vascular assessment.

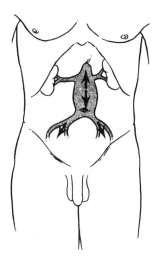

Fig. 8-24. Aortic aneurysm.

3. Peripheral arterial circulation
  a. Arterial occlusion. This may be complete or partial and occurs acutely or gradually.
    (1) Chronic arterial insufficiency. This results from gradual reduction in vessel caliber and is usually due to atherosclerotic or inflammatory processes of the vascular wall (Table 8-4).
      (a) Diminished or absent pulses; audible systolic bruits extending into early diastole heard over major arteries (femoral or subclavian)
      (b) Reduced or absent peripheral hair (over digits and dorsum of hands or feet)
      (c) Atrophy of muscles and soft tissues
      (d) Thickened nails with rough transverse ridges and longitudinal curving
      (e) Coolness on palpation
      (f) Intense grayish pallor on elevation of the extremity. Dependency after 1 or 2 minutes of elevation produces a dusky, plum-colored rubor, which develops gradually (30 seconds to 1 minute) (Burger's sign).

Table 8-4. Causes of Chronic Arterial Insufficiency

Older Patient	Younger Patient
Atherosclerosis	Arteritis
Buerger's disease	Systemic lupus erythematosus
	Polyarteritis nodosa
	Takayasu's arteritis
	Retroperitoneal fibrosis
	Deep venous thrombosis
	Popliteal entrapment

          (g) Delayed venous filling time. Empty the superficial veins by elevating the extremity. Prompt filling (less than 10 seconds) normally occurs with lowering of the extremity.

      (2) Early arterial disease. Assess the effects of exercise. Three important changes, not seen in the resting state, may be elicited:

          (a) Pallor of the skin over the distal limb

          (b) Disappearance of arterial pulses

          (c) Systolic bruits over the major arteries

      (3) Advanced arterial insufficiency: in addition to all of the above features, signs that indicate gangrene is imminent may be seen:

          (a) Bluish-gray mottling of the skin unchanged by position

          (b) Early ulceration between or on tips of digits

          (c) Tenderness to pressure

          (d) Stocking anesthesia

b. Abdominal bruit (known to occur as an isolated finding in young, healthy persons, in whom it may be of no significance) may be signs of other disease.

    (1) Renal artery stenosis. In the presence of hypertension, a bruit heard in the epigastrium or anterior lumbar region may be an important sign.

    (2) Mesenteric arterial disease (abdominal angina). Systolic bruit may be heard.

    (3) Enlarged spleen. Systolic bruit may be heard over a greatly enlarged spleen.

    (4) Cirrhotic liver. Venous hum may be heard over the liver due to torrential flow through venous collaterals.

    (5) Neoplasms. Local arterial involvement may produce abdominal systolic bruits with tumors of the pancreas, stomach, or liver.

c. Aneurysm: a pulsatile swelling along the course of the vessel, most often involving the aorta or popliteal artery. A systolic thrill may be felt over the tumor.

    (1) Aortic aneurysm: usually felt as an expansile mass in the mid-abdomen (Fig. 8-24).

    (2) A lateral film may show calcification in the wall of the aneurysm; the lumbar spine may be eroded.

    (3) Rupture causes severe, constant back pain and is often associated with pain in one or both groins and a mass in the flank.

    (4) A continuous thrill over the mass indicates a possible A-V fistula.

d. Additional vascular syndromes (Table 8-5)

4. Neck

  a. Carotid abnormalities

    (1) Absent carotid pulse

      (a) No pulse on one side. Isolated occlusion often causes neurologic symptoms and signs.

      (b) Causes: arteriosclerosis, arteritis, aortic aneurysm, and congenital anomalies.

    (2) Unequal carotid pulses

      (a) Clear difference in pulse amplitude

      (b) Causes: classic sign of dissecting aneurysm; also partial carotid occlusive disease

    (3) Slow upstroke (pulsus tardus) (Fig. 8-25B)

      (a) Ascending limb delayed, broad summit, pulse pressure may be narrowed; slow upstroke can usually be appreciated, often with thrill

      (b) Causes: valvular aortic stenosis

    (4) Weak pulse (pulsus parvus)

      (a) Normal contour, but low amplitude; feels weak and "thready"

Table 8-5. Additional Vascular Syndromes

Acute Arterial Occlusion[a]	Abdominal Aortic Aneurysm	Leriche's Syndrome
Pain, usually severe, except in a person with diabetes	Expansile abdominal mass	Absent femoral pulses
	Systolic bruit and thrill in abdomen	Intermittent claudication extending into the buttocks
Pallor	Severe lower back pain may reflect rupture[a]	Impotence
Pulselessness		
Paresthesia	Ultrasonography or computed tomography confirms clinical diagnosis	
Paralysis		

[a]Surgical emergency.

- **(b)** Causes: low stroke volume with associated peripheral vasoconstriction—low-output congestive failure, mitral stenosis, acute myocardial infarction, or shock
- **(5)** Brisk upstroke (water-hammer pulse) (see Fig. 8-25C)
    - **(a)** Swift upstroke with increased amplitude and a collapsing quality
    - **(b)** Causes: severe aortic regurgitation
    - **(c)** Swift upstroke with normal amplitude
    - **(d)** Causes: obstructive hypertrophic cardiomyopathy, ventricular septal defect, severe mitral regurgitation
- **(6)** Bounding pulse
    - **(a)** Wide pulse pressure with normal upstroke; when more extreme, it becomes a water-hammer pulse
    - **(b)** Causes: increased stroke volume and diminished peripheral resistance—fever, anemia, hepatic failure, thyrotoxicosis, severe bradycardia
- **(7)** Bifid pulse (pulsus bisferiens) (see Fig. 8-25D)
    - **(a)** Two systolic peaks with an extremely brisk initial upstroke
    - **(b)** Causes: aortic regurgitation, obstructive hypertrophic cardiomyopathy
- **(8)** Alternating pulse (pulsus alternans) (see Fig. 8-25E)
    - **(a)** Alternating large- and small-amplitude beats with regular rhythm; often better appreciated in radial or brachial pulse or with blood pressure cuff
    - **(b)** Causes: severe left ventricular dysfunction
- **(9)** Pulsus bigeminus (bigeminy)
    - **(a)** Coupling of two beats separated by a pause; weak second beat due to reduced diastolic filling time
    - **(b)** Causes: alternating normal and premature beats
- **(10)** Pulsus paradoxus
    - **(a)** An exaggeration of the normal inspiratory decline in systolic blood pressure; often best appreciated in peripheral pulses using blood pressure cuff
    - **(b)** Causes: pericardial effusion with tamponade, constrictive pericarditis (greater than 10 mmHg fall in systolic blood pressure at peak inspiration)
- **(11)** Carotid sinus stimulation
    - **(a)** This is a useful technique for slowing the pulse rate by compression of the carotid sinus at the angle of jaw.

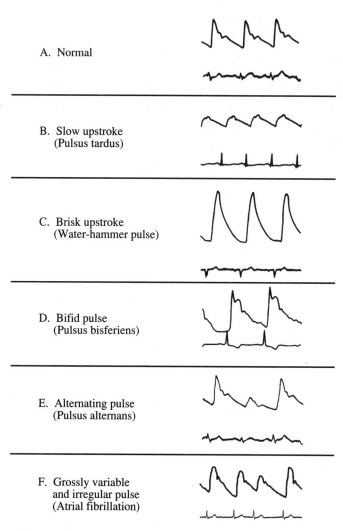

A. Normal

B. Slow upstroke
(Pulsus tardus)

C. Brisk upstroke
(Water-hammer pulse)

D. Bifid pulse
(Pulsus bisferiens)

E. Alternating pulse
(Pulsus alternans)

F. Grossly variable
and irregular pulse
(Atrial fibrillation)

Fig. 8-25. Abnormalities of the carotid pulse (see text).

      (b) Vagal discharge thus produced may slow A-V node conduc-
      tion or depress sinus node function.
      (c) At times cardiac standstill may occur. Be careful and gentle,
      especially in the elderly.
    (12) Grossly irregular and variable pulse (see Fig. 8-25F)
      (a) Common with atrial fibrillation and at times with atrial
      flutter and other rhythm disturbances
      (b) The shorter the interval between beats, the lower the ampli-
      tude (due to reduced diastolic filling); variation affects both
      rate and amplitude
  b. Jugular venous abnormalities

    (1) Abnormal jugular venous pressure
        (a) Estimated from peak venous pulsation with the patient at 45 degrees (see Fig. 8-15); may not be visible in obese persons or those with short, heavy ("bull") necks
        (b) Grading
            (i) To angle of jaw: severe increase
            (ii) To mid-neck: moderate increase
            (iii) To lower third of neck: mild increase or normal
        (c) Causes of distention
            (i) Congestive heart failure; useful for assessing efficacy of treatment day-to-day
            (ii) Cardiac tamponade from pericardial effusion
            (iii) Right ventricular myocardial infarction
            (iv) Mechanical compression, such as intrathoracic neoplasm, aortic aneurysm

    (2) Abnormal jugular venous pulse
        (a) Abnormally prominent A wave (Fig. 8-26A)
            (i) Increased force of right atrial contraction due to loss of right ventricular compliance secondary to hypertrophy or systolic dysfunction; rarely tricuspid stenosis
            (ii) Causes: pulmonic stenosis, primary pulmonary hypertension, right ventricular infarction, congestive heart failure, large or multiple pulmonary emboli, chronic obstructive pulmonary disease (COPD)
        (b) Abnormally prominent V wave (see Fig. 8-26B)
            (i) Significant tricuspid regurgitation
            (ii) Causes: right ventricular failure with dilatation, rheumatic valvular incompetence, COPD
        (c) Cannon waves (see Fig. 8-26C)
            (i) Synchronous right atrial and right ventricular contraction; right atrial contraction against a closed tricuspid valve causes a brisk backward reflux.
            (ii) Causes: atrioventricular dissociation (complete A-V block, VVI pacemaker, ventricular tachycardia), low junctional tachycardia.
        (d) Abnormally prominently descent (see Fig. 8-26D)
            (i) The mean jugular venous pressure is markedly elevated, damping the outward pulsations. The pressure drops abruptly and briefly with tricuspid opening.
            (ii) Causes: chronic constrictive pericarditis, acute pericarditis with tamponade, severe congestive failure, restrictive cardiomyopathy.

5. Precordium
  a. Percussion
    (1) Left cardiac border greater than 10.5 cm from mid-sternal line (or lateral to the midclavicular line) is cardiac enlargement (CE).
    (2) Grading
        (a) Between midclavicular and anterior axillary line: mild CE
        (b) To anterior axillary line: moderate CE
        (c) Beyond anterior axillary line: marked CE
    (3) Good correlation with echocardiogram and x-ray (94.4% sensitivity)
    (4) Shows where to start palpating
  b. Palpation
    (1) This is best done in left decubitus or supine positions in full expiration.
    (2) Time any movement felt against the right carotid upstroke (use two hands) (see Fig. 8-17).

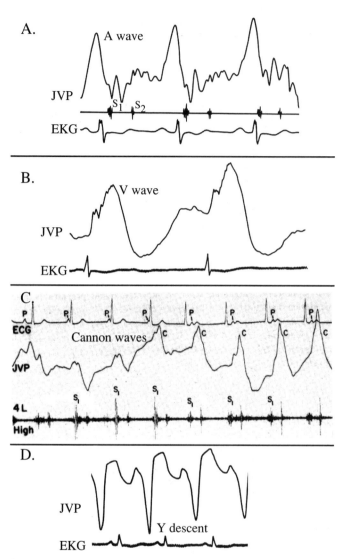

Fig. 8-26. Abnormalities of jugular venous pulse (see text).

    (3) Movement is often visible. Use tongue blade amplifier to analyze
        (see Fig. 8-18).
    (4) Palpable murmurs are called *thrills;* palpable sounds are called
        shocks.
    (5) Abnormal apex impulse
        (a) Left ventricular hypertrophy (Fig. 8-27)
            (i) Best felt in left decubitus position
            (ii) Sustained; small area (dime- to nickel-size)
            (iii) Amplitude usually increased

                (iv) Not necessarily displaced laterally
                (v) Often double due to "atrial kick" causing presystolic distension that correlates with S_4
                (vi) Seems to be synchronous with carotid upstroke rather than to precede it
                (vii) Tongue blade helpful
            (b) Left ventricular dilatation (see Fig. 8-27)
                (i) Multiple causes leading to impaired systolic contractile function, such as cardiomyopathy, advanced valvular or coronary disease
                (ii) Best felt in left decubitus position
                (iii) Sustained (synchronous with carotid)
                (iv) Larger area (quarter-size)
                (v) Increased amplitude
                (vi) Lateral displacement common
                (vii) Sometimes a second movement in early diastole that correlates with an S_3
        (6) Diffuse precordial systolic lift
            (a) Ventricular aneurysm
            (b) Marked left ventricular or right ventricular dilatation
            (c) Amplified by tongue blade
            (d) Often double
        (7) Diffuse precordial diastolic lift
            (a) Constrictive pericarditis
            (b) Must time from carotid or by auscultation
            (c) Often better seen than felt
            (d) Tongue blade helpful
        (8) Parasternal lift (third and fourth left intercostal spaces)
            (a) Right ventricular hypertrophy (pressure overload)
                (i) Sustained
                (ii) Localized
                (iii) Pulmonary hypertension; pulmonic stenosis
            (b) Right ventricular dilatation (volume overload) (Fig. 8-28)
                (i) Not sustained
                (ii) Diffuse
                (iii) Atrial septal defect; tricuspid regurgitation, congestive failure

C. Auscultation
    1. Abnormal heart sounds
        a. First heart sound (S_1)
            (1) Louder with hyperkinetic state: exercise, anemia, sepsis, hyperthyroidism
            (2) Louder with mitral stenosis and short P-R interval (Wolff-Parkinson-White syndrome)
            (3) Softer with low cardiac output or prolonged P-R interval
            (4) Varies from beat to beat with complete A-V block due to variable P-R interval (see Fig. 8-26C)
        b. Second heart sound (S_2)
            (1) Louder with elevation of the systemic or pulmonary artery pressure.
            (2) Softer in aortic or pulmonary stenosis.
            (3) Persistent splitting occurs with delayed pulmonic valve closure (fixed or varying with respiration), atrial septal defect with volume overload causing prolonged right ventricular ejection (fixed), pulmonic stenosis and ventricular septal defects (wide splitting with some respiratory variation), delayed electrical activation of the right ventricle with right bundle branch block (normal respiratory movement).
            (4) Reversed splitting (S_2 split in expiration, single in inspiration) is caused by late aortic valve closure from prolonged emptying time

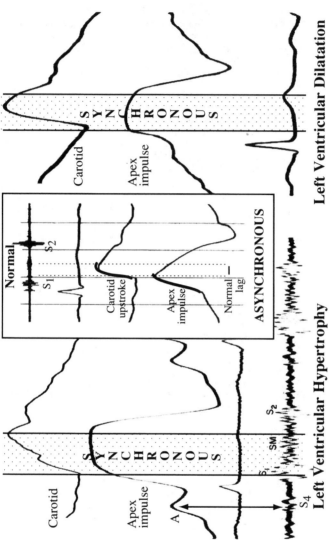

Fig. 8-27. Apical impulse abnormalities with left ventricular hypertrophy and dilatation (see text).

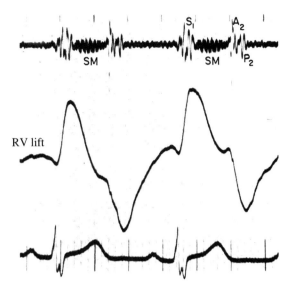

Fig. 8-28. Parasternal (right ventricular) lift in a patient with an atrial septal defect. SM = systolic murmur.

of the left ventricle (aortic stenosis, marked hypertension, poor contractility as seen in cardiomyopathy, myocardial ischemia) or delayed left ventricular ejection (left bundle branch block or artificial pacemaker in right ventricle). In expiration, right ventricular ejection is shortest and pulmonic valve closure precedes the aortic; in inspiration, right ventricular ejection is prolonged and the two closures sound superimposed.

  c. Presystolic extra sound (S_4) (Fig. 8-29A)

    (1) Dull, low-pitched; 0.14 seconds before S_1

    (2) May be more easily felt than heard

    (3) Best heard with bell of stethoscope applied lightly over the apex impulse with patient in left decubitus position

    (4) Left ventricle: caused by vigorous atrial contraction in patients with decreased left ventricular compliance caused by left ventricular hypertrophy or myocardial ischemia; apical S_4 common in patients over age 65 as a result of effects of aging on left ventricular compliance

    (5) Right ventricle: S_4 may be heard along the left sternal border in patients with pulmonary hypertension or pulmonic stenosis; increases with inspiration

  d. Protodiastolic extra sounds (S_3) (see Fig. 8-29B)

    (1) Low-pitched (even lower than S_4); difficult to detect

    (2) Best heard with bell of stethoscope applied lightly over the apex impulse with patient in left decubitus position

    (3) Occur during period of rapid ventricular filling

    (4) Caused by mitral regurgitation, constrictive pericarditis, ventricular failure of varying etiology

    (5) Right ventricular S_3 increase with inspiration; occur with tricuspid regurgitation or right ventricular failure

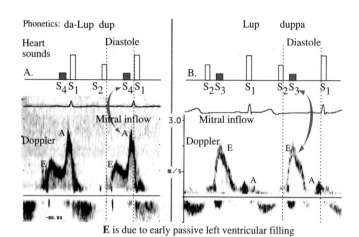

E is due to early passive left ventricular filling
A is due to left atrial contraction

Fig. 8-29. Diastolic extra sounds (see text).

    (6) Occurrence after age 25 or in association with cardiac disease suggestive of congestive heart failure except in aortic or mitral regurgitation with enhanced rapid ventricular filling; to be expected with major mitral regurgitation

  e. Gallop rhythm
    (1) S_3 or S_4 associated with rapid heart rate; third and fourth sounds are superimposed, resulting in a single, loud, prolonged, "summation" gallop; cadence like that of a galloping horse
    (2) Sign of congestive heart failure

  f. Ejection clicks
    (1) Occur in early systole
    (2) Originate in either of the great vessels or their valves; generated by abrupt distention of a dilated great vessel during early ventricular ejection, by upward movement of stiffened deformed valve leaflets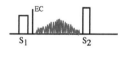
    (3) Congenital valvular pulmonic stenosis: increase in intensity of ejection clicks with expiration and decrease with inspiration
    (4) Pulmonary hypertension: ejection clicks not as likely to vary with respiration
    (5) Pulmonic ejection clicks: best heard at base, high left sternal border
    (6) Aortic ejection clicks: do not vary with respiration; best heard in aortic area, but often over entire precordium

  g. Mid-systolic click
    (1) Due to prolapse of mitral valve leaflets during systole
    (2) Often associated with late systolic murmur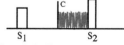
    (3) High-pitched, sharp sound; best heard with bell at apex in left decubitus position
    (4) Occurs earlier in systole in standing position; occurs later in systole in squatting position (see Auscultatory maneuvers for explanation)

  h. Systolic crunch or knock

       (1) Occurs with small, left-sided pneumothorax (noisy pneumothorax); sometimes heard in mediastinal emphysema
       (2) Often audible to patient (and physician) without stethoscope
2. Heart murmurs
   a. Production. Basic factors promote turbulence (see Fig. 8-30A, in which a systolic murmur is used as an example), such as the following:
      (1) Lowering viscosity
      (2) Increasing diameter of a tube
      (3) Changing the caliber of a tube abruptly
      (4) Increasing velocity of flow. Velocity governs intensity and pitch
         (a) Intensity: the faster the flow, the louder the murmur; thus exercise causes most murmurs to become louder
         (b) Pitch: the faster the flow, the higher the pitch; the slower the flow, the lower the pitch
   b. Transmission. Murmurs sound different as the stethoscope is moved over the precordium.

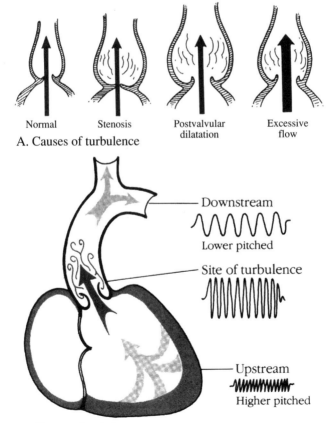

Normal   Stenosis   Postvalvular   Excessive
                        dilatation   flow

A. Causes of turbulence

Downstream

Lower pitched

Site of turbulence

Upstream

Higher pitched

B. Changes in pitch

Fig. 8-30. Production and transmission of systolic murmurs (see text).

(1) Distance: the closer the murmur source to the chest wall, the louder the sound will be.

(2) Interposing tissues: natural damping effect; high-frequency sound reflects backward causing pitch to become lower.

(3) Movement within the cardiovascular system: in moving backward against the stream, low frequencies dampen out; in moving forward with the stream, high frequencies are lost (see Fig. 8-30B).

c. Description. Murmurs are described according to these six terms.

(1) Timing: systolic, diastolic, continuous

(2) Location: point of maximum intensity by anatomic landmarks: apex; left sternal border (LSB); left base (pulmonic area); right base (aortic area); intermediate zones by exact intercostal space

(3) Loudness (Table 8-6): graded on a six-point scale of increasing loudness; grade 1/6 = barely audible; grade 6/6 = audible with stethoscope off chest wall

(4) Pitch: low = 25 to 150 cps; medium = 150 to 350 cps; high = 350 to 600 cps

(5) Duration (Table 8-7)

(6) Quality

(a) Crescendo = increasing in loudness

(b) Decrescendo = decreasing in loudness

(c) Descriptive terms: blowing, harsh, rumbling, musical, cooing, whooping, honking, regurgitant, ejection

3. Heart murmurs—description

a. Systolic murmurs: more variable than diastolic murmurs and occur early, mid-, late, and holosystolic. They fall into two major categories: midsystolic ejection murmurs and holosystolic regurgitant murmurs.

(1) Midsystolic ejection murmurs. These are produced by forward outflow of blood through the pulmonary or aortic valves; they occur in midsystole, are medium-pitched, rise and fall in crescendo-decrescendo fashion, ending before S_2. Causes include valvular or subvalvular stenosis, increased stroke volume, dilatation of the vessel beyond the valve, or a combination of these factors.

(a) Aortic systolic ejection murmurs occur with valvular or subvalvular stenosis (Fig. 8-31), primary dilatation of the ascending aorta, increased left ventricular stroke output. They are best heard in the aortic area, but are often transmitted to the entire precordium where they may seem higher in pitch and more musical, but maintain their ejection quality.

Table 8-6. Murmur Loudness (Six Categories)

	Grade	Description
	I	Heard only after special maneuvers and "tuning in"
	II	Faint, but readily heard; not transmitted elsewhere
	III	Loud, but without a palpable thrill; transmitted elsewhere
	IV	Associated with a palpable thrill, but stethoscope must be fully on chest to be heard
Not clinically useful {	V	Heard with stethoscope partly off the chest; palpable thrill
	VI	Heard with stethoscope entirely off the chest; palpable thrill

Table 8-7. Timing and Duration of Heart Murmurs

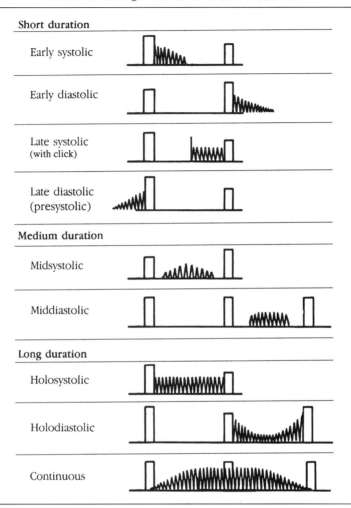

Aortic systolic ejection murmurs are often transmitted to carotid arteries.

(b) Pulmonic systolic ejection murmurs occur with pulmonary valvular and subvalvular stenosis, dilatation of the pulmonary artery, increased pulmonary flow, as with atrial septal defect. Usually, they are localized to second and third intercostal spaces and may be referred to the left upper chest.

(c) Functional systolic murmurs occur when turbulence develops in the absence of any structural abnormality; types include the "hemic" systolic murmur heard with anemia and the basal systolic murmur, often heard with thyrotoxicosis,

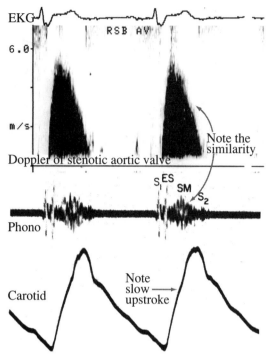

Fig. 8-31. Midsystolic ejection murmur from a patient with aortic valve stenosis. ES = ejection shock; SM = systolic murmur.

fever, or exercise. Elderly patients often have functional murmurs due to the rigidity of their aortas.

(2) Holosystolic regurgitant murmurs. Produced by an escape of blood from a chamber of relatively high pressure (ventricle) into one of relatively low pressure (atrium) through incompetent mitral or tricuspid valve or by flow through a ventricular septal defect (Fig. 8-32A). Regurgitant murmurs are longer in duration and holosystolic and may engulf S_2. They are plateau-shaped and either of constant intensity or increased in late systole. Regurgitant murmurs do not rise and fall in intensity (see Fig. 8-32B).

  (a) Mitral regurgitation (Table 8-8). The systolic murmur varies greatly depending on the pathophysiologic abnormality.

  (b) Tricuspid regurgitation. Murmur is similar to that of mitral regurgitation and is best heard over tricuspid area. It may become louder with inspiration.

  (c) Ventricular septal defect. This murmur has a loud, coarse quality heard in third and fourth left intercostal spaces; it often causes a thrill.

b. Diastolic murmurs

  (1) Aortic and pulmonic regurgitation (Fig. 8-33): high-pitched, decrescendo murmurs

  (a) Aortic regurgitation: high-pitched murmur. This murmur begins immediately with aortic closure and diminishes progressively with diastole. It is heard best in the aortic areas

A.

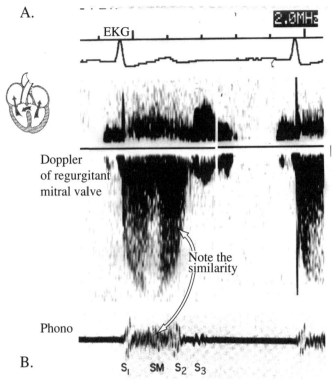

EKG

2.0MHz

Doppler
of regurgitant
mitral valve

Note the
similarity

Phono

B.

S_1 SM S_2 S_3

Fig. 8-32. Holosystolic murmur in a patient with mitral regurgitation. SM = systolic murmur.

and along the left sternal border using a diaphragm end-piece, with the patient sitting and holding the breath in expiration. (Patients with aortic insufficiency may have a low-pitched murmur at the apex that sounds like the murmur of mitral stenosis; this is an Austin Flint murmur.)

(b) Pulmonic regurgitation: similar in pitch, timing, quality, and location to the aortic murmur, but more localized to pulmonic area. It often cannot be distinguished from aortic regurgitation by auscultation. Pulmonic insufficiency from severe pulmonary arterial hypertension causes a Graham Steell murmur. Congenital pulmonic insufficiency occurs with normal pressures in the pulmonary artery and results in a low- to medium-pitched murmur that begins at an interval after the second sound.

(2) Mitral and tricuspid stenosis: lower-pitched murmurs

(a) Mitral stenosis (Fig. 8-34): low-pitched, localized, apical rumble. This is often heard only with the bell and the patient rolled onto left side. Mitral stenosis murmur is only audible precisely over the apical impulse. It is loudest in early and late diastole when the pressure gradient is greatest across the narrowed mitral valve. The murmur is often initiated in early diastole with a sharp click—the mitral opening

Table 8-8. Mitral Regurgitation

Common Etiology	Pathology	Murmur	Diagram
Rheumatic	Leaflet deformity	Holosystolic	S_1 SM S_2 S_3
Hereditary	Mitral valve prolapse	Late systolic (often with click)	S_1 C SM S_2
Coronary disease	Papillary muscle dysfunction	Midsystolic (often with S_4)	S_4 S_1 SM S_2
Idiopathic (often)	Acute chordal rupture	Early systolic (often with S_3 or S_4)	S_4 S_1 SM S_2 S_3
Cardiomyopathy	Ventricular dilatation	Holosystolic (often with S_3)	S_1 SM S_2 S_3

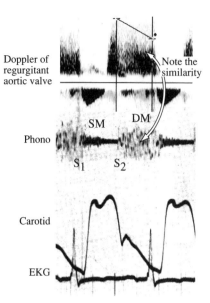

Fig. 8-33. Diastolic murmur in a patient with aortic regurgitation. SM = systolic murmur; DM = diastolic murmur.

snap—heard at the apex, medial to the apex, or along the left sternal border. The higher the left atrial pressure, the closer the opening snap is to the second sound, and vice versa. This 2-OS interval is used to estimate the severity of the stenosis. Decrescendo quality through early and mid-diastole; gradient increases sharply in latter third of diastole owing to atrial contraction, causing a presystolic accentuation of the murmur. With atrial fibrillation, the presystolic accentuation disappears.

   (b) Tricuspid stenosis: similar in timing and quality to mitral murmur but often higher-pitched and localized near the tricuspid area or along the left sternal border. Inspiration usually makes it louder.

  c. Continuous murmurs. These begin in systole and continue into diastole without stopping, but may not occupy the entire cardiac cycle. They occur when flow from a high to a lower pressure chamber is uninterrupted by opening or closing of cardiac valves, as in the Gibson murmur of patent ductus arteriosus that begins in systole, peaks around S_2, spills over into diastole, and may not continue to S_1. It is heard maximally under the left clavicle and in the pulmonic area. Other causes are pulmonary and coronary A-V fistulas. Combined systolic and diastolic murmurs may fill the entire cardiac cycle, but they are separate, not continuous murmurs.

4. Pericardial friction rub—sign of pericardial inflammation

  a. There are three components, corresponding with systolic, early diastolic, and presystolic phases of the cardiac cycle. At least two components should be heard before diagnosing a friction rub.

  b. Rub is often loudest along left sternal border or directly over sternum. It may be loud, or faint, high-pitched, or evanescent; it has a superficial, scratchy, to-and-fro quality suggesting squeaky leather. The

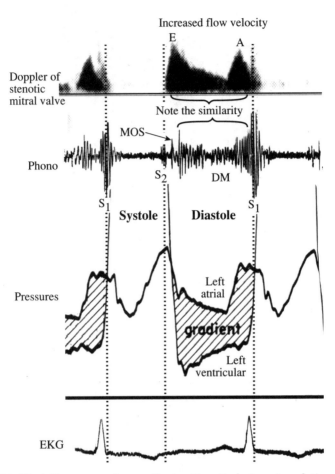

Fig. 8-34. Diastolic murmur in a patient with mitral stenosis: relation among Doppler velocity profile, phonocardiogram, and hemodynamics. DM = diastolic murmur; MOS = mitral opening snap.

sound can be simulated by moving the endpiece on the surface of the skin, particularly on hair.

  (1) Intensity may vary with respiration, but a true friction rub is audible with respiration halted.

  (2) To bring out a friction rub, apply firm pressure with the diaphragm and auscultate with patient sitting up and leaning forward with breath held in expiration.

5. Auscultatory maneuvers (See fig. 8-20C)

  a. Isometric handgrip.

  (1) Increases systemic blood pressure (also cardiac output).

  (2) Louder:

    (i) mitral regurgitation

    (ii) aortic regurgitation

    (iii) ventricular septal defect

  b. Standing.

      (1) Decreases venous return, decreases ventricular volume.
      (2) Louder: obstructive hypertrophic cardiomyopathy
      (3) Softer: innocent murmur
      (4) Longer duration: mitral valve prolapse
  c. Squatting.
      (1) Increases venous return and systemic blood pressure; increases ventricular volume.
      (2) Louder: aortic regurgitation
      (3) Softer: obstructive hypertrophic cardiomyopathy
      (4) Shorter duration: mitral valve prolapse
  d. Sitting, leaning forward, full expiration.
      (1) Thrills better felt.
      (2) Aortic regurgitation is often only heard with this manuever.
  e. Valsalva maneuver (Fig. 8-35).
      (1) Softer: innocent murmur
      (2) Longer: mitral valve prolapse
      (3) Louder: obstructive hypertrophic cardiomyopathy
  f. Amyl nitrite (patient inhales for 15-20 seconds).
      (1) Decreased systemic blood pressure; increased pulse rate, cardiac output, stroke volume.
      (2) Softer:
         (i) mitral regurgitation
         (ii) ventricular septal defect
      (3) Louder:
         (i) aortic stenosis
         (ii) mitral stenosis

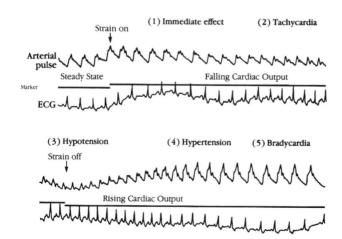

Fig. 8-35. Valsalva's maneuver.

D. Classic physical findings in common cardiovascular disorders

Description   **Heart Sounds Diagrams**

Mitral Stenosis
Small pulse; tapping apex impulse; parasternal lift;
presystolic apical thrill; accentuated S_1 and P_2; mitral
opening snap (OS); mitral distolic rumble; with presystolic
accentuation. Cold hands and feet. Atrial fibrillation (late).

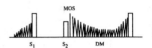

Mitral Regurgitation
Chronic
Normal, brisk, arterial pulse; apical systolic thrill;
sustained apical lift (displaced to left); normal or soft S_1,
apical regurgitant systolic murmur (SM); early diastolic
extra sound (S_3). (Mild forms may show murmur only.)

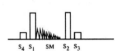

Acute, severe
Usually caused by disruption of supporting structure
apparatus. Varying degrees of congestive heart failure,
loud S_1; harsh decrescendo systolic murmur, S_3 and S_4;
right ventricular lift; increased P_2.

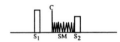

Mitral valve prolapse
Normal S_1 and S_2; one or more midsystolic clicks, and/or a
late systolic murmur or both; frequent arrhythmias; often
associated with slender body habitus and minor musculoskeletal deformities.

Aortic Stenosis
Small, slow-rising pulse; narrow pulse pressure (in severe
cases); sustained apical lift displaced to the left; systolic thrill
in aortic area; decreased or absent A_2; systolic ejection
murmur at base and over carotids; carotid thrill. Cold hands
and feet.

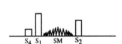

Obstructive Hypertrophic Cardiomyopathy (OHC)
Brisk carotid pulse, often with two waves; thrill at apex or
left sternal border; triple apical impulse (presystolic and two
systolic waves); fourth heart sound; crescendo-descrescendo
systolic murmur at apex and left sternal border.

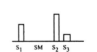

Dilated Cardiomyopathy
Normal or small carotid pulse; jugular A wave; cardiac
enlargement; diffuse sustained apex impulse; soft S_1;
increased S_2; loud S_3 or summation gallop; often apical
systolic murmur; often varying signs of congestive heart failure.

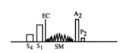

Pulmonary Stenosis
Normal pulse; jugular A wave; parasternal lift; pulmonic
thrill; pulmonary component of second sound absent or soft
and delayed causing widely split S_2; systolic ejection
murmur in pulmonic area; right-sided presystolic extra sound
in tricuspid area (S_4) (severe); pulmonary ejection sound
(mild).

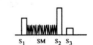

Aortic Regurgitation
Prominent carotid pulsations; watter-hammer or bisferiens pulse. Capillary pulsations of the nail-beds; diffuse, sustained apex impulse displaced down and left; loud M_1, accentuated A_2; decrescendo diastolic murmur (DM) along left sternal border; low-pitched rumbling diastolic murmur at apex (Austin Flint). Systolic flow murmur in aortic area (severe).

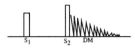

Systemic Hypertension
Elevated blood pressure; carotid usually full; hypertensive funduscopic changes; sustained double apical lift; normal or accentuated S_1, accentuated A_2; presystolic extra sound; aortic ejection murmur (at times).

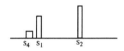

Pulmonary Hypertension
Cyanosis (at times); small pulse; narrow pulse pressure; cold extremities; atrial fibrillation (late); giant jugular A wave; parasternal lift; systolic lift in the pulmonic area; pulmonary ejection sound; pulmonic diastolic murmur (Graham Steell); systolic ejection murmur in pulmonic area; right-sided S_3 and S_4.

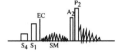

Tricuspid Regurgitation
Jugular V wave; right ventricular parasternal lift; systolic thrill at tricuspid area; tricuspid regurgitant systolic murmur (louder with inspiration); atrial fibrillation; early diastolic extra sound (over right ventricle).

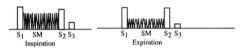

Myocardial Infarction
Tachycardia; pallor; small arterial pulse; narrow pulse   (Varying auscultatory expressions)
pressure; soft heart sounds; presystolic or early diastolic extra sounds; pericardial friction rub; apical systolic murmur (papillary muscle dysfunction); any of the arrythmias.

Atrial Septal Defect
Normal pulse; brisk parasternal lift; lift over pulmonary artery; normal jugular pulse; systolic ejection murmur in pulmonic area; low-pitched diastolic rumble over tricuspid area (at times); persistent wide splitting of S_2.

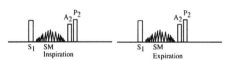

Ventricular Septal Defect
Small pulse; normal jugular pulse; systolic thrill and loud systolic regurgitant murmur in third and fourth interspaces along left sternal border; apical diastolic rumble.

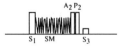

Pericarditis
Tachycardia; friction rub; diminished heart sounds; pulsus paradoxus; neck vein distention, narrow pulse pressure and hypotension (with tamponade).

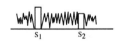

VI. Available Technology for Cardiovascular Diagnosis

Procedure	Suspected Cardiac Condition	Major Sign or Symptom
A. EKG	Arrhythmia	Palpitation, syncope
	CAD	Chest pain
	Ventricular hypertrophy	Abnormal precordial movement, S_4, elevated blood pressure
	Pericarditis	Pleuritic chest pain, friction rub
B. Chest x-ray	Congestive heart failure	Dyspnea, S_3, crackles
	Valvular abnormality	Murmur
	Congenital abnormality	Murmur
	Ventricular dysfunction	CE, S_3, S_4
C. 2-D Echocardiogram with Doppler	Valvular abnormality	Murmur
	Ventricular hypertrophy	Abnormal precordial movement
	Ventricular dysfunction	S_4, elevated blood pressure
	Regional	Chest pain, S_4
	Global	Dyspnea, CE, S_3
	Congenital abnormality	Murmur
	Known arrhythmia (to assess LV function)	
D. Transesophageal echocardiogram	Aortic dissection	Persistent chest pain, murmur, unequal pulses
	Abnormal prosthetic valve	Murmur
	Valvular vegetation	Fever, murmur
	Embolic source	Murmur, dyspnea
	Unsatisfactory transthoracic echo	TIA
E. Standard stress test	CAD	Chest pain
	Arrhythmia	Palpitation, syncope
	Screening	Multiple risk factors
	Functional capacity	Known coronary or valvular disease (follow-up or post-therapy)
	Post-MI risk stratifications	
F. Stress test with imaging	See above	See above, plus: Abnormal EKG (ST-T abnormalities) LBBB, WPW, LVH Digoxin use Pacemaker Female >age 50 (false-positive EKG response)
Thallium preferred	Marked obesity	
	Severe COPD	
	Previous MI	
	Poor echo image	

Echo preferred	Fertile women (radiation) Less expensive Suspected LV dysfunction Suspected associated valvular heart disease	
G. Pharmacologic stress testing Adenosine or dobutamine	Elderly Peripheral vascular and musculoskeletal disease Emphysema Obesity Poorly motivated	Unable to achieve adequate exercise level (85% of age-predicted maximum heart rate)
Adenosine especially useful	Antianginal medication Pacemaker LBBB	e.g., β-blocker
Dobutamine especially useful	Identify viable myocardium	
H. 24-hr ambulatory EKG (Holter)	Arrhythmia	Palpitation, syncope Predisposing ventricular disease Dizzy spells
	CAD (controversial	Silent ischemia
I. Event recorder	Arrythmia	Unexplained recurrent palpitation
J. CT of chest MRI of chest	Chronic pericardial constriction	Edema, dyspnea, S_3 block
	Aortic dissection	Persistent severe chest pain, murmur, unequal pulses
	Cardiac tumor	Dyspnea, TIA
K. Left heart catheterization and coronary angiogram	CAD	Chest pain
	Valvular disease	Murmur and dyspnea
	Ventricular dysfunction	Dyspnea, CE
L. Right heart catheterization (Swan-Ganz)	Shock	Hypotension, pallor, diaphoresis, oliguria
	LV Dysfunction	Dyspnea, CE, S_3
	RV dysfunction	Venous hypertension S_3, clear lungs
	Fluid management	Critical patient
	Transplant evaluation	CE, S_3, dyspnea
M. Electrophysiologic testing	Arrythmia	Syncope, presyncope
	Wide-complex tachycardia	Weakness, presyncope
N. Cardiac biopsy	Myocarditis	Fever, rales, S_3
	Suspected restrictive cardiomyopathy	S_3, edema, venous pressure increase, rales
	Myocardial infiltrative disease	S_3, edema, venous pressure increase, rales
	Transplant evaluation	

CAD = coronary artery disease; CE = cardiac enlargement; COPD = chronic obstructive pulmonary disease; CT = computed tomography; EKG = electrocardiogram; LBBB = left bundle branch block; LV = left ventricular; LVH = left ventricular hypertrophy; MI = myocardial infarction; MRI = magnetic resonance imaging; RV = right ventricular; TIA = transient ischemic attack; WPW = Wolf-Parkinson-White syndrome.

The cost figures cited in this table are **basic direct costs**. The figures are difficult to obtain and change quickly. They include **only** the cost of the test itself (technician, equipment, time, materials). No professional costs (interpretation) are included. Costs vary from region to region based on differences in some components such as labor. However, the relative cost ranking should remain similar.

Procedure	Code
Electrocardiogram (ECG)	$
Chest x-ray	$
2-D-Echocardiogram with Doppler	$$
Transesophageal echocardiogram	$$$
Standard stress test	$$
Stress test with imaging	
Thallium preferred	$$$$$
Echo preferred	$$$
Pharmacologic stress testing:	
Adenosine especially useful	$$$$
Dobutamine especially useful	$$$$
24 hr ambulatory ECG (Holter)	$$
Event recorder	$$
Computed tomography (CT)—chest	$$$
Magnetic resonance imaging (MRI)—chest	$$$
Left heart catheterization and coronary angiogram	$$$$$$
Right heart catheterization (Swan-Ganz)	$$$$
Electrophysiologic testing	$$$$$
Cardiac biopsy	$$$$

$ = $0–$50; $$ = $50–$100; $$$ = $100–$200; $$$$ = $200–$500; $$$$$ = $500–$1000; $$$$$$ = >$1000.

VII. Bibliography

Abrams J. *Essentials of Cardiac Physical Diagnosis.* Philadelphia: Lea & Febiger; 1987.

Braunwald E. *Heart Disease: A Textbook of Cardiovascular Medicine*, 4th ed. Philadelphia: WB Saunders; 1992.

Constant J. *Bedside Cardiology*, 4th ed. Boston: Little, Brown; 1993.

Feigenbaum H. *Echocardiography*, 5th ed. Malvern, PA: Lea & Febiger; 1994.

Grossman W, Baim DS. *Cardiac Catheterization, Angiography and Intervention,* 4th ed. Philadelphia: Lea & Febiger; 1991.

Heckerling PS, Wiener SL, Moseo VK, et al. Accuracy of precordial percussion in detecting cardiomegaly. *Am J Med* 1991;91:328–334.

Lembo NJ, et al. Bedside diagnosis of systolic murmurs. *N Engl J Med* 1988; 318:1572.

Miller G. *Invasive Investigation of the Heart.* Oxford: Blackwell Scientific Publications; 1989.

O'Neill TW, et al. Diagnostic value of the apex beat. *Lancet* 1989;1:410.

Schneiderman H. Do attending physicians really percuss? *Am J Med* 1991;91: 325–327.

Weyman AE. *Principles and Practice of Echocardiography,* 2nd ed. Malvern: Lea & Febiger; 1994.

VIII. Key Search Words

The following key words reflect the content of this chapter. They are provided to assist with an on-line search of computer databases, such as MEDLINE, if you wish to pursue the topic of this chapter further.

Apex cardiography
Arterial occlusive diseases
Arteries
Cardiac output
Cardiovascular diseases
Diagnosis, heart diseases
Heart/anatomy
Heart auscultation
Heart defects, congenital
Heart diseases
Heart murmurs
Heart neoplasms
Heart/physiology
Heart rate
Heart sounds
Heart valve disease
Jugular veins
Myocardial diseases
Myocardial infarction
Myocardial ischemia
Percussion
Pericardium
Peripheral vascular diseases
Physical examination, heart
Pulse
Vascular diseases
Vascular patency
Vascular resistance

9. GASTROINTESTINAL SYSTEM

Joseph C. Kolars

I. Glossary

Anorexia: loss of appetite.

Ascites: free fluid within the peritoneal cavity.

Borborygmi: loud peristaltic bowel sounds easily appreciated without a stethoscope.

Cachexia: profound malnutrition and weight loss.

Choledocholithiasis. Gallstones within the bile ducts.

Colic: acute, cramping abdominal pain occurring in waves or surges.

Constipation: infrequent bowel movements and difficult evacuation of stool because of firm consistency.

Diarrhea: passage of frequent stools (>200g/24 hours) of watery consistency.

Dysentery: bloody diarrhea.

Dyspepsia: upper abdominal discomfort, often related to meals and attributed to indigestion by patients.

Dysphagia: difficulty in swallowing.

Flatulence: passage of gas from the lower bowel.

Guarding: involuntary spasm of the abdominal muscles, frequently localized to an area of underlying pain and tenderness.

Hematemesis: vomiting of blood.

Hematochezia: passage of bright red blood per rectum (BRBPR).

Ileus: dilation and inhibition of motor activity of the intestine; distinguished pathophysiologically from mechanical obstruction in which an anatomic blockage of the intestinal lumen is present.

Jaundice: yellow coloration of the skin, mucous membranes, and sclera due to accumulation of bilirubin pigments in serum and tissues; also referred to as *icterus*.

Malabsorption: inadequate absorption of dietary nutrients from the gut lumen.

Melena: passage of jet-black tarry stool suggestive of bleeding from an upper gastrointestinal source.

Nausea: an unpleasant sensation of impending vomiting, frequently localized to the epigastrium.

Obstipation: failure to pass stool.

Odynophagia: pain with swallowing.

Preprandial and *postprandial*: before and after a meal.

Pyrosis: heartburn, typically attributed to gastroesophageal reflux.

Rebound: abbreviated term for rebound tenderness; abdominal discomfort on sudden withdrawal of the palpating hand.

Scaphoid: a thin, concave-shaped abdomen.

Steatorrhea: excessive fat in the stool (>6 g/24 hours).

Stomatitis: inflammation of the mucous membranes of the mouth.

Tenesmus: the sensation of the need to evacuate the bowels, but without result.

Tympanites: distention of the abdomen, due to presence of gas or air in the intestine or peritoneal cavity.

Water-brash: spontaneous appearance of a bland or salty-tasting fluid in the mouth, which is often associated with gastroesophageal reflux.

II. Techniques of Examination and Normal Findings.

Evaluation of the gastrointestinal system begins with a thorough history and physical examination. Each symptom should be pursued with regard to location, quality, radiation, severity, duration, timing (particularly with regard to meals or defecation), frequency, and palliative or aggravating factors.

A. History. When evaluating any disorder of the gastrointestinal tract, the following questions must be answered:
  1. Are fevers part of the symptom complex?
  2. Has the patient lost weight?
    a. Acute disorders rarely present with weight loss unexplained by dehydration.
  3. Any changes in dietary intake?
    a. Reasons for decreased intake must be defined (e.g., loss of appetite, nausea or pain with eating, poor dentition, limited access to food).
  4. Has the patient noticed a change in bowel habits?
  5. Are extraintestinal symptoms (particularly of the skin, joints, or central nervous system) present?
  6. What is the patient's pattern of alcohol intake?
  7. Is the patient taking medications that affect the gastrointestinal tract?
    a. Nonsteroidal anti-inflammatory drugs (NSAIDs) are a frequent cause of dyspepsia, peptic ulcer disease, and gastrointestinal bleeding.
    b. Prednisone may mask signs and symptoms of inflammation within the abdominal cavity.
    c. Antacids may cause diarrhea (magnesium-based) or constipation (aluminum-based).
    d. Iron tablets or bismuth-containing agents may cause dark stools that could be confused with melena (black, tarry stools caused by blood).
    e. Antibiotics often cause diarrhea and are a risk factor for pseudomembranous colitis.
B. General inspection
  1. Does the patient appear healthy?
  2. Does the patient appear adequately nourished?
    a. Loss of subcutaneous fat, temporal or interosseous muscle wasting, or changes in clothing/belt-size are suggestive of weight loss.
  3. Does the patient appear adequately hydrated?
    a. Increased skin turgor, dry mucous membranes, orthostatic changes in blood pressure or pulse are suggestive of dehydration.
  4. Does the skin appear to be of normal color and without lesions?
    a. Examine carefully for pallor, jaundice, spider angiomata, and excoriations.
  5. Is the patient's behavior during your interaction consistent with his or her symptoms?
    a. Facial expressions, body posturing that limits the pain, tachycardia, or diaphoresis with severe pain
    b. The interface between the gastrointestinal system and the patient's psyche is complex; check for signs of depression, agitation, exhaustion, hostility, fear.
C. Mouth. A brief inspection of the oral cavity is an important part of the gastrointestinal examination.
  1. Inspect the lips, oral mucosa, teeth, gingiva, tongue, and salivation.
  2. Oral ulcers, chelosis (angular stomatitis) should be excluded and distinguished from nonpathologic changes such as cracking of the lips due to exposure, mild gingivitis, or local irritation from poorly fitting dentures.
  3. Oral thrush, a yeast infection manifested by white plaques on an erythematous base must be distinguished from normal variants of papillae on the tongue.
D. Abdomen
  1. Examination process
    a. Position the patient supine with knees slightly raised and arms at the sides. The head should be resting comfortably on a pillow with the abdomen exposed from the costal margin to the symphysis pubis. The patient should be relaxed.

b. Sequence. Inspection, auscultation, percussion, palpation.

c. Topographic anatomy. Dividing the abdomen into topographic sections is a useful way to specify the location of physical signs and symptoms. Two methods are used: four quadrants (Fig. 9-1A), and nine regions (see Fig. 9-1B). The four-quadrant method is most commonly used, but other valuable terms arise from the nine-region method.

d. The inflammatory response, including pain, fevers, and tenderness, is frequently blunted in the elderly or in immunosuppressed patients.

2. Inspection

a. Skin. Observe the color and texture, noting any unusual lesions, striae, or surgical scars. The venous pattern should be barely perceptible.

b. General contour. Check for symmetry, localized bulging or prominence, and the position of the umbilicus in the midline, mid-distance between

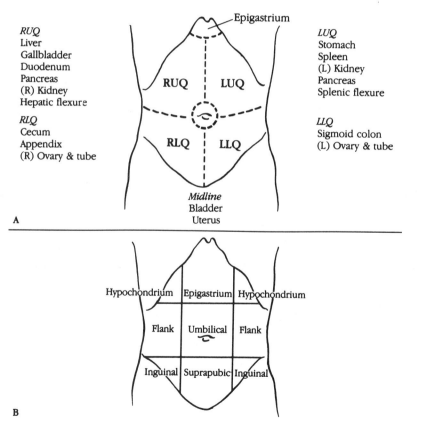

Fig. 9-1. Superficial topography of the abdomen. **(A)** Four-quadrant system. **(B)** Nine-region system.

the xyphoid process and symphysis pubis. Ask the patient to cough or bear down, and note whether this produces any pain or bulging suggestive of a hernia.

   c. Movements. Inspiration normally causes slight protrusion of the abdominal wall due to descent of the diaphragm. Look for visible peristaltic waves and vascular pulsations. Normal aortic pulsations may be evident in the epigastrium of thin persons.

3. Auscultation

   a. Auscultation should take place before palpation of the abdomen and distant in time from recent meals or defecation. Nasogastric tubes should be clamped during the period of auscultation.

   b. The frequency of bowel sounds is highly variable; however, absence of bowel sounds for over 2 minutes is usually abnormal. The localization of bowel sounds to specific quadrants of the abdomen is of relatively little importance. Exaggerated bowel sounds including borborygmi may be a normal finding in arymptomatic patients without other findings.

   c. Auscultation for vascular bruits should take place in the periumbilical region and each of the cardinal four quadrants of the abdomen.

4. Percussion and palpation. If right-handed, approach the examination from the patient's right side. Ask the patient to point with one finger to any areas of pain. The patterns of visceral innervation may limit the patient's ability to specifically localize the pain. Ask "either/or questions" to help the patient localize the pain to a region of greatest intensity (e.g., Is the pain more severe above or below the umbilicus? Is it more prominent on the right or left?). Once this region is identified, approach it last with the percussion and palpation components of your examination.

   a. Your goal is to determine the presence or absence of the following:

      (1) Tenderness (superficial or deep)

      (2) Organ enlargement

      (3) Abdominal mass

      (4) Spasm or rigidity of abdominal muscles

      (5) Ascites

      (6) Exaggerated tympanites

   b. Percussion. Watch carefully for evidence of tenderness. Tenderness to one-finger percussion is commonly seen with peritoneal inflammation. Exquisite tenderness to percussion that was not appreciated with stethoscope placement during auscultation may suggest an exaggerated pain response.

      (1) Percuss all four quadrants, noting degrees of resonance.

      (2) Delineate upper and lower borders of the liver, moving from regions of tympany to areas of dullness in the midclavicular line (although somewhat dependent on body habitus, normal values are generally considered to be ≤ 10 cm).

      (3) Outline Traube's space (gastric air bubble) in left upper quadrant. Splenic dullness may be identified lateral to this region near the left 10th rib, posterior to the midaxillary line.

      (4) The upper border of the urinary bladder may be detected in the suprapubic area in patients with bladder distention.

   c. Light palpation. The purpose is to elicit minor tenderness and guarding, again starting in regions that are farthest from localized areas of pain.

      (1) Rebound tenderness is identified when patients report greater pain with quick release of the hand from its point of maximum descent into the abdominal cavity. Rebound pain that is referred to the area initially identified by the patient as being most painful is suggestive of peritoneal inflammation. Use the flat of the hand, and avoid dragging the hand over the surface when changing positions because this may cause voluntary guarding.

      (2) Areas of focal tenderness should also be examined when the patient has tensed the abdominal wall (e.g., straight-leg raising or flexion of the neck and shoulders). Tenderness that is accentuated by this maneuver is suspicious for abdominal wall origin, whereas tenderness that is diminished suggests an origin within the abdominal cavity.

d. Deep palpation

    (1) Palpation of the liver is performed to assess its contour and texture but is unreliable alone for determining liver size. The patient's body habitus plays a major role in your ability to palpate the liver, even when abnormal. Many patients with a scaphoid abdomen, particularly patients with expanded lung volumes, have an easily palpable, normal liver.

        (a) While standing on the patient's right, place your right hand parallel with the rectus muscle in the right midclavicular line below the percussed border of dullness and press firmly inward (Fig. 9-2A). Ask the patient to take deep breaths. Release your pressure slightly at the height of inspiration, while moving your fingertips gently upward toward the costal margin.

        (b) Attempt to palpate a liver edge that moves with inspiration medially into the epigastrium. Make note of any tenderness,

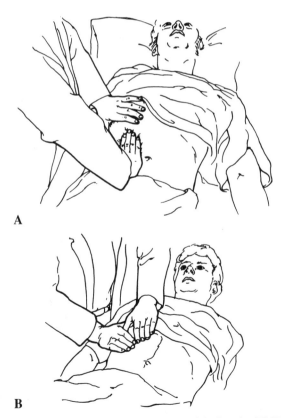

Fig. 9-2. Palpation of the liver. **(A)** Proper position of the hands. **(B)** Hooking.

nodularity, unusual firmness, or pulsations. The "hooking technique" (see Fig. 9-2B) is an alternative approach preferred by some examiners.

(2) Kidneys and spleen are not typically palpable in normal patients except in thin patients with a scaphoid abdomen (see Chapter 11). The spleen is most easily palpated with the patient rolled to the right side (Fig. 9-3).

(3) Masses should be identified as to their location, contour, size, tenderness, movement with diaphragmatic excursion, and relation to other identifiable abdominal organs.

E. The rectal examination is an essential component of the gastrointestinal examination.

1. Position the patient in the left lateral decubitus position with the knees flexed toward the chest. Alternatively, the patient may stand with flexion at the hips while resting elbows on the examining table.

2. Inspect the skin surrounding the anus for inflammation, excoriation, protruding hemorrhoids, or a perianal orifice suggestive of an anorectal fistula. Skin tags are remnants of previous external hemorrhoids. Skin tags in the posterior (or less commonly anterior) midline may be a "sentinel" tag indicative of an underlying anal fissure. Prolapsing mucosa (more common in women and the elderly) may be seen by asking the patient to bear down.

3. Perform a digital examination with a lubricated, gloved index finger while using the opposite hand to spread the patient's buttocks.

a. Insert the finger gently and gradually, allowing time for the patient to relax after insertion. Evaluate the sphincter tone. Spasm due to nervousness can sometimes be minimized by asking the patient to strain while placing the pad of the examining finger on top of the anus before insertion. A local anesthetic suppository may also be used to minimize discomfort.

b. Carefully palpate each wall for palpable masses (e.g., benign polyps, rectal cancer), strictures, and unusual tenderness. The prostate gland should be thoroughly evaluated (see Chapter 11). Internal hemorrhoids are rarely palpable unless thrombosed. A firm, seed-like nodule palpable at the dentate line (3 cm proximal to the anal orifice) is probably a hypertrophic anal papilla and of no clinical significance.

c. The stool should be examined for melena or bright red blood. If the patient has anemia or symptoms of possible gastrointestinal bleeding, the stool should be checked for occult blood (e.g., guaiac test).

III. Cardinal Symptoms and Abnormal Findings

A. Pain. The character, duration, and frequency of gastrointestinal pain are a function of the mechanism of production. The location and distribution of referred pain are related to anatomic site of origin (see Fig. 9-1A). Time of onset, and factors that aggravate or relieve discomfort, such as meals, defecation, or sleep may help in the identification of the underlying causes.

1. Major pain patterns

a. *Colic*—severe pain of relatively acute onset—is typically associated with obstruction of hollow viscera. Common considerations include choledocholithiasis, mechanical bowel obstruction, volvulus (twisting of the bowel on itself), and urolithiasis.

b. Appetite is often diminished *(anorexia)* in disorders of the gastrointestinal tract with a resulting decrease in food intake. Pain aggravated by eating may be associated with mesenteric ischemia, peptic ulcer disease, pancreatitis, and biliary tract disease. Pain relieved by eating may occur with peptic ulcer disease, particularly in patients with duodenal ulcers.

c. Progressive abdominal pain accompanied by a change in appetite and bowel habits is suggestive of acute inflammation of the alimentary canal such as that which occurs with the following:

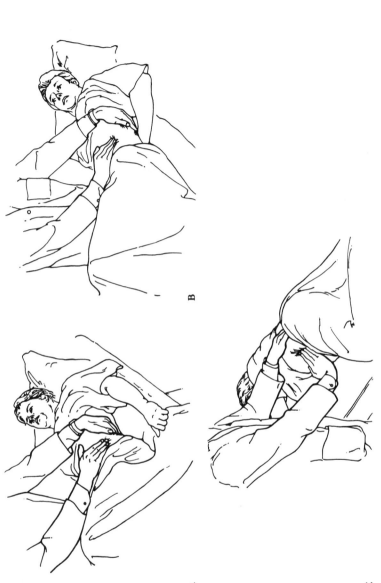

Fig. 9-3. Palpation of the spleen. **(A)** Position of examiner's hands. **(B)** Patient's hand under his back. **(C)** Patient rolled to right side.

(1) Appendicitis (periumbilical pain migrating to the right lower quadrant, decreased stools, nausea, fevers)

(2) Diverticulitis (left lower quadrant-suprapubic region; obstipation, fevers)

(3) Colitis (left lower quadrant pain, often with tenesmus, increased stool frequency, and blood)

d. Pain aggravated by defecation is suggestive of perianal disease (e.g., perianal fissure, abscess, thrombosed hemorrhoid).

(1) Inflammation of the distal small bowel (e.g., Crohn's disease) or colon is often associated with a predefecatory increase in lower quadrant pain.

(2) Pain relieved by defecation is most often suggestive of *irritable bowel syndrome,* a common intermittent problem that is also associated with abdominal bloating, altered bowel habits (loose stools alternating with constipation), and absence of weight loss, fevers, or gastrointestinal blood loss.

e. Pain with deep inspiration may occur with peritonitis or lesions contiguous with the capsule of the liver or spleen.

2. Major sites of localization with disease processes involving the following structures:

a. Esophagus: midline retrosternal pain with occasional radiation to the back at the level of the lesion. Odynophagia is suggestive of an esophageal inflammation of either an infectious etiology (*Candida* species, cytomegalovirus, herpes zoster) or a pill-induced stasis ulcer.

b. Gastric: epigastric; radiation occasionally to the back, particularly left subscapular.

c. Duodenum: epigastric; radiation occasionally to the back, particularly right subscapular.

d. Gallbladder: right upper quadrant or epigastric; radiation to right subscapular or mid-back.

e. Pancreas: epigastric; radiation to mid-back or left lumbar area; relieved with assumption of the fetal position.

f. Small intestine and colon: depending on the location, pain originating in the small intestine may be periumbilical in distribution. Sigmoid pain often localizes to the left lower quadrant with radiation to the sacral region. Rectal pain is localized deep within the pelvis and may be associated with tenesmus.

g. Appendix: periumbilical, migrating later to right lower quadrant.

h. Pain radiating from the abdominal cavity.

(1) Pain radiating straight from the abdomen to the back suggests involvement of the retroperitoneum such as occurs with pancreatitis, pancreatic cancer, duodenal ulcer, aortic aneurysm, and retroperitoneal tumors. Relief from this pain may be obtained with flexion of the knees toward the chest.

(2) Pain radiating from the abdomen to the back in a band-like circumferential pattern on the right side suggests biliary tract disease. Other considerations include pain of musculoskeletal origin or, when unilateral, herpes zoster before development of the classic dermatomal vesicular rash.

(3) Pain radiating from the epigastrium to the chest is suggestive of gastroesophageal reflux and may occur within 60 minutes of eating, when bending over, or when reclining (particularly at night).

(4) Pain radiating to the left subscapular region may be seen in patients with gastric ulcers or tumors.

(5) Pain radiating to the right subscapular region may be seen in patients with biliary tract disease (e.g., cholecystitis, cholangitis, choledocholithiasis).

B. Motor dysfunction

1. Dysphagia (difficulty swallowing) is an important symptom that mandates a structural evaluation with either an esophagram or esophagoscopy to exclude malignancy. Mechanical obstruction of the esophagus (e.g., carcinoma) will present with dysphagia that is more prominent with solids. Dysphagia with both liquids and solids is more suggestive of an esophageal dysmotility syndrome (e.g., achalasia, esophageal spasm).

2. Vomiting may result from structural lesions of the upper gastrointestinal tract, neuropathic disorders of the stomach (including metabolic disorders, sepsis, and other conditions), or disorders within the central nervous system. Diagnostic approaches are guided by the presence of other signs and symptoms. When seen in relative isolation, considerations include the following:

    a. Pregnancy must always be considered in women of childbearing age.

    b. Viral gastroenteritis or "food poisoning" rarely lasts more than 2 to 4 days and may be accompanied by dehydration.

    c. Gastroparesis (delayed gastric emptying) is a subacute or chronic disorder characterized by anorexia, early satiety, or postprandial vomiting, which may be seen in patients with autonomic neuropathy such as diabetes mellitus or uremia.

    d. Hematemesis (blood in the vomitus) may be manifested as contents that are bright red in color or the texture of coffee grounds. Common considerations include peptic ulcer disease, hemorrhagic or erosive gastritis, or gastric blood from a more proximal source (e.g., esophageal varices, epistaxis).

    e. Structural disorders such as peptic ulcer disease, pancreatic malignancy, or dysmotility disorders affecting other regions of the alimentary canal most often are associated with weight loss.

    f. Projectile vomiting unrelated to meals and without a significant prodrome of nausea raise the possibility of an intracranial lesion.

3. Belching is almost always due to subconscious swallowing of air and is rarely a symptom of disease.

4. Altered bowel function. Bowel function varies greatly, and changes from one's baseline pattern are more significant than any well-established pattern. Normal frequency ranges from three movements per day to three movements per week. Answers to the following questions will guide your approach to the patient with altered bowel habits:

    a. How longstanding are the symptoms?

        (1) Diarrhea or "loose stools" of less than 7 to 10 days duration are often due to a self-limited bacterial or viral infection, and diagnostic or therapeutic interventions are rarely required. Patients with underlying illness, dehydration, fevers, gastrointestinal blood loss, a history of recent travel or antibiotic use often require more aggressive intervention. Adult patients, particularly over the age of 40, who present with a distinct decrease in stool frequency without explanation should undergo diagnostic imaging of the distal bowel to exclude a colonic malignancy.

        (2) Diarrhea of more than 2 weeks' duration requires further consideration. Weight loss further supports a more longstanding process. Possibilities include the following:

            (a) Maldigestion, the absence of intraluminal factors necessary for digestion and food assimilation as classically occurs in patients with chronic pancreatitis, gastric acid hypersecretion, and severe impairment of bile flow (i.e., cholestasis). Steatorrhea is a common finding in significant maldigestion or malabsorption.

            (b) Malabsorption, the failure of the small bowel mucosa to facilitate absorption of digested nutrients from the lumen of the alimentary canal as classically occurs in patients with celiac sprue, small bowel bacterial overgrowth, and short-gut syndrome. Commonly overlooked possibilities are diarrhea resulting from the malabsorption of selective dietary components such as lactose, sorbitol, or magnesium-containing antacids.

(c) Persistent infections (e.g., *Entamoeba histolytica,* giardiasis, *Clostridium difficile,* HIV enteropathy, bacterial overgrowth).

(d) Inflammation due to inflammatory bowel disease (Crohn's disease and ulcerative colitis).

(e) Dumping syndrome may occur in patients with a previous partial gastrectomy and vagotomy for management of peptic ulcer disease. Symptoms usually present within 30 minutes of eating and are attributed to the rapid transfer of ingested food into the small bowel. Abdominal pain, nausea, or diarrhea are accompanied by weakness, pallor, diaphoresis, or tachycardia.

(3) Progressive constipation or obstipation mandates diagnostic imaging of the colon to exclude adenocarcinoma, but it may be due to a slowing of gut motility with aging, medications, or metabolic disorders (e.g., hypothyroidism). Other possibilities are colonic narrowing as seen with chronic diverticulitis or strictures secondary to ischemia or previous radiation therapy.

(4) Acholic stools appear white or gray-colored and suggest the recent onset of severe impairment of bile flow into the gut lumen, which may occur with bile duct obstruction (e.g., stone or tumor) or acute hepatitis.

b. Is there blood in the stool?
   (1) Melena is suggestive of an upper gastrointestinal source of bleeding.
   (2) Hematochezia (maroon-colored stools) suggest a lower source of gastrointestinal bleeding unless a large volume of blood from an upper gastrointestinal source stimulates rapid transit.
   (3) Common infections resulting in loss of mucosal integrity and bleeding include those caused by *Campylobacter, Salmonella, Shigella, Entamoeba* species, and selected strains of *Eschirichia coli.*

c. Is the blood uniformly distributed?
   (1) Blood is a cathartic and stimulates evacuation of the more distant bowel, with subsequent mixing of stool and blood.
   (2) Streaking of formed stool with blood is suggestive of a distal (i.e., anal or rectal) lesion such as a neoplasm or perianal disease (which may be associated predominantly with blood on the tissue paper with wiping). Hemorrhoid bleeding is typically painless, whereas bleeding from a perianal fissure is associated with a burning perianal pain at the time of defecation.

d. Can the anatomic site be localized?
   (1) High-volume, watery stools with relatively little pain suggest a source in the small intestine.
   (2) Frequent, small stools with tenesmus suggest a distal colonic site.

C. Abnormal findings detected on general inspection
   1. Skin
      a. Pallor may indicate chronic or acute gastrointestinal blood loss.
      b. Jaundice indicates hepatobiliary disease. Excoriations (or complaints of pruritus) may occur in patients with cholestasis (impaired bile flow) but must be differentiated from dry skin. Xanthomas suggest hyperlipidemia, which is common in longstanding cholestatic disorders such as primary biliary cirrhosis.
      c. Bronze pigmentation may reflect hemachromatosis.
      d. Erythema nodosum, tender red nodules seen most commonly on extensor surfaces, may reflect ulcerative colitis or sarcoidosis.
      e. Flushing raises the possibility of carcinoid syndrome.
      f. Generalized edema may be caused by malabsorption or a manifestation of low-albumin states in patients with chronic liver disease.

g. Spider angiomata and palmar erythema (in addition to gynecomastia and testicular atrophy) are suggestive of chronic liver disease.

h. Ecchymosis suggests abnormal clotting in patients with a prolonged prothrombin time (PT), as occurs with chronic liver disease or impaired vitamin K deficiency due to cholestasis or malabsorption.

i. Nail changes worth noting include koilonychia (spooning) due to chronic iron deficiency, Muerke's nails (paired, parallel white lines) due to hypoalbuminemia, and clubbing seen with malabsorption, inflammatory bowel disease, or cirrhosis.

2. Halitosis may arise from chronic gastroesophageal disease, particularly neoplasms. Fetor hepaticus is a characteristic strong odor associated with severe liver failure. An acid odor may be caused by peptic disease of the stomach and duodenum.

3. Glossitis and stomatitis may accompany deficiency states caused by chronic gastrointestinal disorders such as sprue, with associated malabsorption and depleted body stores of iron, vitamin B_{12}, folic acid, niacin (B_3), thiamine (B_1), and riboflavin (B_2).

D. Abnormal findings detected during examination of the abdomen

1. Inspection.

a. Veins.

(1) Dilated, tortuous superficial abdominal veins radiating from the umbilicus (i.e., caput medusae) are manifestations of portal hypertension, likely due to cirrhosis.

(2) Reversal of flow in the lower abdomen indicates obstruction of the inferior vena cava and reversal of flow in the upper abdomen suggests obstruction of the superior vena cava. (The direction of blood flow is normally away from the umbilicus.)

b. Shape.

(1) A scaphoid abdomen typically accompanies *cachexia* (malnutrition and weight loss).

(2) A distended or protuberant abdomen is usually due to one of the five Fs; fat, flatus, fluid *(ascites)*, fetus, or fatal tumors.

(3) An obese abdomen is worth noting in that pathology within the abdomen may be easily masked.

c. Movement.

(1) Peristaltic waves passing across the abdomen may be seen in intestinal obstruction.

(2) A decrease in abdominal respiratory movements suggests intraperitoneal fluid or acute pain, such as with peritonitis.

d. Ecchymosis in the periumbilical region (Cullen's sign) or flank (Turner's sign) is suggestive of retroperitoneal bleeding and is seen classically (although rarely) in hemorrhagic pancreatitis.

e. Displacement of the umbilicus suggests a mass effect in the opposite direction.

2. Auscultation. Distinguishing abnormal from normal peristaltic sounds requires experience.

a. Absent bowel sounds over a period of at least 2 minutes is suggestive of an ileus or mechanical obstruction. The latter may be accompanied by periodic high-pitched rushing bowel sounds (and cramping pain) suggestive of fluid moving under pressure through a region of partial obstruction. This is a classic (but relatively rare) finding in the right lower quadrant in patients with Crohn's disease of the terminal ileum.

b. In outlet obstruction of the stomach, a succussion splash may be elicited by placing the stethoscope diaphragm over the epigastrium and shaking the patient vigorously from side to side. This splash can also be heard in a normal person who has ingested a large amount of fluid.

c. Cruveilhier-Baumgarten murmur is a venous hum heard in the periumbilical region or in the right upper quadrant caused by the increased collateral blood flow between the portal and systemic venous system that occurs in portal hypertension.

d. Bruits may be heard over the liver in approximately 10% of patients with hepatic malignancies. Vascular bruits are discussed in Chapter 8 and should be distinguished from heart murmurs that are referred into the abdominal cavity.

e. Rubs may be heard over the liver or spleen in patients with tumors, infections, or infarction that involves the capsule.

3. Percussion and palpation

a. Percussion is most useful in distinguishing the cause of a distended or protuberant abdomen.

(1) Bulging flanks with a circumferential region of tympany around the umbilicus that shifts when the patient assumes a decubitus position are suggestive of ascites. Alternative examinations for ascites include the fluid wave (Fig. 9-4), which requires two examiners.

(2) A protuberant abdomen that is tympanitic in most regions is distended with air, whereas an abdomen that is only sparsely tympanitic in the absence of other pathologic signs is obese.

b. Areas of tenderness can be localized by light palpation without causing undue discomfort. To determine whether the cause of pain arises from outside the abdomen (parietal tenderness), have the supine patient contract the abdominal muscles by raising the head or feet. If tenderness on light palpation persists or a mass remains palpable, the cause is more likely to originate within the abdominal wall.

(1) Before beginning active palpation, ask the patient to cough. If peritoneal inflammation is present, coughing may elicit a sharp focus of pain that may help localize the disease process. This area should be palpated last.

(2) Murphy's sign is a sharp increase in tenderness with a sudden arrest in respiratory effort when the patient is asked to take a deep inspiration while the examiner is palpating a region just inferior to the right costal margin between the midclavicular line and the epigastrium. This finding is created when a distended, inflamed

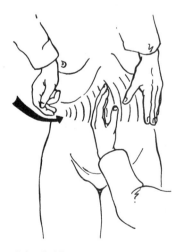

Fig. 9-4. Demonstration of the fluid wave.

gallbladder, as typically found in acute cholecystitis, descends against the examiner's fingers.

(3) McBurney's point is 5 cm from the anterior spinous process of the iliac crest just below a line joining the umbilicus and the anterior superior iliac spine and is a focal point of tenderness in patients with acute appendicitis.

(4) Special maneuvers.

(a) Iliopsoas test involves flexion of the leg at the hip with knee extended observing for pelvic or lower abdominal pain if a focus of inflammation is contiguous with the laterally placed iliopsoas muscle.

(b) Obturator test involves internal/external rotation of the leg flexed at the knee observing for pelvic or lower abdominal pain if a focus of inflammation is contiguous with the medially placed obturator muscle.

c. Localize and describe palpable masses in terms of consistency and contour. Palpable normal structures in many persons include the liver edge, portions of the large bowel filled with stool, the pulsating aorta and iliac arteries, a distended urinary bladder, and the pregnant uterus.

(1) Courvoisier's observation was that of an enlarged, palpable gallbladder in the presence of obstructive jaundice (and often in the absence of pain) and is suggestive of obstructive malignancy of the distal biliary tract, the most common of which is adenocarcinoma of the head of the pancreas.

(2) Ballottement is a technique used to palpate the liver in the presence of ascites. The palpating fingers are quickly thrust into the left upper quadrant of the abdomen and held briefly in place. A mobile solid organ such as the liver will rebound against the fingers; this can be helpful to the examiner who is evaluating the size and consistency of the liver.

(3) A palpable spleen is pathologic in >90% of cases and should first result in an examination for chronic liver disease with portal hypertension or a hematologic malignancy. Palpation of the splenic notch along the medial aspect of the proximal spleen and movement with diaphragmatic excursion help to confirm the identity of this organ in the left upper quadrant.

(4) Hepatic enlargement should be characterized by noting the palpable characteristics below the right costal margin. A hard, somewhat irregular edge is typically seen in cirrhosis (although a cirrhotic liver is often not palpable). A firm nodule or irregular, hard liver suggests the presence of malignancy. Acute distention of the hepatic capsule (as in acute hepatitis, congestion) is tender to palpation.

d. Perianal fissures outside the midline raise the possibility of Crohn's disease or trauma.

IV. Common Clinical Disorders

A. Gastroesophageal reflux disease

1. Gastroesophageal reflux is a common symptom involving reflux of gastric contents into the esophagus. The symptoms are most frequently characterized as pyrosis (heartburn) that occurs when reclining (e.g., in bed at night), when bending over, or after a meal, and occasionally water rash.

2. Refraining from agents that promote reflux such as smoking, ethanol, caffeine, chocolate, and peppermint often leads to relief of symptoms. Reducing meal size, remaining upright for at least 3 hours after a meal, and sleeping with the head of the bed elevated 6 inches will also improve symptoms. An empiric trial of acid reduction therapy with an H_2-blocker (e.g., ranitidine) or omeprazole with improvement in symptoms is further suggestive evidence of gastroesophageal reflux.

3. Refractory symptoms, or more advanced symptoms (e.g., aspiration, dysphagia, gastrointestinal bleeding), are indications for evaluation with esophagogastroduodenoscopy (EGD). Atypical symptoms or symptoms that fail to respond to treatment are indications for evaluation with pH monitoring.

B. Esophageal cancer. Patients with esophageal cancer most frequently present with recent onset of dysphagia associated more with solids than liquids. Patients may also report retrosternal pain, weight loss, or early satiety. A history of chronic ethanol ingestion or smoking is a recognized predisposing factor, as is Barrett's epithelium of the distal esophagus, which is associated with gastroesophageal reflux disease. Evaluation should be directed at imaging of the esophagus, preferably with EGD so that biopsies can be obtained or therapeutic dilation pursued, if indicated. Further staging of the malignancy is performed with a thoracic computed tomography (CT) scan.

C. Peptic ulcer disease

1. Peptic ulcer disease is suspected in patients who present with epigastric burning pain that is most typically relieved by food or antacids (as in duodenal ulcer disease) but may be aggravated with eating.

2. Most ulcers are due either to chronic infection of the gastric mucosa with *Helicobacter pylori* or as a result of injury from non-steroidal anti-inflammatory drug (NSAID) use. Gastric ulcers, particularly when solitary or outside of the antrum, may be due to malignancy and as such must be biopsied and subsequent healing confirmed.

3. Unfortunately, the components of the history or physical examination are unreliable in distinguishing peptic ulcer disease from nonulcer dyspepsia. A common approach to uncomplicated conditions is to discontinue NSAIDs, ask the patient to refrain from smoking, and pursue an empiric trial of acid reduction therapy with either a H_2-blocker (e.g., ranitidine) or omeprazole.

4. Patients with refractory symptoms or a presentation complicated by bleeding, recurrent vomiting, or weight loss should undergo structural imaging with either EGD, which allows biopsies to be taken, or an upper gastrointestinal barium series. Patients with ulcers and *Helicobacter pylori* infection documented by biopsy, serology, or a urease test should undergo a course of antibiotics to eradicate the infection, which will reduce the recurrence rate of peptic ulcer disease.

D. Inflammatory bowel disease

1. Idiopathic inflammatory bowel disease can be attributed to either ulcerative colitis (UC) or Crohn's disease (CD) in over 90% of cases.

2. Patients with UC typically present with a recent onset of dysentery (bloody diarrhea) and abdominal pain but may also report fevers and weight loss. The diagnosis is based on the clinical presentation with a consistent colonoscopy documenting inflammation that extends proximally in a confluent pattern from the anus. Biopsies of the colonic mucosa reveal cryptitis and often crypt abscesses. The inflammatory process spares the small intestine and proximal gastrointestinal tract.

3. Patients with CD present with more insidious symptoms of diarrhea, abdominal pain, and weight loss. Wasting, a palpable right lower quadrant mass or visible perianal inflammation (e.g., fissures, fistulas, abscesses) may be noted on physical examination.

   a. The inflammatory process may involve any region of the alimentary canal but most frequently is focused in the terminal ileum.

   b. Imaging studies such as colonoscopy or a small bowel follow-through illustrate patchy disease (areas of inflammation with intervening normal-appearing mucosa) with biopsies demonstrating crypt inflammation and, on occasion, granulomas.

   c. The inflammation of CD is transmural (in contrast to that of UD), and patients may develop strictures, fistulas, and abscesses anywhere along the alimentary canal.

   d. An abdominal CT scan is often used to evaluate for abscess formation within the peritoneal cavity.
   4. In both UC and CD, gastrointestinal infections must be excluded with stool samples sent for *Clostridium difficile*, ova and parasite examination, and culture. Extraintestinal manifestations involving the joints, skin, eyes, liver, and kidneys may be seen with both disorders.
E. Irritable bowel syndrome
   1. Irritable bowel syndrome is a chronic, intermittent disorder characterized by a stool pattern that alternates between loose stools (often with mucus) and constipation, by abdominal pain, and by abdominal bloating relieved by defecation. As this is a diagnosis of exclusion (currently, no clinical tests are available that confirm the clinical diagnosis), a systematic approach to altered bowel function will determine how aggressive the diagnostic approach should be.
   2. Nocturnal symptoms, weight loss, gastrointestinal blood loss, or fevers are not consistent with a diagnosis of irritable bowel syndrome and warrant further studies.
F. Diverticulitis
   1. Diverticulitis should be suspected in patients who present with lower abdominal pain (particularly in the left lower quadrant), fever, and tenderness to palpation with occasional palpation of a mass. Diarrhea or significant gastrointestinal bleeding is uncommon. Patients who appear toxic should have blood cultures, urinalysis, and plain abdominal x-ray films taken to evaluate for an obstruction or perforation.
   2. Cautious flexible sigmoidoscopy is often performed to exclude the possibility of colitis or ischemia. Broad-spectrum antibiotics should be initiated and abdominal CT studies obtained to exclude the presence of a significant abscess in patients who fail to respond rapidly to hydration and antibiotics.
G. Colonic cancer
   1. Patients with colon cancer may present with a change in bowel habits, gastrointestinal bleeding, occult anemia, unexplained weight loss, or, on occasion, abdominal pain. Two thirds of colonic malignancies are found in the left colon between the anus and the splenic flexure.
   2. The American Cancer Society recommends a screening flexible sigmoidoscopy every 3 to 5 years along with annual screening for fecal occult blood and an annual digital examination at age 50 and older. Most patients who present with colon cancer have not been screened adequately for colonic neoplasms.
   3. Symptomatic patients age 50 or older (or asymptomatic younger patients with affected first-degree relatives) should undergo imaging of the entire colon. Colonoscopy has the greatest predictive accuracy and provides an opportunity to biopsy and remove lesions but is also more expensive than barium contrast radiography.
H. Acute gastrointestinal bleeding
   1. Acute bleeding into the gastrointestinal tract is typically discharged either by vomiting or passage of red, maroon, or melenic stool from the rectum. The physician must stabilize the patient using intravenous fluids and blood product replacement while assessing the site and severity of the bleeding.
   2. Hematemesis is typically indicative of a bleeding source proximal to the ligament of Treitz (as in peptic ulcer disease, erosive gastritis or duodenitis, esophageal varices, Mallory-Weiss mucosal tears at the esophagogastric junction). EGD should be performed promptly both to identify the bleeding site and to arrest selected bleeding vessels with cautery or injection therapy.
   3. Passage of melena is usually indicative of an upper gastrointestinal bleeding source, and a nasogastric tube should be placed to aspirate gastric (and ideally duodenal) contents to inspect visually for gross blood. These patients should first be studied with EGD, and subse-

quently with colonoscopy if the EGD is normal, to evaluate potential bleeding sites.

4. Passage of hematochezia is suggestive of a lower gastrointestinal bleeding site (as in angiodysplasia, colitis, diverticular bleeding, neoplasm, or a perianal source such as hemorrhoids or an anal fissure). Brisk bleeding from an upper gastrointestinal source or a site within the small intestine (as in Meckel's diverticulum) may also occur with hematochezia. Colonoscopy is initially performed, often in unprepped patients, to evaluate the integrity of the colonic mucosa and exclude the presence of a colitis. Further evaluation with an oral purgative may take place later if the patient is stable.

5. Recurrent bleeding in patients with both a negative EGD and colonoscopy is typically pursued with angiography with prior identification of potential sites with a tagged red blood cell (RBC) study.

I. Pancreatitis

1. Acute pancreatitis typically presents with epigastric pain radiating to the back that is often accompanied by nausea and vomiting. The patient may report some symptomatic relief when lying with legs flexed toward the chest (fetal position). Severe cases may present with fevers, peritonitis, or evidence of retroperitoneal bleeding (Turner's or Cullen's sign).

2. Potential risk factors include a history of excessive ethanol use, gallstones, trauma, or hyperlipidemia.

3. An elevated serum amylase and lipase support the diagnosis, and ultrasonography should be an early consideration to exclude gallstones or dilation of the common bile duct, which might warrant a procedure (e.g., ERCP with sphincterotomy) to relieve an anticipated stone at the sphincter of Oddi.

J. Pancreatic cancer. Pancreatic cancer may present either with painless jaundice or epigastric pain with weight loss. A pancreatic mass or distended gallbladder may be palpable. An abdominal CT is usually most useful for defining the presence and extent of the malignancy.

K. Cholecystitis

1. Acute cholecystitis is most commonly caused by obstruction of the cystic duct either with a stone or inflammation. Patients report colicky right upper quadrant pain with radiation to the flanks and occasionally the right shoulder.

2. On physical examination, fevers are commonly present with tenderness in the right upper quadrant, particularly below the right costal margin just medial to the midclavicular line during full inspiration (Murphy's sign). A palpable gallbladder or signs of peritoneal inflammation may also be present.

3. An elevated white blood cell count with abnormal liver chemistries, particularly elevation of alkaline phosphatase, is often noted. A right upper quadrant ultrasound should be obtained to evaluate for stones within the gallbladder and edema or fluid around it. Dilation of the common bile duct is suggestive of choledocholithiasis with cholangitis if the transaminases are significantly elevated.

4. A clinical diagnosis of acute cholecystitis may also be confirmed with a HIDA (hepato-iminodiacetic acid) scan documenting normal uptake and excretion of the isotope into the duodenum without gallbladder pooling.

L. Viral hepatitis

1. Hepatitis implies inflammation of the liver that may occur with toxins (e.g., ethanol, acetaminophen, isoniazid), infections (e.g., hepatitis A, B, C, D, or E viruses), or certain metabolic conditions including steatohepatitis, Wilson's disease, hemachromatosis, and autoimmune hepatitis.

2. Acutely, patients may present with fevers, nausea, and jaundice. Right upper pain or tenderness occurs with distention of the hepatic capsule. The term *fulminant hepatic failure* is reserved for patients who progress from a normal functioning liver to marked hepatocyte destruction with

abnormal synthetic function (prolonged PT) and hepatic encephalopathy in less than 8 weeks.

3. Diagnostically, serology directed at the differential diagnosis cited above is most helpful, and liver biopsy is occasionally helpful in further characterizing the disease process.

M. Chronic liver disease

1. Chronic liver disease is a sequela of ongoing liver inflammation over a course of at least 6 months. Chronic liver disease can be characterized at its extreme with *cirrhosis,* a histologic term referring to hepatic architecture that is replaced with bridging fibrosis and regenerative nodules.

2. Patients may present with symptoms of acute hepatitis, weakness, encephalopathy, or the clinical sequelae of portal hypertension (as in ascites and gastrointestinal bleeding). On physical examination, encephalopathy, asterixis, spider telangiectasias, palmar erythema, gynecomastia, muscle wasting, or testicular atrophy may be present.

3. Patients with cirrhosis are also at risk for the development of a *hepatoma,* which causes abdominal pain or an intraperitoneal hemorrhage. The diagnosis is best directed at the cause of the underlying liver disease.

V. Available Technology

A. *Esophagogastroduodenoscopy* (EGD). This procedure involves passage of a flexible fiberoptic tube through the patient's mouth to the level of the duodenum while under intravenous sedation for purposes of visualizing the mucosal lining of the esophagus, stomach, and duodenum. Biopsy forceps and a variety of therapeutic instruments can be passed through channels within the scope at the time of the procedure. Typical indications for EGD include the following:

1. Evaluation of upper gastrointestinal bleeding and possible therapeutic endoscopic intervention (e.g., hemostasis using injection therapies or cautery)

2. Evaluation of abdominal pain or recurrent vomiting in consideration of possible peptic ulcer disease

3. Evaluation of dysphagia to exclude esophageal malignancy or stricture

B. *Anoscopy.* In patients with pain, bleeding, or palpable abnormalities suggestive of perianal disease on digital rectal examination, anoscopy is performed by passing a metal or plastic anoscope with obturator in place proximal to the dentate line with subsequent removal of the obturator and visualization of the mucosa as the instrument is slowly withdrawn. Hemorrhoids, fissures, perianal lesions, inflamed mucosa, and occasionally fistula openings may be identified. Anoscopy is easily performed but often deferred in favor of more thorough visualization of the proximal bowel using sigmoidoscopy or colonoscopy.

C. *Sigmoidoscopy.* With the patient in the left lateral decubitus position following evacuant enemas, a flexible fiberoptic tube is passed through the anus into the left colon for purposes of visualizing the mucosal lining of the rectum, sigmoid, and descending colon. Typical indications for sigmoidoscopy include the following:

1. Screening for colonic neoplasia in normal patients over the age of 50 and earlier in selected high-risk groups

2. Evaluation of diarrhea or hematochezia in consideration of inflammatory colitis, infectious diarrhea, or ischemia

3. In conjunction with an air-contrast barium enema in evaluation of a positive fecal occult blood test (i.e., an alternative to colonoscopy in asymptomatic patients under the age of 55)

D. *Colonoscopy.* After bowel preparation with an oral purgative regimen, the patient is placed in the left lateral position and sedated with one of several intravenous regimens (most containing a benzodiazepine and an opiate analgesic). A flexible fiberoptic tube is passed via the anus through the colonic lumen to the level of the cecum with cannulation of the terminal ileum if ileitis is suspected, as in CD. Typical indications for colonoscopy include the following:

1. Evaluation for colonic neoplasia (with possible biopsy and removal) in patients with the following
   a. A positive test for fecal occult blood
   b. Lower gastrointestinal bleeding
   c. A change of bowel habits suggestive of mechanical obstruction
   d. Unexplained iron deficiency anemia
   e. Two or more first-degree relatives with a history of colonic adenocarcinoma (particularly with onset at age <50)
2. Surveillance for neoplasia in patients with a previous history of colonic adenomas or colonic adenocarcinoma

E. *Endoscopic retrograde cholangiopancreatography* (ERCP). Under intravenous sedation, a specialized side-viewing fiberoptic tube is passed through the mouth to the level of the mid-duodenum for purposes of visualizing the ampulla of Vater. Once visualized, a cannula is placed into the common bile duct or pancreatic duct with subsequent infusion of radiocontrast dye. Fluoroscopy and roentgenograms are used to evaluate the duct lumens for contour, patency, and possible filling defects such as stones. The duct orifice at the ampulla can be enlarged (sphincterotomy) to facilitate drainage (often with stents) or removal of stones. Typical indications for ERCP include the following:

1. Pancreatitis with choledocholithiasis (i.e., biliary pancreatitis) as a suspected cause
2. Cholangitis with a clinical suspicion of choledocholithiasis or sclerosing cholangitis
3. Symptomatic cholelithiasis and possible choledocholithiasis in a patient scheduled for laparoscopic cholecystectomy
4. Painless jaundice in a patient with possible malignant biliary obstruction and inconclusive CT scans or ultrasonography

F. *Ultrasonography*

1. Real-time ultrasonography is used to evaluate the following:
   a. Liver for masses or cysts
   b. Biliary system for cholelithiasis, pericholic fluid or wall thickening, or common bile duct dilation
   c. Peritoneal cavity for free fluid
   d. Pancreas, when not obscured by overlying bowel gas, for lesions or inflammation
   e. Kidneys for masses or inflammation, the major arteries for aneurysms, the appendix for acute appendicitis, and the pelvic structures
2. Doppler ultrasonography can be used to evaluate the vascular patency and directional flow through the portal vein, hepatic vein, and hepatic artery.
3. Endoscopic ultrasonography is performed with a specialized ultrasound probe on an endoscope. It is used most commonly to evaluate potential pancreatic lesions, chronic pancreatitis, and submucosal lesions of the proximal gastrointestinal tract.

G. Radiographic techniques

1. *Abdominal films* are commonly used to evaluate patients who present with abdominal pain, altered gastrointestinal motility, or abdominal distention. A complete set consists of a supine view (also called a "flat plate") and an upright view, which is used to evaluate the distribution of air throughout the gut and exclude the presence of free air. Soft tissue densities, bony structures, and abnormal patterns of calcification (e.g., chronic calcific pancreatitis) should also be reviewed.
2. Upper gastrointestinal radiography with small-bowel follow-through is performed by having the patient swallow radiocontrast dye (e.g., barium) with serial x-ray films obtained of the lower esophagus, stomach, and small bowel. A barium swallow should be requested if views of the hy-

popharynx or proximal esophagus are required. The indications for an upper gastrointestinal test are similar to those for an EGD. The advantage is that this test is less expensive and does not require intravenous sedation. In contrast to the EGD, it is less sensitive for fine mucosal detail and does not permit the examiner to obtain concomitant biopsies or perform therapeutic maneuvers. The small bowel follow-through is one of the best ways to examine the mucosa of the small intestine. It is ordered most commonly to examine the terminal ileum for CD or to evaluate patients with unexplained weight loss or gastrointestinal bleeding after examination of the stomach and colon for infiltrative disease (as in lymphoma, carcinoid) or ulcerations.

3. *Barium enema radiographic series* is performed after the colon has been evacuated by instilling barium (ideally with air contrast) to the level of the terminal ileum to examine for masses, strictures, or areas of relatively high-grade inflammation. Compared with colonoscopy, this examination is less expensive but often is of lower sensitivity and specificity.

4. *Abdominal CT scanning* is best used to study the contents of the abdomen for masses (particularly in the liver, pancreas, and retroperitoneum), abscess formation, abnormal lymph nodes, ascitic fluid, and to a lesser extent the wall of the alimentary canal. It is almost always imperative that patients ingest a dye (as well as a contrast enema) before this study to allow proper delineation of structures. The mucosa of the alimentary canal is poorly evaluated, if at all, with this imaging technique.

5. *Magnetic resonance imaging* (MRI) of the abdomen is rarely indicated, in part due to artifacts created by normal gut motility and the absence of an adequate bowel contrast agent. MRI of the liver is occasionally performed to evaluate the vascularity of hepatic masses, the hepatic vasculature, and iron deposition in hemachromatosis.

6. *Angiography* of the visceral vasculature is performed to evaluate tumor resectability, to diagnose vascular disease (e.g., vasculitis, mesenteric occlusive disease), or to evaluate the patency and direction of blood flow in the liver in consideration of specific vascular disorders (e.g., Budd-Chiari disease) or in evaluation of patients for potential liver transplantation. Bleeding into the gastrointestinal tract can be identified with active hemorrhage of at least 0.5 mL/min at the time of the procedure.

H. Nuclear medicine studies

1. The *liver-spleen scan,* a measure of hepatic uptake of radiolabeled colloid that provides information on liver size as well as mass defects, has largely been replaced by the abdominal CT. A decrease in hepatic isotope uptake relative to the spleen is suggestive of hepatic dysfunction (e.g., cirrhosis).

2. The *HIDA scan* is based on the extraction by hepatocytes of technetium 99m-dimethylphenylcaramylmethyl-iminodiacetic acid (HIDA) from the blood and excretion into the bile. This study is most useful for the detection of acute cholecystitis, which is detected by the absence of isotope pooling within the gallbladder lumen. The accuracy of this study is compromised in patients with a serum bilirubin >7 mg/dL.

3. The *tagged RBC bleeding scan* depends on the detection of technetium 99m-labeled RBC or technetium 99m sulfur colloid in the extravascular gut lumen. A bleeding source of as little as 0.1 mL/min can be detected. Patients with relatively acute gastrointestinal blood loss and negative endoscopic studies of the upper gastrointestinal tract and colon are the most common candidates for this study. Angiography or surgery can be directed at the region of ongoing blood loss as identified by this study.

4. *Gastric emptying studies* are performed by administering solid food containing a radioactive tracer (technetium 99m) to a fasting patient who complains of early satiety or recurrent vomiting in the absence of other disease processes such as anatomic obstruction. The solid-phase, half-emptying time is calculated and compared with a normal population for the identical meal. Prolonged emptying times are indicative of gastroparesis.

I. *Esophageal pH monitoring* is used to detect gastroesophageal reflux disease in patients with atypical chest pain (or recurrent pulmonary disease that may be attributed to aspiration) that is otherwise not explained by structural studies of the esophagus. Patients have a thin nasogastric tube placed with the pH recording tip positioned in the distal esophagus. This probe remains in place, usually for 24 hours, and is connected to a recorder. The patient is encouraged to continue with usual activities and record in a diary the timing of symptoms. The recording is later evaluated for the intervals of time during which the pH is <4, as well as the activities and symptoms of the patient at that time.

J. *Esophageal manometry* is performed by placing through the mouth a tube with multiple probes that record pressures within the esophagus. This test is reserved for patients with dysphagia and no evidence of anatomic obstructions as occurs with dysmotility syndromes. Although most abnormal motility in the esophagus is attributed to acid reflux, disorders such as achalasia (failure of the lower esophageal sphincter to relax with absence of peristaltic waves in the body of the esophagus) are best made using manometry.

K. *Liver chemistries*
   1. Serum transaminases consisting of aspartate transaminase (AST) and alanine transaminase (ALT) are *hepatocellular parameters* suggesting destruction of hepatocytes, as occurs in hepatitis and acute hepatic inflammation.
   2. Elevations in serum bilirubin and alkaline phosphatase are *cholestatic parameters* and suggest impaired bile flow either at the level of the hepatocyte (e.g., primary biliary cirrhosis) or within the major biliary ductal system (e.g., primary sclerosing cholangitis).
   3. Elevations in PT (without vitamin K deficiency or disseminated intravascular coagulation) with a concomitant low albumin (without nephrotic syndrome or isolated malnutrition) are parameters of impaired *hepatic synthetic function* and are the only commonly used laboratory studies that can be considered liver function tests. Abnormalities typically occur in states of chronic liver disease or cirrhosis and suggest a major loss in functional hepatic parenchyma.

L. *Liver biopsy.* The diagnosis of liver disease is often presumptively based on the history, physical, and selected laboratory or imaging studies. Liver biopsies should be considered when it will provide the patient and clinician with important prognostic information (e.g., tissue confirmation of malignancy) or guide the physician in management decisions that will be influenced by the biopsy results. Diseases that typically require a biopsy before therapy is initiated include chronic hepatitis B, chronic hepatitis C, autoimmune hepatitis, hemachromatosis, and Wilson's disease. Biopsies are often obtained on patients as part of a pretransplantation evaluation for chronic liver failure to ensure the proper diagnosis.

M. The cost figures cited in the table on page 197 are **basic direct costs**. The figures are difficult to obtain and change quickly. They include **only** the cost of the test itself (technician, equipment, time, and materials). No professional costs (interpretation) are included. Costs vary from region to region based on differences in some components such as labor. However, the relative cost ranking should remain similar.

VI. Bibliography

Sapira J. The abdomen. In: Orient JM, Horenstein S, Rosen D, eds. The Art and Science of Bedside Diagnosis. Baltimore: Williams & Wilkins; 3rd ed. 1990:371–390.

Sapira J. The rectum. In: Orient JM, Horenstein S, Rosen D, eds. The Art and-Science of Bedside Diagnosis. Baltimore: Williams & Wilkins; 1990:411–414.

Zakim D, Boyer TD, eds. Hepatology: A Textbook of Liver Diseases, I & II. Philadelphia: WB Saunders; 1996.

Procedure	Code
Esophagogastroduodenoscopy	$$$
Anoscopy	$
Sigmoidoscopy	$$$
Colonoscopy	$$$$
Endoscopic retrograde cholangiopancreatography (ERCP)	$$$$
Ultrasonography	
Real-time	$$
Doppler ultrasonography	$$$
Endoscopic ultrasonography	$$$$
Imaging studies	
Abdominal x-rays: supine view ('flat plate'), upright view	$$
Upper gastrointestinal with small-bowel follow-through	$$$
Barium enema	$$$
Computed tomography (CT)—abdomen	$$$
Magnetic resonance imaging (MRI)—liver	$$$$
Angiography	$$$$$
Nuclear studies	
Liver-spleen scan	*
HIDA scan	$$$$
Tagged RBC bleeding scan	$$$$$
Gastric emptying studies	$$$
Esophageal pH monitoring	$$
Esophageal manometry	$$$
Liver chemistries: serum transaminases: aspartate transaminase (AST) and alanine transaminase (ALT), serum bilirubin, and alkaline phosphatase, prothrombin time	$$
Liver biopsy	$$$

HIDA = hepato-immunodiacetic acid; RBC = red blood cells.
$ = $0–$50; $$ = $50–$100; $$$ = $100–$300; $$$$ = $300–$600; $$$$$ = $600–$1000;
* = highly variable or not available.

Yamada T, Alpers DH, Owyang C, et al. *Textbook of Gastroenterology, I & II*. 2nd ed. Philadelphia: JB Lippincott; 1995.
VII. Key Search Words
The following key words reflect the content of this chapter. They are provided to assist with an on-line search of computer databases, such as MEDLINE, if you wish to pursue the topic of this chapter further.

Abdominal pain
Anorexia nervosa
Aphasia
Ascites
Cachexia
Celiac disease
Cholelithiasis
Constipation
Diarrhea
Dyspepsia
Flatulence

Gastrointestinal hemorrhage
Heartburn
Hematemesis
Intestinal obstruction
Jaundice
Malabsorption syndromes
Melena
Nausea
Obstipation
Tenesmus

10. ACUTE ABDOMEN

Gerald B. Zelenock

I. Glossary

Acute abdomen: a clinical disorder of sudden onset with signs and symptoms focused in the abdominal area.

Guarding: the voluntary or involuntary tensing of abdominal muscles in response to a noxious stimulus.

McBurney's point: located one third of the way along a line from the right anterior superior iliac crest to the umbilicus; point tenderness at McBurney's point is a classic sign of appendicitis.

Murphy's sign: pain in the right upper quadrant that occurs when the examining hand is placed along the right costal margin and the patient inspires; this moves the liver and gallbladder into contact with the examining fingers.

Pain: the subjective complaint of discomfort voiced by the patient; it can be generalized or very well localized.

Peritoneal signs: signs of peritoneal irritation, typically due to localized or generalized inflammation. Palpable rigidity, and rebound and referred tenderness are peritoneal signs.

Psoas and obturator signs: pain occurring with manipulations that cause contact between an inflammatory process and the muscle; signs of retroperitoneal irritation.

Rigidity: palpable spasm in the abdominal musculature.

Rebound tenderness: sign of peritoneal irritation; elicited by compression and sudden release of the abdominal wall; may be localized or generalized.

Referred tenderness: tenderness that occurs remote from the area being palpated; for example, pain at McBurney's point when one presses remote from this area is a sign of localized peritoneal irritation consistent with appendicitis (Rovsing's sign).

Tenderness: the physical finding elicited by the examiner during the course of an examination; can be generalized or very well localized.

II. General Approach to the Patient

A. All clinicians, regardless of clinical specialty, will encounter patients with an acute abdomen (sudden onset of abdominal symptoms always including pain). This is a common, serious, and urgent situation that requires a rapid, accurate diagnosis. The symptoms and signs may or may not be secondary to an abdominal disorder; they often suggest a need for surgical management. Consultation may be required in the best interest of the patient and can shorten hospitalization and decrease patient morbidity and mortality.

B. The directed evaluation (Fig.10-1; Table 10-1). A timely diagnosis cannot be accomplished by obtaining an extensive laundry list of information.

1. Use discrimination. Your evaluation must be limited or expanded using logical clues, such as the patient's age, sex, and race. (A 16-year-old is unlikely to have a ruptured aortic aneurysm, men do not have ectopic pregnancies, and a sickle cell crisis is unlikely in a blond, blue-eyed Scandinavian.)

2. Localizing symptoms and a knowledge of regional anatomy may help to limit the diagnostic possibilities. For example, a person with appendicitis would be unlikely to present with left upper quadrant pain.

3. The presence or absence of significant findings in the physical examination may dictate further evaluation and analysis. Thus, a patient with abdominal pain who lacks localized tenderness to palpation may have

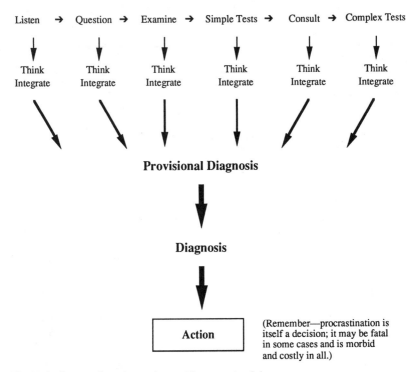

Fig.10-1. Approach to the patient with an acute abdomen.

appendicitis, but it is much less likely than in a patient with abdominal pain and point tenderness at McBurney's point. The former may benefit from a 2- to 6-hour period of observation and reexamination; the latter needs prompt appendectomy).

4. The examiner must incorporate every clue from the history and physical examination and integrate that information with *simple* laboratory and x-ray studies (and occasionally more sophisticated studies) to arrive at a diagnosis.

5. In certain circumstances, a short, purposeful observation period with repeat evaluation may be helpful, but there is no virtue to procrastination. Once a diagnosis has been made, appropriate treatment is usually straightforward (see Chapters 7, 9, and 13).

III. **History.** The standard history may need modification if the patient is suffering from acute, severe pain. Direct questions asked of the patient may be supplemented by information gathered from accompanying family or friends. Even an abbreviated history must include sufficient information to develop an adequate working diagnosis.

   A. History of present illness
      1. Note precise time and mode of onset of symptoms.
         a. Did the pain begin abruptly, or was it progressive over a period of time?
         b. Was the onset of pain preceded or followed by symptoms such as anorexia, nausea, vomiting, diarrhea, or constipation? Has there been a change in bowel habits? Is blood or mucus in the stool?
      2. Note precise location, including radiation of pain.
      3. Note duration of pain.

Table 10-1. Assessment of the Patient With Acute Abdomen

Detailed history
Physical examination
  Attitude in bed
  Vital signs
  General physical examination
  Abdominal examination
    Inspect.
    Auscultate.
    Palpate.
      Be gentle.
      Palpate all hernia sites/orifices.
      Note spasm referred/rebound.
      Note hyperesthesia.
    Percuss (lightly).
      Referred/rebound
  Pelvic and rectal examinations

    4. Note character of pain (cramping, burning, aching, tearing). Is it constant or intermittent?
    5. Note other symptoms.
      a. Women of childbearing age should be asked whether there is any possibility that they are pregnant. A detailed gynecologic history must be obtained.
      b. Urologic history. Inquire about sexually transmitted diseases, voiding patterns, and changes in urine (color, frequency, and volume).
  B. Past medical history. Ask about significant elements, including history of previous pain.
  C. Family history. Ask about significant elements.
  D. Review of systems. Ask about significant elements. Keep in mind possible extra-abdominal causes of the acute abdomen.
IV. Physical Examination. In stable patients, the importance of a thorough general physical examination cannot be overemphasized.
  A. Technique
    1. The patient should be fully disrobed, in a gown, and properly draped.
    2. Follow the sequence of a standard abdominal examination, including inspection, auscultation, palpation, and percussion.
    3. Note vital signs. Even a low-grade fever, mild tachycardia, and tachypnea have strong correlative significance in the proper setting. More pronounced abnormalities, including significant hypotension or shock, are always significant.
    4. Note patient response to abdominal symptoms. The patient who is pacing the room or intermittently writhing in pain from a ureteral stone or some other cause of colicky abdominal pain looks and acts differently from a patient who is lying in bed, barely moving, and taking very shallow respirations so as not to aggravate an inflamed peritoneum.
  B. Inspection
    1. Gross visual inspection. The surface projection of abdominal contents extends from the nipple line to the perineum. The presence or absence of distention, surgical scars, and protuberant masses are readily appreciated.
    2. Causes of protuberant abdomen: intestinal obstruction, ascites, pregnancy, obesity, and intra-abdominal and retroperitoneal masses can often be distinguished.
  C. Auscultation. Auscultation of the abdomen for bowel sounds and abdominal bruits is routinely performed. Except in unusual circumstances, it has little diagnostic sensitivity or specificity.

1. Total absence of bowel sounds. This is consistent with diagnosis of generalized peritonitis, but other signs and symptoms must be present to make this diagnosis.
2. High-pitched, "tinkly" bowel sounds. These may have clinical significance in a patient with a distended abdomen and a history of not having passed stool or flatus for 72 hours. Without distention or obstipation, these sounds are not particularly specific.
3. Abdominal bruits. These sounds can support a diagnosis of renal artery stenosis, superior mesenteric or celiac artery stenosis, or significant obstruction of the aortoiliac bifurcation, but only in the context of other significant signs and symptoms suggesting renovascular hypertension, intestinal angina, or peripheral vascular occlusive disease. An isolated abdominal bruit is nonspecific.

D. Palpation
1. Avoid causing unnecessary discomfort. In a patient with an acute abdomen, tenderness is certain and severe discomfort is common. Significant modification of standard palpation techniques may be necessary. Assure the patient that you will be careful and delicate with the examination. Ask the patient to point with one finger to the area of maximum discomfort, and examine this area last. This is especially important in children, who are often uncooperative after they have been hurt.
2. Technique. Palpation is gentle yet firm, not jabbing, poking, or prodding. Use the fleshy pads of the distal phalanges, not the fingertips. Slow, purposeful, and deliberate movements are helpful. Having the patient flex the hips and knees relaxes the abdominal muscles and may allow better examination.
   a. Begin with very light palpation, merely resting the flat of your hand on the abdominal wall. This reassures the patient and allows palpation of underlying muscle spasm (rigidity), which may be an important clue to peritoneal irritation.
   b. Progress to light palpation.
   c. Deep palpation may require a slight to-and-fro motion, often timed with the patient's respirations. This is not a massage or a heavy, jerky, kneading type of movement.
3. In an overly responsive patient (one who is very suggestible or one in whom there is the possibility of secondary gain), palpation with a stethoscope can be very helpful. The findings should be consistent; if the patient is nontender when palpating with the stethoscope, but palpation with the examining hand produces guarding or a vigorous withdrawal response, one has reason to consider secondary gain.

E. Percussion
1. Avoid causing unnecessary discomfort. Standard percussion may produce excruciating pain in a patient with an acute abdomen due to localized or generalized peritoneal irritation. Use the modified percussion technique outlined below (E3 and E4).
2. Purpose. Unlike the routine examination, percussion is used in the evaluation of a patient with an acute abdomen to demonstrate *peritoneal signs* suggesting irritation, and to distinguish gassy distention from other causes of a protuberant abdomen.
3. Technique. Very light percussion (a gentle "finger tweak" rather than deep palpation and abrupt release) can demonstrate tympany or rebound tenderness.
4. Avoid unnecessary percussion. A patient who describes sharp right lower quadrant pain every time the car hits a bump on the drive to the emergency room or who clutches the right lower quadrant when coughing has provided a spontaneous demonstration of rebound tenderness. These findings can be used as confirmation of clinical suspicion and may negate the need for percussion. Their very spontaneity lends credence, and the absence of such confirmatory evidence suggests caution.

F. Specialized signs of peritoneal or retroperitoneal irritation. Certain physical findings are so common and reproducible in the evaluation of patients with acute abdominal complaints that they have received eponymous designations as a tribute to their usefulness.

   1. *Murphy's sign.* Place the examining hand in the right upper quadrant several centimeters below the right costal margin. Ask the patient to inhale; this pushes the diaphragm down, moving the liver and gallbladder into the range of the palpating finger. A catch in the respiration is a positive finding, strongly suggestive of an acute inflammatory process involving the gallbladder.

   2. *Rovsing's sign:* tenderness at a site remote from the area being palpated. Press in the left lower quadrant. Discomfort at McBurney's point in the right lower quadrant is a sign of localized peritoneal irritation.

   3. *Psoas and obturator signs:* signs of retroperitoneal irritation. These signs may indicate a retroperitoneal inflammatory process, such as retrocecal appendicitis.

      a. Obturator sign. Flex the patient's hip and knee upon the chest; internally and externally rotate the hip. Discomfort indicates a positive test result.

      b. Psoas sign. Extend the leg on the trunk. This stretches the iliopsoas muscle. Discomfort indicates a positive test result.

G. Pelvic and rectal examination (see Chapters 9 and 13). Evaluation of a patient with an acute abdomen is not complete until a pelvic or rectal examination or both has been performed. These examinations add important confirmatory evidence to the abdominal examination and may be the only way to elicit important signs of pelvic pathology.

H. Repeat examination. In some cases, a repeat examination after a short period of observation can clarify clinical signs of illness or determine how the patient's symptoms have evolved. However, it is vitally important to make a considered decision—either by making the diagnosis or by deciding that ongoing care and evaluation is the appropriate course. Procrastination is in itself a decision with important consequences; delayed diagnosis of appendicitis can increase the risk of perforation with attendant morbidity. Moreover, missing a ruptured aneurysm ensures a mortality.

I. Consultation. Early and appropriate consultation is proper and cost-effective and has enormous potential for patient benefit, particularly when matters of urgent surgical, obstetric, or gynecologic concern are being considered. There is no merit to avoiding consultation when a specialist will ultimately be required to deal with the problem or will aid in the diagnosis or ongoing care of the patient. In patients with persistent symptoms refractory to diagnosis, a careful consideration of a pathophysiologic classification system of the multiple causes of abdominal pain may be helpful (Table 10-2).

V. Special Situations

A. Abdominal apoplexy. This ancient term refers to cardiovascular collapse secondary to an intra-abdominal cause. In contemporary practice, this is often due to a ruptured abdominal aortic aneurysm.

   1. Abdominal aortic aneurysm

      a. Unstable patient. A hypotensive patient with a tender, pulsatile abdominal mass does not benefit from a prolonged evaluation, but should go directly to the operating room. There is no time (and no need) for a detailed history or physical examination; laboratory or x-ray studies are irrelevant and unnecessary. Ultrasonography, CT scans, chest x-rays, and electrocardiograms (ECGs) are superfluous. Admitting laboratory studies and a sample to cross-match 6 to 10 units of blood can be drawn while starting an intravenous line for fluid and blood administration.

      b. Stable patient. A patient with abdominal pain and *equivocal* findings suggesting an abdominal aortic aneurysm may benefit from further diagnostic study.

Table 10-2. Pathophysiologic Classification of Abdominal Pain[a]

Pain Arising From Abdomen	Extra-abdominal Causes	Metabolic, Toxic, Infectious, Other Causes	Neurogenic Causes
INFLAMMATION "____itis" disorders (appendicitis, cholecystitis, hepatitis, gastritis, pancreatitis, Meckel's diverticulitis, colonic diverticulitis, and so on) Pelvic inflammatory disease (PID) Inflammatory bowel disease	THORAX Acute MI Pneumonia Pulmonary embolism Aortic dissection (and so on) SPINE Fracture Potts disease	Uremia Ketoacidosis Sickle cell anemia Porphyria Hemolytic crisis C'1 esterase deficiency (angioneurotic edema) Familial Mediterranean fever	Herpes zoster Tabes dorsalis Causalgia Functional Malingering
MECHANICAL OBSTRUCTION Small bowel obstruction Large bowel obstruction Biliary tract Genitourinary obstruction	GENITOURINARY Ectopic pregnancy PID Ovulatory pain (and so on) Renal, ureteral and/or urethral calculi (stones) Pyelonephritis	Hyperlipoproteinemia Food poisoning, Lead poisoning, other toxicities Spider bites Medications Amebiasis Tuberculosis Typhoid Malaria Primary peritonitis	
VASCULAR Aortic aneurysm; other vascular ruptures Superior mesenteric artery embolus, thrombosis			
ABDOMINAL WALL Hernia Muscular tears, strains, and so on Rectus sheath hematoma			

MI = myocardial infarction.
[a]Partial list.

2. Rupture of other arteries or occult problems involving other organs. Visceral artery aneurysms, Ehlers-Danlos syndrome, spontaneous or delayed rupture of the spleen, and a perforated viscus in an elderly patient can produce symptoms of abdominal apoplexy. In general, these require urgent surgical intervention. When in doubt, an unstable patient can be rapidly transported to an operating room for further resuscitation, a surgical team can be assembled, and additional diagnostic studies (e.g., chest x-ray, ECG, laboratory studies) can be performed.

B. Evaluation of the hard-to-examine or compromised patient with an acute abdomen (Tables 10-3 and 10-4). Thoughtful, thorough, and meticulous evaluation is essential for timely diagnosis and appropriate treatment. These complicated patients are commonly encountered.

VI. Clinical Vignettes

A. Case 1: Right lower quadrant abdominal pain

1. History. A 24-year-old man complains of right lower quadrant abdominal pain. His symptoms began 24 hours ago with vague and diffuse abdominal discomfort, anorexia, and a mild sensation of nausea but no vomiting. Over the last 12 hours, the pain has localized to the right lower quadrant. He has never had similar symptoms and denies any other gastrointestinal or genitourinary symptoms. His general health has been excellent. His past medical history, family history, and review of systems are noncontributory.

2. Physical examination: temperature 100.8° F pulse 80 and regular, respirations 12, blood pressure 110/70 mmHg. The general physical examination is entirely unremarkable except for the abdominal examination. The patient's abdomen is not visibly distended, and there are no surgical scars. Bowel sounds are present. He has point tenderness at McBurney's point and rebound and referred tenderness to McBurney's point. There are no herniae and the genitourinary examination is normal. Rectal examination reveals a vague fullness and tenderness in the right lower quadrant.

3. Laboratory studies. A complete blood cell count (CBC) and urinalysis are obtained. Hematocrit is 44%. White blood cell (WBC) count is 11,200 with a left shift. Urinalysis is negative.

4. X-rays and diagnostics. A chest x-ray and abdominal series are normal except for a single sentinel loop in the right lower quadrant.

5. Preliminary diagnosis: appendicitis.

6. Action: preoperative preparation for an appendectomy.

7. Discussion. Although the differential is theoretically large, practically it is virtually certain appendicitis.

B. Case 2: Right lower quadrant abdominal pain

1. History. A 24-year-old previously healthy woman complains of 24 hours of abdominal discomfort localized to the right lower quadrant. She is in excellent general health except that for the last 2 years she has noticed

Table 10-3. Factors Making an Abdominal Examination More Difficult

Pregnancy	Mechanical ventilation
Extremes of age	Body cast
Morbid obesity	Malingering
Massive abdominal musculature	Drug-seeking behavior or other secondary gain
Previous operations	
Immediate postoperative period	Immunosuppression/neutropenia
Retroperitoneal source of pain	Drugs (corticosteroids, analgesics, anesthetics)
Coma, paraplegia, quadriplegia, prior cerebrovascular accident	

Table 10-4. Caveats for the Examiner

---

1. Accurate diagnosis is the key to appropriate treatment.
2. Refine or expand your diagnosis by careful considerations of the age, sex, race, and associated medical illnesses of your patient.
3. Use all available diagnostic clues.
4. The abdomen extends from the nipple line to the perineum.
5. The abdominal examination is never complete until pelvic and rectal examinations have been performed.
6. Recognize and be very careful with hard-to-examine patients.
7. Pain out of proportion to physical findings suggests a vascular etiology.
8. Simple laboratory tests and radiologic examinations confirm diagnostic suspicions in most patients. Shotgun laboratory and radiologic examinations are only occasionally helpful, are always expensive, and may be dangerous.
9. Think and rethink. Use anatomic, physiologic, and pathophysiologic algorithms.
10. Common things occur commonly.
11. Uncommon things happen now and then.
12. A person ill enough to come to the emergency room at 4 AM is usually sick. A person who returns to the emergency room having previously visited is virtually always sick.
13. Be aware that manipulative, drug-seeking, and secondary gain behaviors are real, but do not be overly suspicious. Appendicitis is much more common than Munchausen syndrome.
14. Even manipulative, unpleasant individuals get sick.
15. Early and appropriate consultation is not a sign of weakness.
16. Always act in your patient's best interest.

---

occasional crampy abdominal pain, sometimes associated with diarrhea. She is sexually active with a single partner, who usually wears a condom. Her menstrual periods are usually normal every 28 days. Her last period was lighter than normal and occurred 6 weeks ago. Her past medical history, family history, and review of systems are unremarkable.

2. Physical examination: temperature 99° F, blood pressure 110/70 mmHg, heart rate 100, respirations 20. The patient's general physical examination is unremarkable. Abdominal examination reveals slight bilateral lower quadrant abdominal distention, active bowel sounds, and tenderness to direct palpation in the right lower quadrant. There is no evidence of rebound or referred tenderness. Pelvic examination reveals tenderness in the right lower quadrant and a trace amount of blood at the cervical os.

3. Laboratory studies. Laboratory studies reveal a CBC with a hematocrit of 24%, WBC count of 11,000, and a normal urinalysis. HCG (pregnancy test) is positive.

4. X-rays and diagnostics. A diagnostic ultrasound text was obtained in the emergency room, which revealed a 6×10 cm right lower quadrant mass with a surrounding hematoma.

5. Preliminary diagnosis: ectopic pregnancy

6. Action: consult an ob-gyn; preoperative preparation for salpingo-oophorectomy (removal of tubal pregnancy usually requires removal of tube and ovary)

7. Discussion. The differential diagnosis of abdominal pain is considerably larger in women than in men. Possible pregnancy should always be con-

sidered in women of childbearing age. An ectopic pregnancy is a potentially life-threatening problem; delay in diagnosis is avoided by careful history, physical examination, and pregnancy test. The portable ultrasound examination confirmed the clinical diagnosis.

C. Case 3: Left lower quadrant pain

1. History. A 65-year-old man has fever, chills, diarrhea, and left lower quadrant crampy abdominal pain of 36 hours' duration. He has not had similar symptoms in the past. A detailed inquiry regarding gastrointestinal symptoms reveals that he has never had blood or mucus in the stool and has only occasionally (once or twice a year) been troubled by gas and constipation. His past medical history is significant for a myocardial infarction 5 years ago. The remainder of his family history, review of systems, and social history are unremarkable.

2. Physical examination: temperature 101.2° F, heart rate 110, blood pressure 110/70 mmHg, respirations 20 and unlabored. The patient's general physical examination is unremarkable. Abdominal examination reveals minimal distention. Bowel sounds are present with occasional hyperactive rushes. On palpation, the patient is slightly tender in a diffuse pattern but markedly tender in the left lower quadrant. A palpable but vague fullness is present in the left lower quadrant; his tenderness precludes precise definition. There is slight rebound and referred tenderness. Rectal examination causes discomfort referred to the left lower quadrant.

3. Laboratory studies. CBC demonstrated a hematocrit of 44%, WBC of 14,800 with a left shift. Urinalysis is normal. The stool obtained during the rectal examination is trace-positive for blood.

4. X-rays and diagnostics. An abdominal series revealed gassy distention of the small bowel with air-fluid levels in the left lower quadrant and gas in the colon including the rectum.

5. Preliminary diagnosis: diverticulitis

6. Action: intravenous hydration, bowel rest, and antibiotics. If the patient fails to respond to this regimen or if a complication such as a perforation with peritonitis develops, perform surgery. When the symptoms become quiescent, additional diagnostic studies including barium enema or endoscopy (colonoscopy) would be appropriate to confirm the diagnosis of diverticulitis.

7. Discussion. Diverticulitis is likely. The treatment that is undertaken is appropriate and conservative and allows assessment of cardiac status. A precipitous operation is not necessary and may be harmful. Failure to respond to this treatment plan or a complication may subsequently require an operation.

D. Case 4: left-sided abdominal pain

1. History. An 18-year-old black man presents to the emergency room with a 3-day history of progressive abdominal pain. Initially mild, the pain is now severe and localized to the left side of the abdomen. His general health has been excellent except that 10 days ago he had an upper respiratory infection, which resolved without specific treatment.

2. Physical examination: temperature 100° F, pulse 110, respirations 20, blood pressure 110/70 mmHg. The sclerae are slightly icteric. The patient has some mild aching in his elbows and knees and significant abdominal discomfort. The abdomen is slightly distended. Bowel sounds are present. He has guarding in the left upper and left lower quadrant. Rectal examination is unremarkable.

3. Laboratory studies. Laboratory evaluation reveals a hemoglobin of 12, hematocrit of 36%, WBC 11,200 with a leftward shift. Urinalysis is negative.

4. X-rays and diagnostics. The abdominal series and chest x-ray are within normal limits.

5. Preliminary diagnosis: sickle cell crisis

6. Action: Admission, rehydration, and additional laboratory studies to confirm suspected hemoglobinopathy. Surgery would be contraindicated.

7. Discussion. Surgery does not usually benefit a patient with sickle cell crisis. Likewise many of the toxic, metabolic, and infectious causes of abdominal pain (see Table 10-2) are best treated nonoperatively.

VI. Available Technology

A. Routine tests and studies. In most cases, the evaluation of an acute abdomen is straightforward. Often, a focused history and physical examination and routine tests suffice to make the diagnosis.

1. CBC
2. Urinalysis
3. Pregnancy test (sexually active females of childbearing years)
4. Liver panel, amylase, lipase, prothrombin time (patients with upper abdominal or hepatobiliary symptoms).
5. Admitting chemscreen panel (clearly indicated if patient requires hospitalization and in many instances, the panel is less expensive than the sum of the individual components).
6. Blood type and cross-match (if blood loss is suspected or likely to occur or an operation is probable).
7. Radiologic examination; abdominal x-ray series. These can help to identify free air, suggesting a hollow viscus perforation, or dynamic and distended loops of bowel compatible with bowel obstruction. On occasion, air in the bowel wall or the biliary tree can suggest a diagnosis. Edema of the bowel wall or ascites is usually readily recognized. Ectopic calcifications are sometimes noted with ureteral or biliary stones or in the presence of an abdominal aortic aneurysm.

B. Other diagnostic procedures. The more serious the nature of the illness, the more frail or chronically ill the patient, and the wider the diagnostic possibilities, the more likely that detailed testing will be helpful.

1. Hematologic studies
2. Biochemical studies
3. Serologic analyses
4. Imaging studies (for selected cases):
   a. Standard contrast studies
   b. Abdominal and pelvic ultrasonography
   c. CT
   d. Intravenous pyelogram
   e. Angiography
5. Peritoneal lavage (only in selected cases and by a skilled practitioner)
6. Culdocentesis (only in selected cases and by a skilled practitioner)
7. Laparoscopic evaluation (only in selected cases and by a skilled practitioner)
8. Endoscopy (adds little to the evaluation of the acute abdomen). It is much more useful in cases of acute gastrointestinal bleeding or in patients with chronic abdominal complaints.

C. The cost figures cited in the table on page 209 are **basic direct costs**. The figures are difficult to obtain and change quickly. They include **only** the cost of the test itself (technician, equipment, time, and materials). No professional costs (interpretation) are included. Costs vary from region to region based on differences in some components such as labor. However, the relative cost ranking should remain similar.

VII. Bibliography

Silen W. *Cope's Early Diagnosis of the Acute Abdomen*, 19th ed. New York and Oxford: Oxford University Press; 1996.

VIII. Key Search Words

The following key words reflect the content of this chapter. They are provided to assist with an on-line search of computer databases, such as MEDLINE, if you wish to pursue the topic of this chapter further.

Abdomen, acute
Abdominal pain

Procedure	Code
Routine tests and studies:	
Complete blood count	$
Urinalysis	$
Pregnancy test	$
Liver panel, amylase, lipase, prothrombin time	$$
Admitting panel	$$
Blood type and crossmatch	$$
Abdominal x-rays: supine view (flat plate), upright view	$$
Other diagnostic procedures:	
Hematologic studies	$$
Biochemical studies	$$
Serologic analyses	$$
Imaging studies studies (for selected cases):	
Abdominal and pelvic ultrasonography	$$
Computed tomography (CT)	$$$
Intravenous urogram	$$$
Angiography	$$$
Peritoneal lavage	$$$
Culdocentesis	$$$$
Laparoscopic evaluation	$$$$
Endoscopy	$$$

$ = $0–$50; $$ = $50–$100; $$$ = $100–$200; $$$$ = $200–$500.

11. GENITOURINARY SYSTEM

William D. Belville

I. Glossary

Anuria: complete cessation of urinary output.

Bacteriuria: presence of bacteria in the urine; not equivalent to clinical infection.

Balanoposthitis: inflammation of the glans penis and prepuce.

Bulbocavernosus reflex: reflex elicited by squeezing the glans penis, which results in constriction of the bulbocavernosus muscle and the anal sphincter.

Chordee: bowing of the penis during erection secondary to fibrotic plaques in the corpora cavernosa or to congenital hypoplasia of the corpus spongiosum.

Cryptorchidism: failure of one testis or both testes to descend properly into the scrotum; may be undescended or ectopic.

Cystitis: inflammation of the urinary bladder.

Dysuria: painful micturition.

Enuresis: involuntary voiding during sleep (*nocturnal enuresis* more specific).

Hematuria: blood in the urine; blood detected visually in the urine is *gross hematuria*, detected only microscopically, *microscopic hematuria*; may be *painless* or *painful, initial* or *terminal*.

Hydrocele: cystic scrotal mass containing clear, amber-colored fluid.

Nephrocalcinosis: deposition of calcium in the renal parenchyma.

Neurogenic bladder: dysfunction of bladder secondary to abnormality of its innervation.

Oliguria: urinary output less than 400 mL/24 hours.

Paradoxical incontinence: involuntary dribbling of urine secondary to chronic urinary retention (also called *overflow incontinence*).

Paraphimosis: the inability to replace a retracted foreskin over the glans penis.

Phimosis: tightness of the prepuce preventing retraction to uncover the glans penis.

Pneumaturia: voiding of urine containing free gas.

Polycystic kidney: congenitally abnormal kidney that contains numerous cysts of various sizes.

Priapism: prolonged painful erection of the penis unassociated with sexual excitement.

Proteinuria: protein in the urine; *orthostatic proteinuria,* presence of protein in a urine specimen taken while the patient is upright, which is absent from specimen taken while patient is supine.

Pyuria: leukocytes in the urine.

Residual urine: urine that remains in the bladder after micturition.

Spermatocele: a cystic scrotal mass containing cloudy fluid with spermatozoa.

Stress incontinence: involuntary loss of urine during period of increased intravesical pressure, such as can be produced by coughing, straining, or lifting.

Urge incontinence: involuntary loss of urine caused by an uninhibited bladder contraction.

Varicocele: dilated veins of the pampiniform plexus in the scrotum.

II. Techniques of Examination and Normal Findings

A. Kidneys and ureters.

    1. Examination techniques for kidney. Patient lies supine with knees flexed and slightly raised.

    a. Inspection. Inspect upper abdomen for obvious asymmetry or bulg-
ing, particularly in the flanks. Observe during patient's deep inspiration and expiration.

    b. Palpation. Palpate the right kidney from the right side, and the left
kidney from the left side. Place one hand posteriorly beneath the
costal margin, and press directly upward (Fig. 11-1). Place other hand
below the costal margin at about the midclavicular line. Ask patient
to take a deep breath; this depresses the diaphragm and pushes the
kidney downward. Press hand inward and upward toward costal margin. Normal kidneys often cannot be palpated.

        (1) When pathology is suspected, have patient lie on side; this causes
the uppermost kidney to fall downward and medially, making it
more accessible to palpation.

        (2) Renal tenderness and pain. The kidney is nearest to the skin sur-
face at the costovertebral angle; deep pressure by the examiner's
fingers may elicit pain due to intrinsic renal parenchymal disease
(i.e. inflammation). This must be differentiated from muscle tenderness, which is much more likely and can be demonstrated by
deep palpation directly over the back muscles that lie medial to
the costovertebral angle.

    c. Percussion is not used routinely; however, large masses in the renal
area may be outlined.

    d. Auscultation may detect bruits originating in the renal arteries. Lis-
ten over the costovertebral angles posteriorly and in both upper
quadrants of the abdomen.

    e. Transillumination may occasionally be useful in small light skinned
children. Darken the room and press the light source into the costovertebral angle posteriorly.

    f. Renal ultrasonography has largely replaced detailed physical exami-
nation of the kidneys.

  2. Ureters are not generally accessible to physical examination.

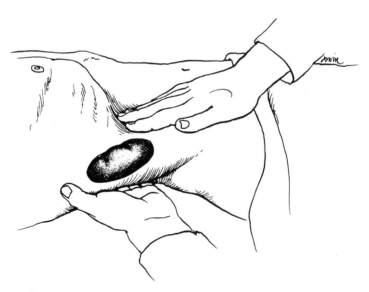

Fig. 11-1. Palpation of the kidney.

B. Urinary bladder. The empty bladder is not accessible to physical examination, but may be felt with bimanual examination (especially in females).
  1. Inspection. When distended, the bladder produces a bulging mass in the lower abdomen, and it can be mistaken for lower abdominal tumor.
  2. Percussion. Dullness may be elicited over a distended bladder, which may extend up as far as the umbilicus.
  3. Palpation. Palpate the symphysis region carefully. Bladder pain is usually elicited by direct palpation over the suprapubic area.
    a. Bimanual examination in men is performed at the time of rectal examination in the lithotomy position; place one finger in rectum pressing upward, the opposite hand on the lower abdominal wall (Fig. 11-2).
    b. Bimanual palpation of the bladder in women is done at the time of pelvic examination.
    c. The empty bladder feels much like a thick-walled, collapsed balloon; not tender, freely movable, no lateral extensions or palpable discrete masses.
  4. Pelvic ultrasonography has become an integral part of the pelvic examination in females and is very useful to measure residual urine in both sexes.
C. Male genitalia (remember your gloves).

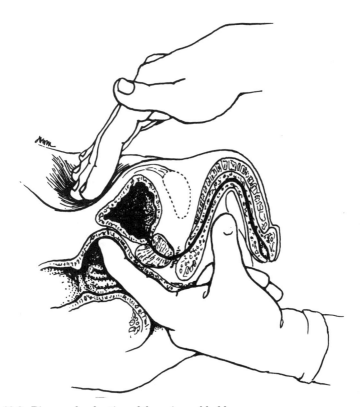

Fig. 11-2. Bimanual palpation of the urinary bladder.

1. External meatus. Ask patient to retract foreskin (if uncircumcised) to expose the glans penis. Place thumbs on either side of glans penis; separate and examine the external meatus.
2. Shaft. Palpate, searching for areas of tenderness or induration. Normally, no masses or tenderness are palpable. Be alert for any urethral discharge.
3. Scrotum. Inspect skin. Palpate scrotal contents. Use two hands.
   a. Testes. Palpate each testis between thumb and first two fingers. The testes should move freely in the scrotum. In the average man, they are 4 × 3 × 2.5 cm in size and correspondingly smaller in boys.
   b. Epididymis. Gently palpate the soft, comma-shaped structure on the posterolateral surface of each testis. Normally, no tenderness is present. The spermatic cord extends upward from the epididymis to the external ring.
   c. Vas deferens. Palpate this small, hard, solid cord between the thumb and index finger, using the opposite hand to exert gentle downward traction on the testis.
   d. Transillumination should be used to examine a scrotal mass. It can be diagnostic if done correctly in light-skinned persons.
   e. Scrotal ultrasonography is highly accurate to characterize scrotal pathology.
D. Prostate gland (Fig. 11-3). The prostate is assessed during rectal examination (see Chapter 9). Digital examination is best done with patient standing and bending over an examining table or chair, or, if unable to stand, in the Sims' position.

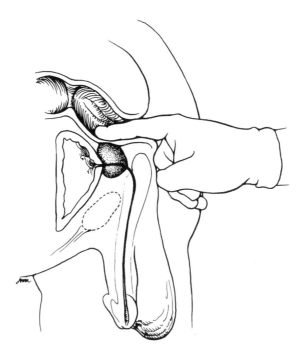

Fig. 11-3. Examination of the prostate.

1. Gently but firmly introduce the lubricated index finger into the anal canal, pointing toward the umbilicus. Assess the muscle tone of the anal sphincter, which is normally not lax.
2. The bulbocavernosus reflex can be used to document an intact sacral arc. With a finger in the patient's anus, ask him to relax as much as possible, then *after warning* the patient, squeeze the glans penis with the opposite hand. Normally, this stimulus will produce an involuntary contraction of the anal sphincter. (Voluntary contraction may produce a false-positive test.) The presence of this reflex signifies an intact sacral arc, which also innervates the urinary bladder. The reflex can also be elicited by clitoral pressure, but requires care and forethought.
3. Prostate gland. Outline the upper limits, lateral margins, and medial sulcus. Palpate each lobe, searching for areas of irregularity or enlargement. The prostate varies greatly in size, usually increasing with age. It is smooth and rubbery in consistency, and normally not tender. Palpate the anterior wall of the rectum.
4. Seminal vesicles. The region of the seminal vesicles extends upward and laterally along the upper margin of the prostate gland. The seminal vesicles usually are not palpable.

E. Expected findings in elderly (age >75)
1. Prostatic enlargement (benign prostate hypertrophy [BPH]) is very common. If symmetric, smooth, and without nodules or induration, it is of little clinical concern.
2. Small, soft testicles (atrophy) are common and if symmetric, not worrisome.

III. Cardinal Symptoms and Abnormal Findings

A. Irritative bladder symptoms. Frequency, urgency, and dysuria often occur alone or together and may be secondary to disease of the bladder, prostate, or urethra as well as a common functional complaint.

B. Prostatism. Symptoms historically said to be produced by an enlarged prostate gland are classified into two types.
1. Irritative symptoms. See A above.
2. Obstructive symptoms characterized by a urinary stream delayed in starting (hesitancy) or decreased in size and force of streams, with interruption of the stream during voiding. These symptoms may also be produced by any obstruction (urethral stricture, such as bladder neck hypertrophy and urethral valves) as well as by common cold medications.

C. Incontinence. Careful history-taking is mandatory to properly identify the type of incontinence and therefore the appropriate treatment. Inappropriate surgery may make some incontinence worse.
1. Stress urinary incontinence (SUI): involuntary loss of urine caused by straining, coughing, or lifting. This occurs most often in multiparous women, is often associated with a cystourethrocele, and can be corrected surgically by any type of suspension procedure.
2. Urge incontinence: involuntary loss of urine cause by the sudden urge to void. This usually occurs from inflammation of the bladder, urethra, or prostate as well as neurogenic and idiopathic causes. Urge incontinence is typically a drenching incontinence. (These patients are more wet than pure SUI.)
3. Dribbling incontinence: *constant* loss of urine in varying amounts with or without stress. This occurs from vesicovaginal or ureterovaginal fistula or ectopic ureter or after exuberant prostatectomy when sphincteric controls have been damaged. Typically, such individuals are *never* dry.
4. Paradoxical overflow incontinence: involuntary dribbling of urine due to longstanding urinary retention. This may occur with obstruction of the urethra in the male, or it may be secondary to a neurogenic bladder.

D. Pain.
1. Renal pain is usually present in the costovertebral angle; may radiate anteriorly. It may be due to pyelonephritis, calculi, renal, or perinephric

abscess, tumor, acute glomerulonephritis, or intermittent hydronephrosis. Renal pain may be *referred pain,* consisting of the following two types:

   a. Renal: afferent autonomic nerves carrying sensation from the kidneys to the spinal cord through the 10th, 11th, and 12th thoracic nerves. The patients feel referred pain over the somatic distribution of these nerves in the abdominal wall.

   b. Ureteral: fibers supplying the ureter enter the spinal cord from the 12th thoracic and first three lumbar nerves. Pain is referred over the somatic distribution of the subcostal, iliohypogastric, ilioinguinal, and genitofemoral nerves, depending on which portion of the ureter is affected. Pain often radiates to the testicular, scrotal, and vulvar areas.

   2. Vesical pain is usually present in the suprapubic region. It may be intermittent with bladder distention, and relieved by voiding (as in interstitial cystitis), or it may be continuous (as in urinary retention or acute cystitis).

   3. Testicular pain is usually due to torsion, epididymal infection, trauma, or occasionally tumor. Pain can be referred to this region from ureters (e.g., calculus).

   4. Prostatic and urethral pain may be referred to the low back area, often claimed to be perineal.

E. Mass.

   1. Renal. A palpable mass in this area may be produced by hydronephrosis, neoplasm, renal cysts, or multicystic kidney in the neonate.

   2. Suprapubic. A palpable mass in this area is usually secondary to bladder distention, but occasionally may be due to a neoplasm (bladder or rarely urachus). In women, it is more likely uterine or ovarian process.

   3. Scrotal. A palpable scrotal mass may be inflammatory or neoplastic or secondary to trauma. If it can be transilluminated, it probably represents either a spermatocele or a hydrocele. If intratesticular, there is a high likelihood of malignancy. A left-sided soft mass simulating a "bag of worms" is a varicocele (dilated pampiniform plexus).

F. Pneumaturia. Occasionally develops from infection due to gas-forming bacteria, or more often from an enterovesical fistula due to inflammatory or neoplastic disease of the gastrointestinal tract.

G. Hematuria. Neoplasm must be ruled out when hematuria, either microscopic or gross, is present. Initial or terminal hematuria is usually associated with disease of the lower urinary tract. Blood throughout urination (total hematuria) may come from kidney, ureter, or bladder. Calculi, infection, trauma, acute glomerulonephritis are often associated with hematuria.

H. Nocturia. Usually a common symptom of the elderly of both sexes and seen in association with benign prostatic hypertrophy, diabetes mellitus, urinary tract infections, and often due to mobilization of dependent extracellular fluid.

I. Gastrointestinal symptoms.

   1. Acute renal or ureteral obstruction may cause nausea, vomiting, abdominal distention.

   2. Hydronephrosis. Symptoms may suggest gallbladder disease or duodenal ulcer when the right kidney is affected, or a lesion of the colon when the left kidney is affected.

   3. Chronic renal insufficiency (azotemia) may present with nausea and vomiting.

IV. Common Clinical Disorders

A. Kidneys and ureters.

   1. Acute pyelonephritis. Fever is usually present; patient may look quite ill. The entire flank region may be tender, with tenderness to deep palpation or percussion in the costovertebral angle. Signs of peritonitis may be present when the peritoneum overlying the kidney is affected by the inflammatory reaction, including abdominal distention, muscle spasm, rebound tenderness, hypoactive bowel sounds. Urinalysis consistent with infection. Ultrasound may show enlargement (swelling), intravenous urogram (IVU) needed if obstruction is suggested.

2. Perinephric or renal abscess. Signs may include low-grade or septic fever, exquisite tenderness on affected side often with bulging mass palpable in the flank, scoliosis of the spine with concavity pointing toward the affected side (due to irritation of psoas major and quadratus lumborum muscles), elevated diaphragm somewhat fixed on the affected side, basilar rales due to inflammatory reaction, or edema of the skin over the abscess. Ultrasound may be suggestive but CT diagnostic.

3. Obstructive uropathy. Obstruction initially causes hypertrophy of the musculature of the renal pelvis; if the obstruction persists, decompensation and dilatation occur and the resultant enlarged kidney can often be palpated on bimanual examination. As back pressure increases, the renal blood supply is compromised producing ischemia; eventually the renal parenchyma is destroyed, leaving a thin-walled cystic mass. Ultrasound is an excellent diagnostic modality for this diagnosis whereas IVU shows the site and probable source of obstruction (given adequate renal function).

4. Tumor.
   a. Benign tumor is rare, usually too small to be palpated.
   b. Embryoma (Wilms' tumor) is malignant, usually occurs in children under 5 years; presenting sign often is a palpable mass in one or both flanks. Ultrasound helpful but CT imaging usually necessary for staging.
   c. Renal cell carcinoma (hypernephroma) is the most common renal malignant neoplasm; it is occasionally palpable in the flank if of sufficient size. Tumor extension into renal vein and inferior vena cava may produce (collateral) dilated veins in the abdominal wall. The left spermatic vein may be obstructed by tumor growing into the renal vein which produces a varicocele on the left side that does not decompress when the patient is supine. An acute right varicocele requires urgent retroperitoneal imaging. Ultrasound may be diagnostic. CT best for staging. MRI best to demonstrate large vessel invasion.

5. Renal calculi may produce costovertebral-angle tenderness, especially with associated pyelonephritis. Acute renal colic often produces abdominal distention and hypoactive or absent bowel sounds (ileus). IVU diagnostic.

6. Hypertension due to a stenotic lesion of the renal artery may produce a bruit heard anteriorly in upper quadrants of the abdomen. Diagnosis made by a high index of clinician suspicion. Arteriography best diagnostic choice.

7. Polycystic kidneys are usually bilateral and contain multiple cysts; as cysts enlarge, palpable masses (usually not tender unless infected) are produced and may be of considerable size. Ultrasound diagnostic.

8. Renal ectopia produces a palpable mass in the lower part of the abdomen, mandating preoperative urologic imaging. IVP diagnostic.
   a. Crossed renal ectopia. Both kidneys are on same side and are often fused, giving rise to a rather large mass which suggests neoplasm.
   b. Horseshoe kidney. The lower poles of the kidneys are fused, producing an isthmus of renal tissue across the midline, occasionally palpable in a thin person.

9. Ureter disorders.
   a. Ureterocele, retrocaval ureter, congenital stricture of ureter do not produce physical findings, unless the lesion causes hydronephrosis.
   b. Ectopic ureter. In the male, it always opens proximal to the external sphincter, and produces no characteristic physical findings. In the female however, it may empty into the uterus, cervix, vagina, or ves-

tibule, resulting in dribbling incontinence. The orifice can often be found on inspection, particularly after intravenous injection of indigo-carmine which colors the urine blue.

c. The ureter usually is involved in the inflammatory process of tuberculosis and may be shown to be severely strictured on imaging studies.

d. Chronic ureteritis. The ureter becomes fibrotic and shortened; rarely may be palpated on rectal examination in the male or vaginal examination in the female.

10. Ureteral calculi originate in kidney, pass into ureter, commonly become arrested in one of three narrowed areas: the ureteropelvic junction, the pelvic brim where the ureter crosses the iliac vessels, and the ureteral vesical junction. Ureteral colic produces *severe* pain, agitation, great tenderness in costovertebral angle, and often has associated abdominal distention, nausea, and vomiting with hypoactive bowel sounds (ileus).

B. Bladder.

1. Exstrophy of the bladder is a rare, serious, congenital anomaly, easily identified from inspection of the lower abdominal wall, and accompanied by inguinal hernias and epispadias. The rami of the symphysis pubis are separated, and if untreated the patient's gait is a "duck waddle."

2. Cystitis is the most common disorder of the bladder, particularly in females. Palpation over the suprapubic region often elicits tenderness.

3. Obstruction below the bladder may be due to vesicle neck hypertrophy or to hypertrophy of the prostate or rarely, congenital urethral valves. Chronic obstruction produces trabeculation, cellules, and diverticula. A decompensated bladder may follow as residual urine and bladder capacity increase; it may be palpated in the midline of the suprapubic region. Large diverticula also may be palpated. Pelvic ultrasound is diagnostic.

4. Bladder tumors and calculi are common, both producing irritative symptoms. Tumors occur particularly in smokers which usually produce no physical findings unless large.

5. Neurogenic bladder dysfunction results from various causes, which may produce pathognomonic physical findings.

a. Sensory paralytic bladder. Produced by a lesion affecting the sensory side of the reflex arc; saddle anesthesia, no bulbocavernosus reflex; suprapubic mass may be palpated when bladder decompensates.

b. Motor paralytic bladder. Produced by a lesion affecting the motor side of the reflex arc; no saddle anesthesia, no bulbocavernosus reflex; large distended bladder may be palpated. Patient is unable to initiate a bladder contraction.

c. Autonomous neurogenic bladder. Produced by a lesion affecting sacral segments 2, 3, 4; saddle anesthesia, no bulbocavernosus reflex; pressure in suprapubic region can force urine from bladder since the bladder neck is open.

d. Reflex neurogenic bladder. Produced by transverse myelitis or traumatic spinal cord injury; hyperactive bulbocavernosus reflex and urethral sphincter. Associated neurologic findings due to paraplegia.

e. Uninhibited neurogenic bladder. Occurs after cerebrovascular accidents, and in normal infants before myelinization of the spinal cord; normal bulbocavernosus reflex.

Sorting these "pure" dysfunctions into types is often not clinically realistic nor the critical patient management factor; the key is maintenance of urine storage at low pressure (bladder compliance) since loss of compliance leads to high bladder storage pressure which may be transmitted upstream and produce renal failure.

C. Penis and urethra.

1. Anomalies. Congenital anomalies are uncommon, but must be recognized to save the foreskin for later reconstruction if needed.

    a. Hypospadias (not uncommon). The urethral meatus is present on the ventral surface of the penis; classification is dependent on location of the external urethral meatus. Hypoplasia of the corpus spongiosum often causes an associated chordee.

    b. Epispadias (rare). The upper wall of urethra is absent and is often associated with exstrophy of the bladder; urinary incontinence is often present.

    c. Phimosis. Inability to retract the prepuce over the glans. A normal finding in young children. May occur as a result of recurrent infection or diabetes in adults.

    d. Paraphimosis. The prepuce is retracted behind the glans penis and cannot be returned to normal position; painful swelling of glans may occur. A urologic emergency.

    e. Priapism. Painful prolonged erection not associated with sexual stimulation. Corpus spongiosum and glans *not* involved. A urologic emergency.

    f. Peyronie's disease. An idiopathic fibrosis of the corpora cavernosa that produces a bent penis to the ipsilateral side when erect.

    g. Balanoposthitis. Painful infection of prepuce and glans penis in uncircumcised men, showing erythema, tenderness, sometimes a purulent discharge.

  2. Lesions and ulcers.

    a. Primary lesion of syphilis. *Painless* ulcer with indurated borders and relatively clean base; appears 2 to 4 weeks after infected sexual contact. Inguinal lymph nodes are often palpable, especially with superinfection.

    b. Chancroid. *Painful* ulcer with less sharp borders and dirty base.

    c. Lymphogranuloma venereum. Begins with small papular or vesicular penile lesion; buboes (painful enlarged inguinal lymph nodes) may ulcerate and drain.

    d. Granuloma inguinale. Painful superficial ulceration, erythematous and velvety in appearance (rare in northern climates).

    e. Epidermoid carcinoma. Painless ulceration that fails to heal; often begins under prepuce; almost always found in uncircumcised men. Palpable lymph nodes may indicate metastatic extension of neoplasm or superinfection.

    f. Stenosis of the external urethral meatus may produce a serious obstructive lesion. Meatal stenosis is often over-diagnosed in children since calibration is necessary for the diagnosis.

    g. Urethritis. The urethra may be tender to palpation, purulent discharge may occur. Wear gloves. Do not allow purulence near your eyes.

D. Scrotal contents.

  1. Epididymitis.

    a. Acute epididymitis (common). Inflammation of the epididymis results in a painful swelling in the scrotum; if progressive it may not be possible to distinguish the epididymis from the testis. Early in the process, globus minor (lower pole) first involved area.

    b. Chronic epididymitis. The epididymis is enlarged and indurated, may result from recurrent epididymitis and is often found only as a slightly tender globus minor.

    c. Tuberculous epididymitis may resemble acute or chronic epididymitis; the vas deferens may contain a group of beadlike enlargements (beading). The infection may fistulize through the scrotal skin.

  2. Acute orchitis (rare). Enlarged, painful testis; scrotal skin erythematous. May occur with any infectious disease process, most commonly mumps parotitis.

  3. Testicular tumor. Enlarged or heavy testis. Painless, nodular area must be regarded as tumor. Secondary hydroceles may develop; fluid will help ultrasound characterize mass. Simple hydroceles are common and transmit light readily, and also are an excellent acoustic window.

4. Torsion of the spermatic cord can result in acute ischemia to the distal epididymis and testis; this occurs commonly among prepubertal boys. The scrotum contains a painful, high-riding testicle. Acute testicular pain in children is a torsion until proved otherwise. Doppler ultrasound helpful in good hands.

E. Prostate and seminal vesicles

1. Prostatitis.

   a. Acute bacterial prostatitis causes fever, often urethral discharge and a very tender, enlarged prostate gland. It may progress to abscess. Gentle transrectal ultrasound is diagnostic for abscess, but not indicated unless clinical course is atypical.

   b. Chronic bacterial (or granulomatous) prostatitis may be asymptomatic; may cause the prostate to be boggy or irregular or with large areas of fibrous tissue simulating neoplasm. Biopsy required for diagnosis.

2. Benign prostatic hypertrophy. Very common in men over 50; overall prostate size not critical since the intraurethral protrusion produces obstruction. The gland is symmetric, with smooth rubbery consistency; median sulcus can be identified, well-defined lateral borders.

3. Carcinoma of prostate is very common in men over 60. Clinically detected lesions usually involve the posterior lobe where nodule on the posterior surface is readily palpable at rectal examination. More advanced malignant lesions usually are stony hard, irregular, and painless on palpation. Biopsy safe and necessary to determine clinical significance since grade and stage are critical.

V. **Available Technology**

A. Urinalysis (U/A). This is a key study. Too often it is done simply by dipstick which has a high false positive rate (especially blood). Much information can be obtained from a urinalysis when properly performed.

   Both the male and female urethra harbor bacteria and leukocytes. After careful cleansing of the urethral meatus and with the foreskin retracted in males and the labia separated in females, a clean mid-stream specimen is collected in a sterile container. Prompt examination of the urine specimen is important. The only clinically reliable voided urine from females is a normal one. Catheterized specimens are necessary for reliable diagnosis otherwise. Catheterization in the male may also be done with little risk.

B. Ultrasound. Excellent modality to screen both upper and lower urinary tracts. Noninvasive and requires no ionizing radiation.

C. Plain film of the abdomen. Shows the kidney, ureter and bladder (KUB) area. This is very helpful in the diagnosis of genitourinary disease. The position, shape and size of the kidneys can often be determined on the plain film. Evidence of bony abnormalities and soft-tissue densities may be identified, as may calcification in the region of the adrenals, kidneys, ureter, bladder, and prostate.

D. Intravenous urogram (IVU). Begins with a KUB which is the most important film. This visualizes the upper urinary tract in a physiologic manner. It is extremely valuable in the diagnosis of a wide variety of renal processes provided that renal function is adequate for safe excretion.

E. Cystogram. This is made by instilling radio-opaque fluid into the bladder via a catheter. Voiding cystourethrograms allow observation of the vesical neck and urethra. The presence or absence of reflux into one or both ureters may be observed. A critical trauma study often proceeded by urethrography.

F. Cystoscopy. Various optical systems which allow the examiner to directly observe the urethra, bladder neck, and bladder. Accessory instruments are available for ureteral catheterization, biopsy, fulguration, laser, and many operative procedures.

G. Retrograde urography. This is done by passing a catheter into the ureter at the time of cystoscopy. Contrast medium is injected to outline the collecting system and ureter. This procedure is particularly useful when sufficient outline of the collecting system is not obtained by intravenous urography or when renal function is inadequate to allow safe excretion of the contrast material.

H. CT scanning. Excellent modality to *ultimately* determine size, extent, and probable etiology of many urologic processes. Not necessary in most clinical cases.

I. MRI imaging. Noninvasive and no ionizing radiation. Complementary to CT scanning in many ways, but shows intravascular extension of diseases without invasive techniques.

J. Radionuclide studies. Imaging done with radiolabeled tracers that are useful assessments of *function*. Not good anatomic detail. Best used for determining degree of renal obstruction by provocative testing (using potent diuretic in conjunction with scanning).

K. Selective renal arteriography. This study is done with percutaneous puncture of the femoral artery; a catheter is inserted into the aorta just above the take off of the renal arteries. An aortic injection of contrast material is first made to show the position, health, and the number of the renal arteries. Each renal artery may be selectively catheterized to visualize the blood supply to its parenchyma. This procedure may be useful in the diagnosis of renal mass lesions or preparatory for parenchyma during surgery, parenchyma sparing surgery as well as the study of renal vascular disease (RVD).

L. The cost figures cited in this table are **basic direct costs**. The figures are difficult to obtain and change quickly. They include **only** the cost of the test itself (technician, equipment, time, materials). No professional costs (interpretation) are included. Costs vary from region to region based on differences in some components such as labor. However, the relative cost ranking should remain similar.

Procedure	Code
Urinalysis, not by dipstick	$
Ultrasonography	$$
Plain x-ray of the abdomen	$$
Intravenous urogram (IVU)	$$$
Cystogram	$$$
Cystoscopy	$$
Retrograde urography	$$$
Computed tomography (CT)	$$$
Magnetic resonance imaging (MRI)	$$$$
Radionuclide studies	$$$$$
Renal arteriography	$$$$$

$ = $0–$50; $$ = $50–$100; $$$ = $100–$200; $$$$ = $200–$500; $$$$$ = $500–$1000.

VI. Bibliography

Gillenwater JY, Grayhack JT, Howards SS, et al (eds). *Adult and Pediatric Urology*, 2nd ed. St. Louis: Mosby-YearBook; 1991.

Pollack HM (ed). *Clinical Urography: An Atlas and Textbook of Urological Imaging*. Philadelphia: WB Saunders; 1990.

Skinner DG, Lieskovsky G. *Diagnosis and Management of Genitourinary Cancer*. Philadelphia: WB Saunders; 1988.

Smith RB, Ehrlich RM. *Complications of Urologic Surgery: Prevention and Management*, 2nd ed. Philadelphia: WB Saunders; 1990.

Walsh PC, Retik AB, Stamey TA, et al (eds). *Campbell's Urology*, 6th ed. Philadelphia: WB Saunders; 1992.

VII. Key Search Words

The following key words reflect the content of this chapter. They are provided to assist with an on-line search of computer databases, such as MEDLINE, if you wish to pursue the topic of this chapter further.

Anuria
Bacteriuria
Dysuria
Enuresis
Hematuria
Priapism
Prostatic hypertrophy
Prostatic neoplasms
Pyuria
Oliguria
Testicular neoplasms
Urinary incontinence
Varicocele

12. HERNIA

Lisa M. Colletti

I. Glossary

Diaphragmatic hernia: occurs from defects in the diaphragm that allow the abdominal viscera to protrude into the thoracic cavity; they may be congenital or acquired.
Congenital
  Bochdalek's hernia: occurs through the posterolateral portion of the diaphragm.
  Morgagni's hernia: occurs through the anteromedial portion of the diaphragm.
Acquired
  Traumatic: may be secondary to either blunt or penetrating trauma.
  Hiatal and paraesophageal hernias
    Type I: "sliding hiatal hernia." The gastroesophageal junction moves up into the thoracic cavity.
    Type II: the gastroesophageal junction retains its normal position within the abdominal cavity, and part or all of the stomach herniates into the chest through the esophageal hiatus in the diaphragm. This is a true hernia and is enclosed by a peritoneal covering or sac.
    Type III: a combination of type I and type II; that is, the gastroesophageal junction moves up into the chest cavity and is accompanied by some or all of the stomach. This is also a true hernia and is covered by a peritoneal sac.
    Type IV: a type II or type III hernia in which additional organs besides the stomach have herniated up into the chest cavity.
Direct inguinal hernia: passes through Hesselbach's triangle in the inguinal region.
Epigastric hernia: protrudes through a defect in the linea alba, somewhere between the xiphoid and the umbilicus.
Femoral hernia: an abdominal wall defect that lies along the femoral canal, with the hernia sac presenting deep to the inguinal ligament. The structures of the femoral canal, from lateral to medial, include the femoral nerve, femoral artery, femoral vein, an "empty space," and some lymphatics: nerve, artery, vein, empty space, lymphatic (NAVEL). A femoral hernia lies within the empty space and therefore typically lies medial to the femoral artery and vein.
Hernia: a defect in the muscular enclosure of the abdominal or thoracic cavity.
Hesselbach's triangle: area in the inguinal region through which a direct inguinal hernia occurs. It is bounded by the inguinal ligament, the inferior epigastric vessels, and the lateral border of the rectus muscle.
Hydrocele: a cystic structure or mass, typically arising as a result of incomplete obliteration of the processus vaginalis. These are common in infancy and are often bilateral. Hydroceles may also occur in the scrotum in proximity to the testicle, within the labia, or anywhere along the inguinal canal. A hydrocele typically occurs adjacent to the spermatic cord when it lies within the inguinal canal in males.
Incarcerated hernia: the contents of the hernia sac cannot be returned to the abdominal cavity. There is no interference with the blood supply to the intestine and therefore no associated ischemia or inflammation.
Incisional hernia: hernia that occurs through a previous surgical incision.

Indirect inguinal hernia: a hernia that passes through the internal inguinal ring. It typically descends adjacent to the spermatic cord and may extend into the scrotum or labia.

Internal hernia: occurs within the peritoneal cavity.

Littre's hernia: contains a Meckel's diverticulum.

Lumbar hernias

Petit's triangle hernia (inferior lumbar hernia): the borders of this hernia are formed anteriorly by the external oblique muscle, posteriorly by the anterior border of the latissimus dorsi muscle, and inferiorly by the iliac crest.

Hernia of the superior triangle of Grynfeltt-Lesshaft: superior and anterior to a Petit's triangle hernia. The hernia's borders are formed superiorly by the 12th rib, inferiorly by the inferior margin of the serratus posticus muscle, anteriorly by the posterior border of the internal oblique muscle, and posteriorly by the anterior border to the erector spinae muscle.

Obturator hernia: protrudes through the obturator foramen. The Howship-Romberg sign is pathognomonic of this hernia and consists of pain along the obturator nerve—that is, pain radiating down the medial aspect of the thigh to the inner border of the knee. Obturator hernias are often palpable on rectal or vaginal examination along the lateral wall of the rectum or vagina, respectively.

Pantaloon or saddlebag hernia: a combined indirect and direct inguinal hernia that derives its name from the fact that the hernia sac becomes draped over the inferior epigastric vessels and is therefore somewhat "tented up" in the middle of the hernia sac, resembling saddlebags or a pair of pantaloons.

Perineal hernia: protrudes between the muscles or fascia forming the pelvic floor.

Reducible hernia: the contents of the hernia sac are able to be returned to the abdominal cavity.

Richter's hernia: only the antimesenteric border of the bowel wall is caught within the hernia defect. Strangulation usually occurs, with resultant localized gangrene. This may occur without signs or symptoms of bowel obstruction or only with signs of partial bowel obstruction. Richter's hernias are most commonly seen in association with femoral or obturator hernias.

Sciatic hernia: emerges through the greater or less sacrosciatic foramen. Patients often have pain that radiates down the sciatic nerve.

Sliding hernia: typically occurs in the inguinal location. The large intestine or bladder slips retroperitoneally between the leaves of its mesentery to protrude through the defect in the abdominal wall.

Spigelian hernia: occurs at the semilunar line of Douglas at the lateral margin of the rectus sheath, typically in the lower abdomen where the posterior rectus sheath is absent.

Strangulated hernia: an incarcerated hernia in which the blood supply to the bowel has been compromised, with resultant inflammation and possible gangrene of the involved viscera.

Umbilical hernia: a hernia that protrudes through the umbilical ring.

II. Anatomy and Risk Factors

A. All abdominal hernias are composed of a sac lined with peritoneum, which protrudes through a defect in the abdominal wall. The contents vary and may include omentum, small or large bowel, bladder, or any of the contents of the abdominal cavity (Figures 12-1 through 12-4).

B. Risk factors for the development of hernias include any factor that increases intra-abdominal pressure. Common risk factors are obesity and chronic constipation urinary straining (need to rule out benign prostatic hypertrophy and prostate cancer), chronic cough (common in smokers), pregnancy, and ascites. Always perform a rectal examination and guaiac test of the patient's stool because a change in bowel habits with new-onset straining, thus precipitating a hernia, may be a presenting pattern for a sigmoid or rectal cancer.

III. Techniques of Examination

A. Inguinal canal. In both men and women, perform the examination with the patient in both the standing and supine positions. It is almost always easier

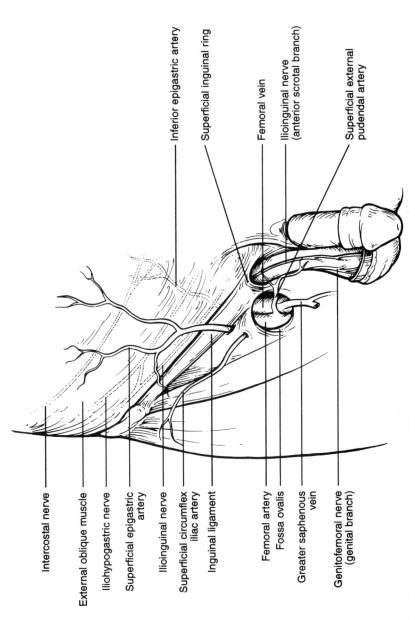

Fig. 12-1. Superficial groin anatomy of the male.

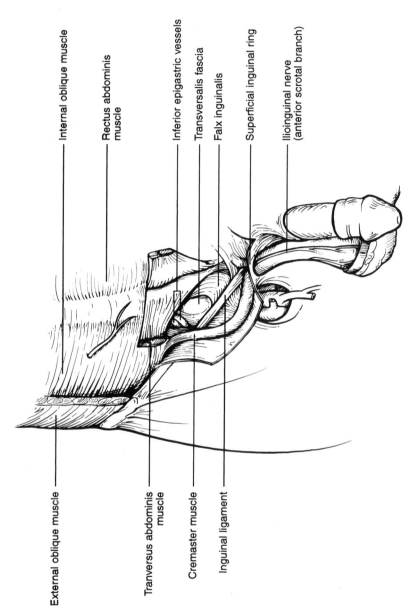

Internal oblique muscle

Rectus abdominis muscle

Inferior epigastric vessels

Transversalis fascia

Falx inguinalis

Superficial inguinal ring

Ilioinguinal nerve (anterior scrotal branch)

External oblique muscle

Tranversus abdominis muscle

Cremaster muscle

Inguinal ligament

Fig. 12-2. Deep groin anatomy of the male.

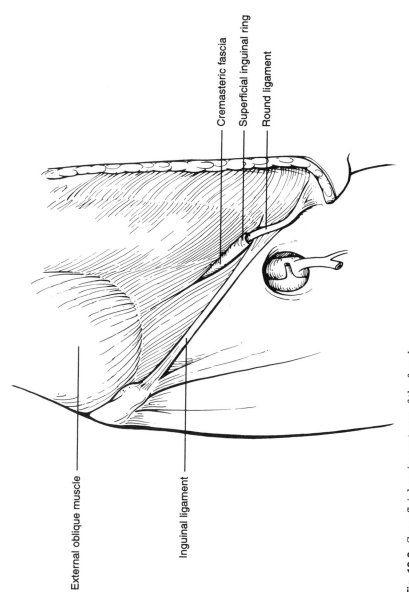

Fig. 12-3. Superficial groin anatomy of the female.

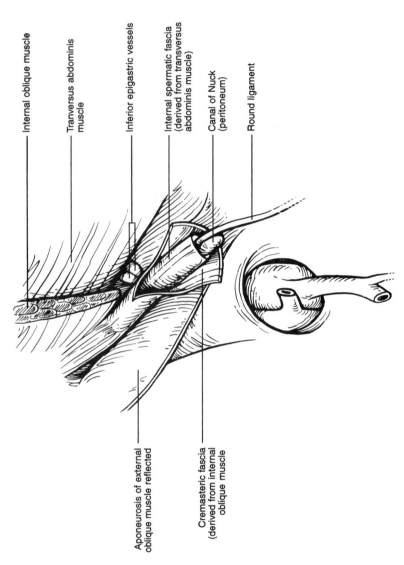

Internal oblique muscle

Tranversus abdominis muscle

Inferior epigastric vessels

Internal spermatic fascia (derived from transversus abdominis muscle)

Canal of Nuck (peritoneum)

Round ligament

Aponeurosis of external oblique muscle reflected

Cremasteric fascia (derived from internal oblique muscle

Fig. 12-4. Deep groin anatomy of the female.

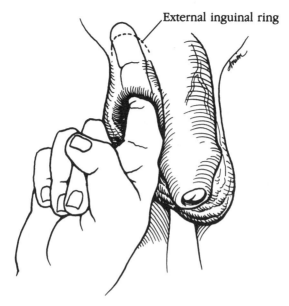

External inguinal ring

Fig. 12-5. Technique of examination of inguinal hernia.

to detect an inguinal hernia with the patient upright. Having the patient cough or perform a Valsalva's maneuver may also be helpful in detecting smaller hernias.

1. Examination of the male (Fig. 12-5). Slowly and gently insert the examining finger in the lower portion of the scrotum; invert the scrotum so that the examining finger passes up along the inguinal canal and palpates the external inguinal ring. The following structures are then identified:

   a. Extent of the os pubis

   b. The spermatic cord within the inguinal canal

   c. Size and boundaries of the external inguinal ring; enlargement of the external inguinal ring not diagnostic of hernia

   d. Hesselbach's triangle medial to the deep epigastric vessels

2. Examination in the female

   a. Identify the inguinal ligament and os pubis; locate the external inguinal ring. Having the patient cough or strain at this point may aid in the detection of a bulge.

   b. Place the palmar surface of the hand over the area of the internal inguinal ring and again ask the patient to cough or strain. This may allow you to feel a bulge or impulse.

   c. A small bulge may be visually detected by observing the inguinal area when the patient coughs or strains.

B. Femoral region

1. The external opening of the femoral canal is just medial to the femoral artery and deep to the inguinal ligament. The structures of the femoral canal from lateral to medial are nerve, artery, vein, empty space, lymphatic (NAVEL). A femoral hernia passes through the empty space.

2. The structures of the femoral canal can be visualized if the examiner is on the right side of the patient and places the right index finger on the patient's right femoral artery. Thus, the middle finger will overlie the

femoral vein and the ring finger will overlie the femoral canal—the area through which a femoral hernia will occur.

3. A femoral hernia often flips upward to overlie the inguinal ligament, thus presenting a somewhat confusing picture. Therefore, it is important to perform a careful examination of the inguinal canal to diagnose this problem properly.

C. Expected findings in elderly (>75 years)

1. Physical findings should be similar in the elderly to those seen in the rest of the population.

2. Systemic signs of sepsis may be very subtle in elderly patients. Therefore, the development of incarceration and especially strangulation may be recognized late in elderly patients.

3. *Worldwide, hernias are the most common cause of small bowel obstruction.* This diagnosis is an important consideration in an elderly patient with signs and symptoms of bowel obstruction, particularly in a person who has not had prior abdominal surgery.

III. Cardinal Symptoms and Abnormal Findings

A. Inguinal hernia

1. If a mass is felt within the inguinal canal, the presumptive diagnosis of hernia may be made.

2. This diagnosis is confirmed by the ability to completely reduce the hernia into the abdominal cavity.

3. Common inguinal pathology that may be confused with a hernia includes enlarged inguinal lymph nodes, a psoas abscess, varices of the main saphenous venous system, hydroceles, and femoral artery aneurysms.

4. Differentiation between direct and indirect hernias can be difficult. When a direct and indirect hernia occur simultaneously in the same patient, it is referred to as a *saddlebag* or *pantaloon hernia.*

5. Types of inguinal hernia

a. *Indirect inguinal hernias* are the most common type of inguinal hernia in both men and women and are the most common type of hernia in infants, children, and young adults. They have a congenital origin and result from a failure of the processus vaginalis to obliterate (Fig. 12-6).

(1) An indirect inguinal hernia passes through the internal inguinal ring, traverses the inguinal canal in proximity to the spermatic cord, and may also pass through the external inguinal ring. The hernia sac may extend into the scrotum or labia.

(2) The sac lies anterior and medial to the spermatic cord; this is usually not detectable at the time of physical examination, but is clearly obvious during surgical repair. In addition, the neck of the sac is lateral to the deep inferior epigastric vessels and passes through the internal inguinal ring.

(3) An indirect hernia can be differentiated from a direct hernia if it is palpable above Hesselbach's triangle, passing through the internal inguinal ring.

b. *Direct inguinal hernias* are more common in persons over age 40. They result from a weakness in the transversalis fascia forming the floor of Hesselbach's triangle.

(1) A direct inguinal hernia protrudes through Hesselbach's triangle, and the neck of the sac is medial to the deep inferior epigastric vessels.

(2) This hernia does not lie in close proximity to the cord and may pass through the external inguinal ring.

(3) The boundaries of Hesselbach's triangle are the inguinal ligament, the inferior epigastric vessels, and the lateral border of the rectus muscle.

B. Femoral hernia (common location for a Richter's hernia)

1. Femoral hernias are more common in women than men.

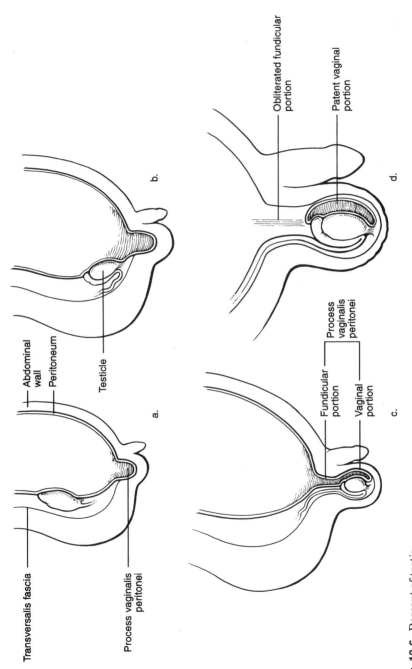

Fig. 12-6. Descent of testis.

2. They must be distinguished from enlarged lymph nodes, a saphenous varix, femoral artery aneurysms, and psoas abscesses.

3. Large femoral hernias are often directed upward and then overlie the inguinal ligament, often making diagnosis difficult. In these cases, the sac lies lateral to, and below the level of the symphysis pubis.

4. *Strangulation* may be difficult to detect, particularly in elderly patients, since local signs may be minimal. Systemic signs indicate the need for careful inspection of the inguinal canals, and potential urgent operation.

   a. Systemic signs: tachycardia, tachypnea, fever, and leukocytosis.

   b. Local signs: erythema and edema of the overlying skin and pain and tenderness at the site.

   c. Most common sites for the development of a Richter's hernia: the femoral and obturator canals.

   d. Localized gangrene of the bowel wall without frank intestinal obstruction may lead to bowel perforation and abscess formation just below the inguinal ligament. This may be difficult to differentiate from a psoas abscess or femoral lymphadenitis.

C. Sliding hernia. This hernia typically occurs in the inguinal location. On the right side, the cecum is often the presenting organ. On the left side, the sigmoid is often involved. The bladder may be involved on either side and typically forms the medial wall of the hernia sac. Sliding hernias may be difficult to reduce.

   1. The large intestine or bladder slips retroperitoneally between the leaves of its mesentery to protrude through the defect in the abdominal wall.

   2. At least a portion of this hernia is not contained within a peritoneal sac in that the retroperitoneal portion of the bowel or bladder makes up one of the walls of the hernia sac.

   3. During repair, care needs to be taken not to injure the bowel or bladder wall during excision of the sac and repair of the defect.

D. Incarcerated and strangulated hernias. Differentiation is often difficult. The patient is always at risk for the development of ischemic or gangrenous bowel.

   1. An incarcerated hernia cannot be reduced; its contents cannot be returned to the peritoneal cavity. It is reasonable to attempt nonoperative reduction of a recently incarcerated hernia, as long as the patient lacks signs of strangulation—no redness of the skin overlying the hernia, no significant pain or edema in the area of the hernia, and no fever, tachycardia, tachypnea, or leukocytosis.

      a. Nonoperative reduction. With the patient lying down, gentle pressure is applied to the hernia in an attempt to return the sac and its contents through the muscular defect. Other maneuvers that can aid in this process are the administration of a mild sedative to the patient, lowering the head of the bed, and flexing the leg on the affected side to relax the abdominal musculature.

      b. Surgical reduction. If any signs of strangulation are present (see preceding section on strangulation), operative reduction and repair should be urgently performed after the patient has been adequately resuscitated.

   2. Strangulated hernia. Strangulation occurs when the blood supply to the viscera within the hernia sac has been interrupted. If there is any question of strangulation, nonoperative reduction should *not* be attempted.

      a. Local signs of inflammation: pain, edema, and erythema

      b. Systemic signs of inflammation (in more advanced cases): fever, tachycardia, tachypnea, and leukocytosis

E. Hydrocele. If the processus vaginalis is not completely obliterated, fluid may accumulate within the involved segment, producing a cystic mass in the inguinal, labial, or scrotal region.

   1. In males, hydrocele of the testicle may occur in the scrotum, whereas hydrocele of the cord presents within the inguinal canal. Transillumination

can often help to differentiate a hydrocele from an incarcerated hernia or testicular tumor. Hydroceles are particularly common in infancy and are often bilateral. They may spontaneously regress; however, hydroceles may also indicate the presence of an indirect inguinal hernia if the processus vaginalis has continued to remain patent.

2. In females, hydroceles may develop anywhere between the internal inguinal ring and the labia majora. A hydrocele of the canal of Nuck is characterized by a cystic, irreducible, translucent appearance.

F. Umbilical hernia. An umbilical hernia passes through the umbilical ring.

1. Newborns. These hernias are particularly common in newborns and often spontaneously close by age 2 years.

   a. A congenital umbilical hernia results from incomplete closure of the abdominal wall.

   b. An *omphalocele* is a hernia of the umbilical cord that is not covered by skin.

2. Infants and children. True umbilical hernias are common; increased abdominal pressure due to trauma, coughing, or constipation may be precipitating factors.

3. Adults. Umbilical hernias are more common in women; they are associated with diastasis or separation of the rectus muscles in the midline.

   a. Contributing factors include obesity, pregnancy, ascites, and preexisting congenital defects.

   b. Size varies widely, but the neck of the sac is often small, thereby increasing the risk of incarceration and strangulation.

   c. The hernia sacs often contain omentum, but may also contain large or small bowel or other abdominal viscera.

G. Epigastric hernia. An epigastric hernia protrudes through a weakness in the linea alba between the xiphoid and pubis and is usually related to a developmental defect.

1. These hernias are most frequently seen in young adult males.

2. Contributing factors include trauma, obesity, constipation, pregnancy, chronic coughing, and urinary straining.

3. The sac is usually small and contains omentum. Intestine is rarely present within the sac and strangulation is rare.

H. Incisional hernia. This type of hernia is the result of previous surgical incisions.

1. Contributing factors include infection, poor wound healing, faulty wound closure, postoperative vomiting, ileus, partial wound disruption, obesity, and poor nutrition.

2. Incisional hernias are often quite large, with the abdominal viscera adherent to the undersurface of the peritoneum.

3. Strangulation is uncommon.

I. Spigelian hernia. Located in the semilunar line of Douglas at the lateral margin of the rectus muscle, spigelian hernias are usually in the lower abdomen below the umbilicus where the posterior rectus sheath is absent.

J. Diaphragmatic hernia. This hernia results from defects in the diaphragm; the abdominal contents protrude into the chest cavity. The hernia may be detectable on physical examination by auscultation of bowel sounds within the chest cavity and dullness to percussion of the chest wall. Diagnosis of diaphragmatic hernia is often made with a plain chest x-ray

1. Congenital: some portion of the diaphragm absent

   a. Morgagni's: anteromedial defect

   b. Bochdalek's: posterolateral defect

2. Traumatic: may be related to either blunt or penetrating trauma

3. Acquired: most commonly include hiatal and paraesophageal hernias; diagnosis suggested on history, but cannot be made on physical examination

   a. Type I: sliding hiatal hernia. This hernia is commonly associated with gastroesophageal reflux and is very common in the general population. The gastroesophageal junction slides up into the thoracic cavity.

      b. Type II: a paraesophageal hernia, which is a true hernia and is contained within a peritoneal sac. Some or all of the stomach herniates through the esophageal hiatus, up into the chest cavity. The gastroesophageal junction retains its proper position below the diaphragm within the abdominal cavity.

      c. Type III: a combined type I and type II hernia. The gastroesophageal junction slides up into the chest cavity, and some or all of the stomach herniates within a true peritoneal hernia sac up into the chest cavity.

      d. Type IV: additional abdominal contents herniated through the esophageal hiatus into the chest.

K. Rare hernias

   1. *Sciatic hernias* emerge through the greater or lesser sciatic foramen. Patients may have pain radiating down the sciatic nerve.

   2. *Perineal hernias* protrude between the muscles or fascia of the pelvic floor.

   3. *Lumbar hernias* protrude through the inferior triangle of Petit or the superior triangle of Grynfeltt-Lesshaft (see Glossary).

   4. *Obturator hernias* present through the obturator foramen. Patients often present with a Howship-Romberg sign, which is pain along the obturator nerve (pain radiating down the medial aspect of the thigh to the knee). These hernias are difficult to detect and may be palpable on rectal or vaginal examination as a tender swelling along the lateral aspect of the rectal or vaginal wall. Obturator hernias commonly incarcerate; they are one of the most common locations for the presentation of a Richter's hernia.

   5. *Internal hernias* occur within the peritoneal cavity and commonly present with signs and symptoms of small or larger bowel obstruction, including nausea, vomiting, obstipation, and abdominal distention.

V. Available Technology

The most important technique for the diagnosis of a hernia remains the history and physical examination. In most cases, the diagnosis of a hernia can be made without the need for additional tests. However, in more difficult or subtle cases, the following additional modalities of testing may be helpful to confirm or exclude the diagnosis of hernia.

A. Ultrasonography. This inexpensive, easy test can often confirm or refute the presence of a hernia, especially in a slender person.

B. Computed tomography (CT) scanning. A more expensive test, it is probably the most sensitive method of detecting a hernia that is not clear-cut on physical examination or in an obese person.

C. Herniography.

D. The cost figures cited in this table are **basic direct costs**. The figures are difficult to obtain and change quickly. They include **only** the cost of the test itself (technician, equipment, time, and materials). No professional costs (interpretation) are included. Costs vary from region to region based on differences in some components such as labor. However, the relative cost ranking should remain similar.

Procedure	Code
Ultrasonography	$$
Computed tomography (CT)	$$$$
Herniography	*

$$ = $50–$100; $$$$ = $200–$500; * = highly variable or not available.

VI. Bibliography

Cameron JL, ed. *Current Surgical Therapy,* 4th ed. St. Louis: Mosby-Year Book; 1992;34-36,526–543.

Ekberg O, Abrahamsson PA, Kesek P. Inguinal hernia in urological patients: the value of herniography. *J Urol* 1988;139:1253–1255.

Ekberg O, Fritsdorf J, Blomquist P. Herniographic appearance of contralateral inguinal hernia. *Acta Radiol: Diagn* 1984;25:125–128.

Greene WW. Bowel obstruction in the aged patient: a review of 300 cases. *Am J Surg* 1969;118:541–545.

Gullmo A. Herniography. The diagnosis of hernia in the groin and incompetence of the pouch of Douglas and pelvic floor. *Acta Radiol* 1980;361(Suppl):1–76.

Lo CY, Lorentz TG, Lau PW. Obturator hernia presenting as small bowel obstruction. *Am J Surg* 1994;167:396–398.

McVay CB, ed. *Anson and McVay Surgical Anatomy 1984*. Philadelphia: WB Saunders; 1984;484–584.

McVay CB, Read RC, Ravitch MM. Inguinal hernia. *Curr Probl Surg* 1967;1–50.

Nyhus LM, ed. *Shakelford's Surgery of the Alimentary Tract, V*. Philadelphia: WB Saunders; 1991;99–151.

VII. Key Search Words

The following key words reflect the content of this chapter. They are provided to assist with an on-line search of computer databases, such as MEDLINE, if you wish to pursue the topic of this chapter further.

Abdominal muscles
Groin
Hernia
Hernia, diaphragmatic
Hernia, femoral
Hernia, hiatal
Hernia, inguinal
Hernia, obturator
Hernia, umbilical
Hernia, ventral
Inguinal canal
Physical examination

13. FEMALE REPRODUCTIVE SYSTEM

Mel L. Barclay

I. Glossary

Abortion: spontaneous, medical, or surgical interruption of pregnancy with fetal death before the time of fetal viability (usually before 20 weeks of gestation).

Adnexa: ovaries, fallopian tubes.

Amenorrhea: absence of menses.

Cystocele: hernial protrusion of the urinary bladder though the anterior vaginal wall.

Dysmenorrhea: painful menses.

Hypermenorrhea (menorrhagia): abnormally increased volume of menstrual flow.

Menarche: the beginning of menstrual function.

Menopause: termination of menses at the end of a normal reproductive span of years.

Miscarriage: a nonmedical term for premature expulsion of a fetus.

Multipara: a woman who has borne more than one child.

Polymenorrhea (metrorrhagia): abnormally increased frequency of menstrual flow.

Primigravida: a woman pregnant for the first time.

Primipara: a woman who has borne one viable infant.

Rectocele: hernial protrusion of rectal wall into the vagina.

II. Gynecologic History
  A. General medical history
  B. Catamenial information including the last normal menstrual period.
   1. Age of first menstrual period
     a. Typically around 12.5 years in North America
     b. Other pubertal events that precede menarche:
       (1) Prepubertal growth spurt
       (2) Thelarche: appearance of breasts
       (3) Adrenarche: development of pubic and axillary hair
     c. Delayed menarche—usually constitutional but may be associated with the following:
       (1) Male genotype or other genetic abnormality
       (2) Endocrine abnormalities
       (3) Abnormal or absent genital structure
       (4) Vigorous and protracted exercise
       (5) Bulimia or anorexia
   2. Age at time of cessation of menses if past climacteric
     a. Usually around 55
     b. Patient defined as menopausal after 12 months of amenorrhea
     c. Presence or absence of menopausal symptoms
       (1) Hot flushes
       (2) Sleep disturbances
       (3) Vaginal discomfort with or following intercourse
       (4) Decreased vaginal lubrication with sexual stimulation
       (5) New onset of stress or urge urinary incontinence
   3. Frequency (interval) of menstrual flow (Treolar et al, 1967)
     a. Normal range in human females is 21 to 35 days.
     b. Interval may be irregular at both early and late extremes of menstrual life.

      c. Interval is most regular with least variation between 25 and 38 years of age.

      d. Some variation is customary and normal with occasional anovulatory cycles.

      e. Acute stress either physical or psychological may disturb normal cyclicity.

      f. Changes occur with *abnormal pregnancy,* anovulation, endocrinopathies, pelvic tumors, and ovarian malignancy.

    4. Duration of flow

      a. Usually less variable than duration of flow

      b. Average between 3 and 5 days

      c. Normal pattern of flow:

        (1) Begins slowly with spotting

        (2) When ovulatory, may be associated with physiologic premenstrual symptoms:

          (a) Breast tenderness

          (b) Fluid retention

          (c) Mood change

          (d) Appetite changes

          (e) Dysmenorrhea

          (f) Change in nature of vaginal discharge

        (3) Rapidly becomes heavy requiring tampons or menstrual pads

        (4) Tapers off rapidly with only spotting on last several days

      d. Changes indicative of *abnormal pregnancy,* uterine leiomyomata, menopause, uterine malignancy, and anovulatory dysfunctional bleeding

    5. Character of flow

      a. Usually no clots

      b. Commonly dark in color

      c. Changes possibly reflective of *abnormal pregnancy,* increased uterine surface area (tumors), lack of normal maturation (anovulation), or cervical or vaginal malignancy particularly with postcoital variant

C. Obstetric history

    1. Gravidity: number of times pregnant

    2. Parity: number of viable pregnancies delivered

    3. Abortions: spontaneous, elective losses before 20 weeks' gestation

    4. Living children

    5. Premature deliveries: earlier than 37 weeks

    6. Major complications

      a. Hemorrhage

      b. Infection

      c. Toxemia of pregnancy

      d. Surgical or instrumental delivery

      e. Significant obstetrical lacerations

III. Examination Techniques and Normal Findings

A. Equipment and personnel necessary for examination

    1. Examination table that permits lithotomy position

    2. Portable white light source that can be focused

    3. Stool for examiner

    4. Assortment of sizes of vaginal specula

    5. Materials for collection of Papanicolaou (Pap) smears:

      a. Clean glass slides

      b. Ayers-type spatula for cervical sampling

      c. Spray fixative for immediate fixation of slides

      d. Cotton-tipped applicator moistened with saline for collection of endocervical sample

    6. Rubber gloves (clean, not necessarily sterile)

    7. Culture tubes for gonorrhea, *Chlamydia*

    8. Instruments for biopsy of lesions observed

9. A patient gown and sheet for proper draping during the examination
10. A chaperone (for *both* male and female examiners) to assist with collection of specimens and function as a patient advocate (Buchta, 1986)

B. General considerations

1. The appropriate medical approach to pelvic examination is *circumspect.* The examiner should be sensitive to the patient's need for privacy and the special nature of the examination. The examination should be gentle, thorough, and respectful. An approach that fosters patient education and patient-examiner cooperation produces significantly more positive attitudes toward the examination (Willard et al, 1986).

   First-time pelvic examination experiences should include a discussion of the procedure and a demonstration of the instruments and how they work (Koadlow, 1990; Vella, 1991; Hein, 1984).

2. All physicians should be prepared to carry out pelvic examinations or to refer their patients for such examinations.

3. All women of reproductive age (ages 15 to 45) and beyond, especially those who are sexually active, should have regular pelvic examinations. Regular examination of prepubertal females may also be valuable. Reassurance without examination is inappropriate (Balk, et al, 1982).

4. The patient should disrobe privately and be provided with a gown, preferably tied in the back. She should empty her bladder before the examination to minimize discomfort and facilitate uterine palpation. An additional linen or paper sheet is necessary for draping the patient.

5. The patient is placed in the lithotomy position with the buttocks at the end of the examining table. This may be facilitated by assisting the patient when she places her feet in the foot supports. By placing the back of the examiner's hand at the end of the table and asking the patient to slide down until she feels contact, the proper examination position can be obtained without repeated adjustment by the patient or the examiner (Fig. 13-1A).

C. Examination of the external genitalia

1. Before exposing the perineum, ask the patient to allow her legs to fall apart. The examiner can demonstrate this by showing the patient hands together and then falling apart as the pages of a book (Fig. 13-2). This provides a very neutral and precise description of the position required for perineal and pelvic examination and illustrates for the patient precisely what is needed. Expose the perineum by lifting the drape.

2. Inspect the vulvar structures including the escutcheon, clitoris, labia majora, labia minora, urethral meatus, and vaginal introitus (Fig. 13-3). This may be facilitated by applying lateral traction on the pudendum lateral to the labia majora. Before applying such traction, however, the examiner should announce the intention to touch and make first contact

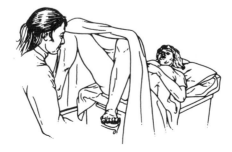

Fig. 13-1. The proper examination position.

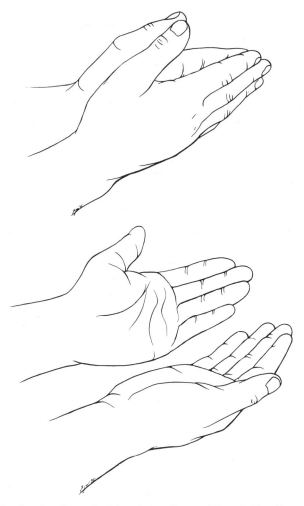

Fig. 13-2. By showing the patient hands together and then letting them fall apart like the pages of a book, the examiner can demonstrate the position required for perineal and pelvic examination.

with the back of the hand on the medial thigh away from the genital area. With the labial structures retracted laterally, asking the patient to bear down or cough will permit observation of cystocele or rectocele (Fig. 13-4). If the bladder is full of urine, this may demonstrate stress urinary incontinence. Also, the perineal "wink," which this touching elicits is a normal reflex that is integrated at S2-S4.

3. Inspect the perineal and perianal areas for evidence of episiotomy scars, condylomata, hemorrhoids, and dermatologic lesions. Note the presence or absence of pediculi on the pubic hair, any vaginal discharge present that is obvious on the perineum, and the appearance of any vulvar abnormalities, particularly evidence of white dystrophic lesions or signs of

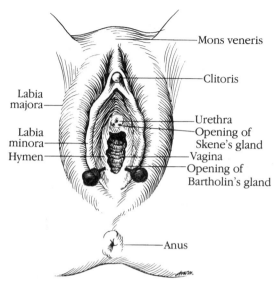

Fig. 13-3. External female genitalia.

chronic scratching in menopausal women. Note the general configuration of the vaginal introitus. Does it gape as in parous women, or is it closed as in young nulliparous women?

    4. Palpate (after announcing your touch as above) the area of Bartholin's glands. Normal glands are not palpable (Fig. 13-5). Gently attempt to express purulent material from Skene's periurethral glands.

D. Examination of the internal genitalia

    1. Speculum insertion

        a. After lubricating the speculum with warm water, hold the speculum by the handle so that the blades are between the index and middle fingers.

        b. While separating the labia with the other hand, introduce the speculum with the blades oblique and the pressure largely against the posterior fourchette (Fig. 13-6). This avoids the sensitive anterior structures.

        c. When the blades have passed the introitus, rotate the speculum so that the blades are horizontal and the handle is at approximately 45 degrees off a line perpendicular to the surface of the examining table.

        d. The tip of the speculum should be directed posteriorly toward the table surface in the axis of the vagina until the blades of the instrument are completely within the vagina.

        e. Once completely inserted, open the blades of the speculum by pressing gently on the thumbpiece attached to the upper blade in order to expose the cervix and vaginal walls. Tighten the knurled knob to maintain this exposure.

    2. Inspection

        a. Note the presence of normal or abnormal vaginal secretions including the color, transparency or opacity, and amount. Depending on the phase of the menstrual cycle, these secretions may be copious or scant, crystalline and stretchable, or thick and tenacious.

        b. The vaginal walls are normally pink and rugose in the woman of reproductive age. In prepubertal, menopausal, and lactating women,

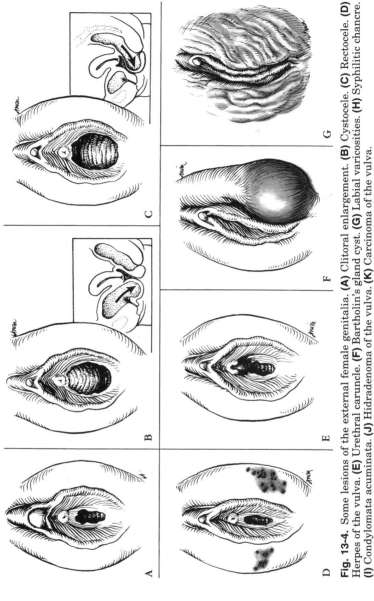

Fig. 13-4. Some lesions of the external female genitalia. **(A)** Clitoral enlargement. **(B)** Herpes of the vulva. **(E)** Urethral caruncle. **(F)** Bartholin's gland cyst. **(G)** Labial varicosities. **(H)** Syphilitic chancre. **(I)** Condylomata acuminata. **(J)** Hidradenoma of the vulva. **(K)** Carcinoma of the vulva.

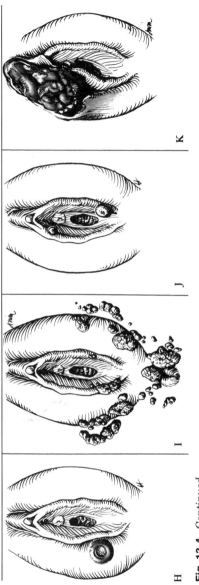

Fig. 13-4. *Continued*

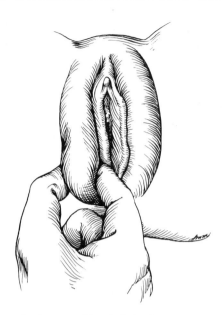

Fig. 13-5. Technique of palpation of Bartholin's glands.

the rugosity is diminished or absent, and the vaginal walls are thin and more pale.

  c. The squamocolumnar junction is most often visible in young nulliparous women and those of reproductive age. In the nulliparous woman, the cervical os is circular, whereas in parous women it may be more slit-like or have a stellate appearance resulting from obstetric injury. The cervical os and endocervix may be more and less visible as the speculum opens and closes in the parous woman. Observe and note the presence of polyps, surface vessels, and lesions, particularly in the area of the squamocolumnar junction. Nabothian inclusion cysts on the vaginal surface of the cervix are also common (Fig. 13-7).

  d. The axis of the cervix, whether pointing anteriorly, posteriorly, or centrally in the vagina, gives some indication of the position of the uterine fundus.

3. Collection of materials for microscopic examination including the Pap smear is most efficiently done during this phase of the examination.

  a. Where materials for hanging drop or wet mount are secured using cotton-tipped applicators, they should be suspended in 2 to 3 mL of warmed, normal saline in a small test tube. A normal wet mount will show vaginal epithelial cells, bacteria (classically gram-positive *Lactobacilli,* and other organisms) and menstrual detritus if the patient is bleeding at the time. In vaginitis produced by pathogens such as *Trichomonas hominis, Candida albicans*, and bacterial vaginosis, the findings will differ. Vaginal pH may also be determined by applying the secretions obtained onto standard pH paper.

  b. The Pap smear is accomplished by scraping the external os of the cervix with an Ayers-type spatula and applying the obtained scrapings to a clean glass slide (Fig. 13-8). The endocervical canal is sampled next by insertion of a saline-moistened cotton-tipped applicator

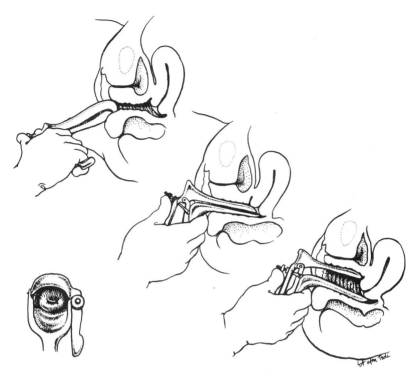

Fig. 13-6. Insertion of the vaginal speculum (see text).

into the endocervical canal. This may be smeared on the same glass slide. To prevent drying artifact and to ensure proper adhesion to the slide, it is important that the materials be fixed *immediately* either by spraying with an alcohol-containing fixative or by immersing them in ether-alcohol.

4. Bimanual internal digital examination. Intravaginal and abdominal manipulation assist in bringing pelvic structures into a position in which they can be palpated either vaginally or through the abdomen.

a. Remove the speculum carefully, examining the vaginal walls in their entirety by rotation of the blades of the speculum while removing it from the vagina. The examiner should be careful to have the speculum mostly closed while it exits the vagina so that it does not snap open, traumatizing the urethral meatus and the labia minora.

b. Lubricate the first two fingers well with water-soluble material. Announce your touch, and then place the index finger at the posterior vaginal fourchette and press posteriorly. Wait for the perineum to relax and then advance the finger gently along the posterior vaginal wall all the way into the vagina until the cervix becomes palpable. Manipulation of the cervix should not produce pain or discomfort (Fig. 13-9).

c. Vaginal fornices. Placing one finger into the lateral vaginal fornices, note whether they are of equal depth. Obstetric injuries with tearing of uterine supports may cause the fornices to be unequal in depth, as

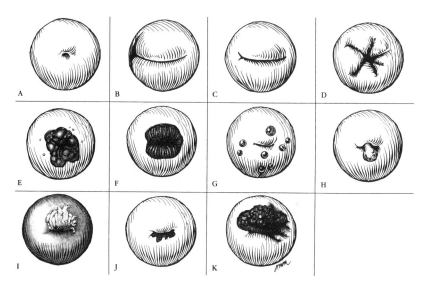

Fig. 13-7. Some cervical lesions. **(A)** Virgin. **(B)** Parous. **(C)** Minor tear. **(D)** Stellate tear. **(E)** Erosion. **(F)** Eversion. **(G)** Cysts. **(H)** Polyp. **(I)** Leukoplakia. **(J)** Early cancer. **(K)** Advanced cancer.

may the presence of uterine anomalies, tumors, and adnexal masses. Similarly assess the anterior and posterior fornices.

d. Positioning intravaginal fingers for internal examination. Remove the single finger from the vagina and depress the perineum with two fingers. Wait for perineal relaxation and advance two fingers into the posterior vaginal fornix. Push upward and anterior to elevate the uterine fundus toward the abdominal wall. If the uterus is retroverted or in midposition, other maneuvers may be necessary such as placement of fingers in the anterior vaginal fornix.

e. Uterus. Place the abdominal hand halfway between the umbilicus and the symphysis pubis and press downward toward the pelvis while pressing upward with the intravaginal fingers. The uterine fundus should be palpable with the abdominal hand. Assess mobility, size, symmetry, and consistency. It is often possible to capture the uterus between the vaginal and abdominal hand. Most of uterine palpation and assessment is done with the abdominal hand.

f. Uterine ligaments and fallopian tubes (parametria). Generally, these structures are not palpable unless there is some pathology present. Place two fingers lateral to the cervix on one side of the uterus and then the other while palpating the lateral portions of the uterus. Sausage-shaped, tender masses lateral to the uterus suggest tubal ectopic pregnancy, broad ligament leiomyomata, or pyo- or hydrosalpinges.

g. Ovaries (adnexa). Place the vaginal fingers high in the lateral vaginal fornix and, with the fingers of the abdominal hand, sweep the area lateral to the uterus downward toward the inguinal ligament. The ovaries, which are difficult to palpate under normal conditions, are usually more palpable with the vaginal than the abdominal fingers. The patient may express discomfort as the ovary moves past the examining fingers.

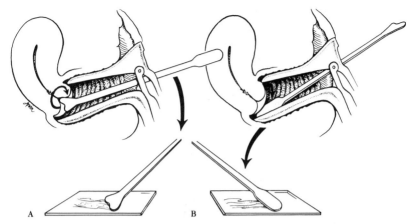

Fig. 13-8. Technique of the Papanicolaou smear. **(A)** Cervical scraping. **(B)** Vaginal pool sampling.

h. Rectovaginal. This area is done last because it is the most uncomfortable portion of the examination. Change gloves to prevent passage of potential pathogens from the vagina and cervix to the rectum. Lubricate the first and second fingers well. Place the first finger in the vagina and the second at the anal verge. Press on the perineum with the vaginal finger while asking the patient to bear down as if having a bowel movement. The perineum and the anus will relax simultaneously. Advance the rectal finger in an anterior and upward (ventral) direction at the same time as you advance the vaginal finger. The rectovaginal septum is palpable between the two fingers. Normally, this septum is supple and without nodularity. With the rectal finger, assess for the presence or absence of internal hemorrhoids or masses in

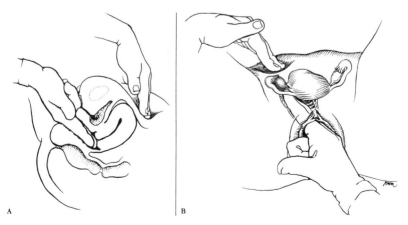

Fig. 13-9. Technique of bimanual pelvic examination. **(A)** Lateral view. **(B)** Perineal view.

the anal canal and rectal ampulla. Assess the posterior aspect of the cervix and the posterior *cul-de-sac* for nodularity, which is characteristic of endometriosis. If the uterus is in a retroverted position, the fundus may be more easily palpated by combined rectovaginal and abdominal examination (Fig. 13-10).

    i. Stool obtained on the rectal examination may be assessed for the presence of blood using a standard guaiac test.

  5. After the examination is completed, dispense with the gloves, encourage the patient to push back with her feet, and offer assistance in sitting up at the end of the table.

E. Special techniques applicable to pregnancy

  1. Physical findings diagnostic of pregnancy

    a. Cyanosis of the cervix and upper vagina (Chadwick's sign).

    b. Softening of the cervical isthmus: the segment of the uterus connecting the cervix with the uterine fundus becomes very soft in pregnancy, producing a sensation of separation between the upper and lower portions of the uterus (Hegar's sign).

    c. Asymmetric softening of the uterine fundus (Piskacek's sign).

  2. Physical examination techniques for the identification of fetal position in a known pregnancy (Leopold's maneuvers [Leopold and Sporlin, 1894]) (Fig. 13-11)

    a. Leopold's first maneuver. Facing the mother's head, gently palpate the uterine fundus with the fingers to ascertain the contents. The breech position is soft and irregular. The fetal head is firmer, more regular, and ballotable.

    b. Leopold's second maneuver. Facing the mother's head, determine which side of the uterus the fetal back is on. The back is smooth and firm, and at times the washboard-like feeling of fetal ribs can be palpated. The opposite side containing the fetal small parts (arms, legs, knees, and elbows) will feel irregular.

    c. Leopold's third maneuver. Facing the mother's head and using the thumb and forefingers, grasp the lower portion of the maternal ab-

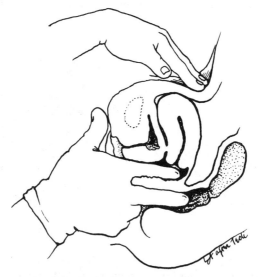

Fig. 13-10. Technique of rectovaginal examination.

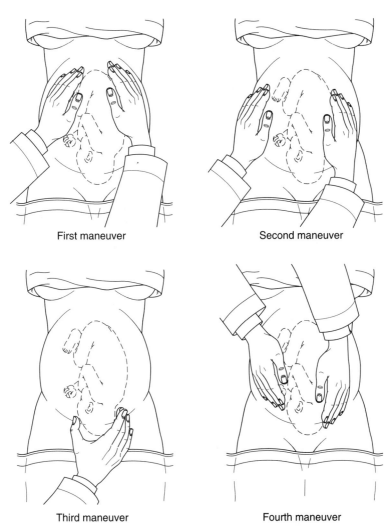

First maneuver

Second maneuver

Third maneuver

Fourth maneuver

Fig. 13-11. Longitudinal lie. Palpation in left occiput anterior position (LOP) (maneuvers of Leopold). (Adapted from Cunningham. *William's Obstetrics,* 19th ed. Norwalk, CT: Appleton & Lange.)

domen just above the symphysis pubis. If the presenting part, usually the head, has passed through the pelvic inlet, it will not move laterally. If the presenting part is not the head, this maneuver provides additional evidence.

d. Leopold's fourth maneuver. Facing toward the mother's feet, use fingers to make deep pressure downward and in the direction of the pelvic inlet. If the head is presenting, the fingers of one hand will meet a rounded firm body before the fingers of the other hand. The rounded body is the occiput of the fetal head or cephalic prominence.

This aids in determining fetal presentation in association with the findings of the other maneuvers.

IV. Cardinal Symptoms and Abnormal Findings

A. Pain on examination is usually a reflection of inflammatory processes. Normally, pelvic examination, like intercourse, is not especially uncomfortable. The uterus is usually mobile without eliciting discomfort.

B. Cervical motion tenderness. Manipulation or induced movement of the cervix that causes severe pain or discomfort is usually a reflection of pelvic peritonitis or the presence of some irritating fluid, such as blood or ovarian cyst contents.

C. Fullness or bulging of the *cul-de-sac* (posterior vaginal fornix) may indicate the presence of blood, fluid, or purulent material. A fluctuant mass suggests a tumor or abscess.

D. Voluntary guarding on abdominal or pelvic examination may make complete assessment of the pelvic organs impossible. A patient's inability to cooperate during a pelvic examination when she has been able to do so previously is a significant finding.

E. Presence of a pelvic mass in the absence of pregnancy should be correlated with history and symptoms. Irregular, sometimes very large, midline masses that move with the cervix are commonly uterine leiomyomata. Mobile or fixed masses lateral to the midline may be ovarian or tubal in origin. Cystic masses in any pelvic location are likely ovarian. A mobile, cystic mass anterior to the uterus suggests the possibility of a cystic teratoma of the ovary. Imaging that shows teeth or other well-developed bony or cartilaginous structures confirms this diagnosis.

F. Cervical dilatation and bleeding, with or without passage of formed material or fluid, suggests the possibility of some accident of pregnancy such as spontaneous or incomplete abortion.

V. Available Technology

A. Imaging permits visualization when palpation is uncertain or difficult.
1. Ultrasonography in gynecology
   a. Useful in the obese patient or where examination is difficult or impossible
   b. Useful for confirmation of physical examination findings
   c. Differentiates cystic from solid; particularly useful in ovarian neoplasms
   d. Useful in diagnosis of ectopic pregnancy
   e. Increases diagnostic accuracy when used in association with pelvic examination (Carter et al, 1994; Chadha et al, 1994)
2. Ultrasonography in obstetrics
   a. Diagnosis of intrauterine pregnancy
   b. Diagnosis of viability as reflected by fetal heart activity; fetal heart motion obvious at 8 weeks with vaginal ultrasonography
   c. Location of placenta as in placenta previa
   d. Determination of gestational age and fetal growth
      (1) Measurement of biparietal head dimensions
      (2) Measurement of femur length
      (3) Measurement of abdominal circumference
   e. Early diagnosis of fetal anomalies
   f. Early diagnosis of multiple gestation

B. Imaging permits evaluation of metabolic activity.
1. Doppler uterine artery blood flow
2. Tumor blood flow patterns
3. Nuclear magnetic resonance studies of tumors

C. The cost figures cited in this table are **basic direct costs**. The figures are difficult to obtain and change quickly. They include **only** the cost of the test itself (technician, equipment, time, and materials). No professional costs (interpretation) are included. Costs vary from region to region based on differences in some components such as labor. However, the relative cost ranking should remain similar.

Procedure	Code
Ultrasonography	$$
Doppler uterine artery blood flow	$$
Tumor blood flow patterns	$$
Nuclear magnetic resonance studies of tumors	$$$$$

$$ = $50–$100; $$$$$ = $500–$1000.

VI. Bibliography

Balk SJ, Dreyfus NG, Harris P. Examination of genitalia in children; the remaining taboo. *Pediatrics* 1982;70(5):751–753.

Buchta RM. Adolescent females' preferences regarding the use of a chaperone during a pelvic examination. *J Adolesc Health Care* 1986;7(6):409–411.

Carter J, Fowler J, Carson L, Carlson J, Twiggs LB. How accurate is the pelvic examination as compared to transvaginal sonography? A prospective, comparative study. *J Reprod Med* 1994;39(1):32–34.

Chadha P, Puri M, Gupta R. A comparative evaluation of clinical examination, pelvic ultrasound and laparoscopy in the diagnosis of pelvic masses. *Ind J Med Sci* 1994;48(7):158–160.

Hein K. The first pelvic examination and common gynecological problems in adolescent girls. *Women Health* 1984;9(2-3):47–63.

Koadlow E. The pelvic examination. The first pelvic examination for a healthy young woman. *Aust Fam Physician* 1990;19(5):665–669.

Leopold G, Sporlin. Conduct of normal births through external examination alone. *Arch Gynaekol* 1894;45:337.

Treolar AE, Boynton RE, Borghild GB, Brown BW. Variation of the human menstrual cycle through reproductive life. *Int J Fertil* 1967;12:77.

Vella PV. A survey of women undergoing a pelvic examination. *Aust NZ J Obstet Gynaecol* 1991;31(4):355–357.

Willard MD, Heaberg GL, Pack JB. The educational pelvic examination. Women's responses to a new approach. *J Obstet Gynecol Neonatal Nurs* 1986;15(2):135–140.

VII. Key Search Words

The following key words reflect the content of this chapter. They are provided to assist with an on-line search of computer databases, such as MEDLINE, if you wish to pursue the topic of this chapter further.

Abortion
Amenorrhea
Fertility
Genital diseases, female
Genital neoplasms, female
Genitalia, female
Gynecology
Infertility
Menopause
Obstetrics
Pregnancy
Pregnancy complications
Pregnancy, high risk
Pregnancy trimester, first
Pregnancy trimester, second
Pregnancy trimester, third
Reproduction
Reproductive medicine

14. BREAST

Vernon K. Sondak
Carolyn M. Johnston

I. Glossary

Atypical hyperplasia (either lobular or ductal): severely abnormal cells within the ductal or lobular unit that do not qualify for a diagnosis of carcinoma *in situ*. These lesions are associated with an increased risk of a subsequent invasive breast cancer, particularly in women with a family history of breast cancer.

Cystosarcoma phyllodes (phyllodes tumor): an uncommon tumor that arises from the stromal (as opposed to the glandular) elements of the breast, which may be either benign or malignant. In some cases, the ultimate behavior (i.e., benign or malignant) can be difficult to determine histologically.

Dominant mass: a palpable breast mass that is discrete from the surrounding glandular breast tissue, in contrast to the nondiscrete areas of prominence or thickening seen in some women with fibrocystic changes. Most palpable breast cancers present as a dominant mass; therefore, in most cases a dominant mass must be considered cancerous until proved otherwise by some type of biopsy.

Ductal carcinoma in situ (DCIS): noninvasive form of ductal adenocarcinoma of the breast. It is usually unilateral, but may be multifocal within the breast. DCIS can be detected mammographically as a cluster of calcifications, or it can present as bloody nipple discharge, nipple erosion (see *Paget's disease*) or, most rarely, as a palpable mass (also referred to as *intraductal carcinoma*).

Fibrocystic changes (disease): term given to a broad group of benign breast conditions, most related to cyclic maturation and involution of glandular breast tissue during the menstrual cycle. Studies show that virtually all women of reproductive age have some fibrocystic changes on breast biopsies; the condition becomes a disease only when it causes signs or symptoms that require medical intervention. This category includes a variety of histologic conditions including cysts, fibrosis, adenosis, and proliferative changes (lobular and ductal hyperplasia).

Gynecomastia: hypertrophy of the normally insubstantial ductal elements of the male breast, such that there is palpable or visible presence of glandular breast tissue.

Inflammatory breast cancer: locally advanced breast cancer that can simulate an infectious or inflammatory process. It is characterized histologically by dermal lymphatic invasion in many cases; it presents clinically with erythema, warmth, and edema of the breast skin. A palpable mass may not be present; sometimes the entire breast is diffusely thickened without a discrete mass (see also *peau d'orange*).

Intraductal papilloma: a benign growth that occurs within the ductal system of the breast. It is the most common cause of a bloody nipple discharge, which can also be caused by breast cancer.

Intramammary lymph node: the normal breast, particularly the axillary tail, may harbor one or several lymph nodes. These may be palpable in the slender patient or in any situation associated with lymphadenopathy, including breast and extramammary cancers or consequent to infection or inflammation in the region.

Lobular carcinoma in situ (LCIS): noninvasive form of lobular adenocarcinoma of the breast. It is primarily a disease of premenopausal women and is usually multifocal, clinically unapparent either by examination or mammography, and an incidental finding on biopsy. Women with LCIS are at increased risk for the subsequent development of invasive breast cancer, which may be in either breast and may be either invasive ductal or lobular histologic type.

Mastitis: inflammation of the breast, usually caused by bacterial infection but also occasionally part of autoimmune inflammatory conditions such as systemic lupus erythematosus. Infectious mastitis is most commonly seen during lactation (puerperal mastitis). Mastitis must always be differentiated from inflammatory breast cancer. A biopsy is often required for definitive diagnosis (see also *periductal mastitis*).

Mastodynia (mastalgia): breast pain, which may be cyclic (i.e., varying with the menstrual cycle) or noncyclic in nature. Cyclic mastodynia is virtually always secondary to fibrocystic changes; noncyclic mastodynia may represent a more severe form of fibrocystic changes or may be secondary to some other process.

Mondor's disease: superficial thrombophlebitis of a breast vein (usually the thoracoepigastric vein extending straight down from the nipple). It presents with a palpable, tender cord and may occur spontaneously or as a consequence of a breast biopsy. It resolves spontaneously in most cases; management is directed toward relief of symptoms.

Paget's disease: ductal carcinoma *in situ* involving the surface of the nipple, usually a manifestation of underlying carcinoma *in situ* deeper within the breast ductal system. Its presentation is an eczematoid or scaling lesion of the nipple, which may spread to involve the entire areolar complex and even the surrounding breast skin. Paget's disease is associated with an underlying invasive ductal cancer (as opposed to carcinoma *in situ*) in about one third of cases.

Peau d'orange (pronounced "poe dor-ahnj" from the French words for peel of an orange): breast edema from any cause, but particularly from inflammatory breast cancer. In this condition, the breast skin is thickened, erythematous, and pock-marked (at the points of cutaneous fixation of Cooper's ligaments) and looks remarkably like an orange peel.

Periductal mastitis: a benign condition most often found in postmenopausal women (also called mammary duct ectasia). It presents clinically as nipple retraction (which may mimic a subareolar breast cancer), usually along with a thick, whitish, creamy, or purulent nipple discharge. It may be a cause of chronic subareolar infections.

II. Techniques of Examination and Normal Findings

A. General considerations. A thorough breast examination should be part of every complete physical examination, regardless of whether the patient has noted any particular signs or symptoms. Breast cancer is the most common malignancy among women today, and a good breast examination is an important screening tool that complements (but is definitely not replaced by) imaging techniques such as mammography. During the breast examination, it is important to be sensitive to the patient by maintaining coverage of areas not actually being examined, by using appropriate but not excessive pressure in palpating the breasts, by limiting the number of times the patient must recline and rise, and by minimizing the number of maneuvers the patient must perform. It is also important to address the patient's anxiety as the examination progresses by describing what you are doing and why and, *in the asymptomatic patient*, by educating the patient to perform breast self-examination.

B. Inspection (Fig. 14-1). Begin with the patient sitting, disrobed to the waist but dressed in a gown that opens in the front. Compare each side to the other. Both breasts must be examined at once during this part of the examination.

1. Symmetry. Normally, the right and left breasts vary by as much as 10% in size; note larger degrees of asymmetry.

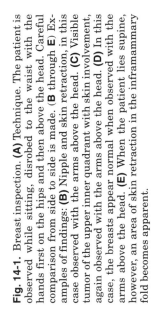

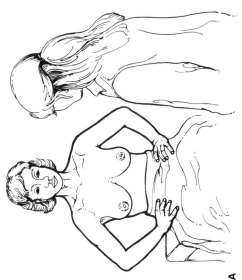

A

Fig. 14-1. Breast inspection. **(A)** Technique. The patient is observed while sitting, disrobed to the waist with the hands first on the hips and then above the head. Careful comparison from side to side is made. **(B** through **E)** Examples of findings: **(B)** Nipple and skin retraction, in this case observed with the arms above the head. **(C)** Visible tumor of the upper inner quadrant with skin involvement, again observed with the arms above the head. **(D)** In this case, the breasts appear normal when observed with the arms above the head. **(E)** When the patient lies supine, however, an area of skin retraction in the inframammary fold becomes apparent.

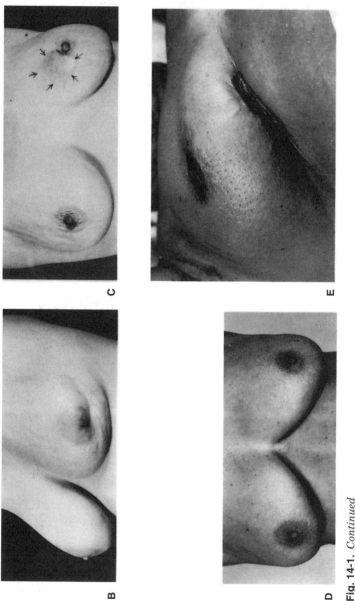

Fig. 14-1. *Continued*

2. Accessory breast tissue. Accessory nipples (polythelia) occur in about 1% to 2% of the population; accessory breast tissue is less common. Look for both in the axillary tail, above the breast mound, and below the breast along the milk line (midclavicular line from clavicle to groin). Accessory nipples often look like benign moles unless inspected closely.

3. Breast skin (Fig. 14-2)

    a. Look for areas of edema, erythema, or an altered venous pattern.

    b. Look for skin retraction in two positions.

        (1) Patient seated, hands on hips

        (2) Patient seated, hands overhead

4. Nipples

    a. Inversion or retraction of the nipple

    b. Erosions or other lesions of the nipple

    c. Visible evidence of nipple discharge

5. Regional nodes; only massive axillary adenopathy is visible, but lesser degrees of supraclavicular or cervical adenopathy may be seen in the thin patient.

C. Palpation. Establish a systematic pattern that thoroughly covers all parts of the breasts and the regional lymph nodes. Begin palpation as inspection ends: with the patient seated and facing the examiner. The breast not being examined should be covered.

    1. Neck and supraclavicular region. Out of convenience, first palpate the lymph nodes of the neck and supraclavicular region and the thyroid gland. Shrugging the shoulders slightly forward facilitates palpation of the supraclavicular fossa.

    2. Bimanual palpation. First palpate each breast with the upper hand while supporting it with the lower hand, moving from medial to lateral (Fig. 14-3). This provides a feel of the general amount of glandularity of the breast; in the woman with atrophic or pendulous breasts, this may be the best way to detect a small mass.

    3. Supine palpation. Ask the patient to recline and place both arms above her head. Begin this part of the examination in the upper outer quadrant of the breast; for the symptomatic patient start with the uninvolved breast. Use the pads (not the tips) of the fingers to feel for nodularity or masses. Proceed systematically—one entire quadrant at a time—from the edges of the breast to the areola. Include the axillary tail (but not the axillary nodes, yet) in the upper outer quadrant palpation. After all four quadrants of the breast have been examined, palpate the areola and *gently* squeeze the nipple at the base to elicit a discharge. Vigorous squeezing of the nipple is never indicated. Proceed to the opposite breast in the same manner.

    4. Skin. Note the texture of the skin, feeling for any thickened or abnormal areas.

    5. Glandularity. Note how glandular (lumpy) or fatty the breast tissue feels. Note any areas of thickening contiguous with the surrounding breast tissue. Assess which quadrants have the most glandular breast tissue, and note any areas of tenderness to palpation and whether these correspond to any symptomatic areas. Compare carefully from side to side as needed.

    6. Dominant masses. Feel carefully for any palpable masses discrete from the surrounding breast tissue.

    7. Axillary regions. Defer palpation of the axillae to the end of the examination, after the patient has returned to a seated position. The breasts should be covered, but the axillae must not be examined through clothing.

        a. To relax the shoulder muscles, support the patient's arm at the wrist or elbow with your same hand (e.g., patient's left arm held by examiner's left hand); carry out the axillary examination with your other hand (Fig. 14-4). Begin by inserting the tips of the fingers high into the apex of the axilla; this may be uncomfortable to the patient but

Lesion	Cause
Peau d'orange	Lymphedema due to obstruction of lymphatic drainage by tumor

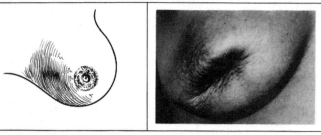

Retraction of the skin	Tumor involvement of Cooper's ligaments

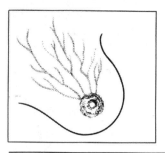

Increased venous pattern	Tumor obstruction of normal venous drainage

Erythema	Inflammatory tumor infiltrating skin or infection

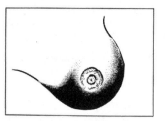

Fig. 14-2. Visible signs of breast cancer and their underlying cause.

Lesion	Cause
Paget's disease	Tumor originating in nipple

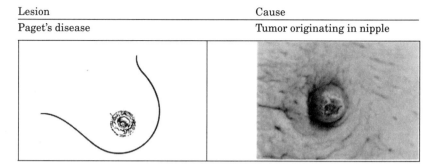

Fig. 14-2. *Continued.*

should not hurt. Feel the chest wall at the apex and palpate for nodes by pulling the fingers down to the base of the axilla along the chest wall. A palpable lymph node will be felt as it pops beneath the fingertips. It is critical that the muscles of the shoulder be relaxed during the axillary examination for maximal sensitivity.

b. Normal axillary nodes. In the obese patient, normal axillary nodes cannot generally be felt. In the slender person, normal nodes—up to 1 cm in size—can be felt and will be mobile and rubbery ("shotty") in consistency. Intramammary lymph nodes may occasionally be palpable in the slender patient along the lateral edge of the breast near the axillary tail.

c. Abnormal axillary nodes. Lymph nodes larger than 1 cm in size, firm or hard in consistency, fixed to the chest wall, or matted to one another are abnormal.

d. Other findings. The axilla is a relatively common site of breast tissue, which is usually contiguous with the main breast mass (axillary tail) but may be entirely separate (accessory breast tissue). Note the pres-

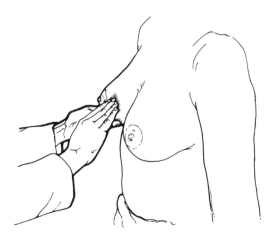

Fig. 14-3. Technique of bimanual palpation of the breast with the patient seated.

ence of such accessory tissue, and carefully assess for nodularity or masses, just as with the breast itself. Lipomas, sebaceous cysts, and hidradenitis suppurativa (chronic infection of the sweat glands) all can occur within the axilla and should be noted.

8. Completion of the examination. Allow the patient to fully cover herself, and explain all the findings and their significance. If the examination is normal, instruct the patient in the techniques of breast self-examination (see following section). If the examination is abnormal, invite the patient's spouse, significant other, relative, or friend into the examination room at this time to hear the explanation of the findings.

D. Self-examination of the breast. About 80% of all breast cancers—90% of all palpable tumors—are discovered by the patient. A well-informed and motivated patient can significantly increase the chance of early detection of breast cancer by the combination of monthly self-examination and yearly mammography (see Mammography). Self-examination ideally should begin when the patient reaches 20 years of age and should be performed monthly during the week immediately following the menstrual period, when the breasts are generally at their least nodular and least tender. It should be stressed to the patient that she is not trying to determine what abnormality she is feeling, but rather to identify any changes out of the ordinary for further evaluation by her physician. Teaching self-examination of the breast is an important part of the breast examination.

1. Observation. The patient should place herself before a mirror with her arms at her sides. She should carefully examine her breasts in the mirror for symmetry, size, and shape, searching for any evidence of puckering, dimpling of the skin, or retraction of the nipple. She should then raise her arms above her head and again study her breasts in the mirror, looking for the same physical signs. She should also be alert for any evidence of fixation of the breast tissue to the chest wall. This may be displayed as she moves her arms and shoulders.

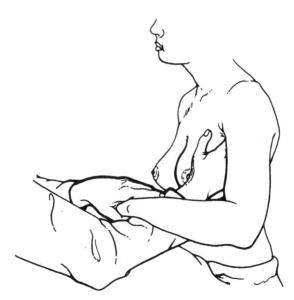

Fig. 14-4. Technique of examination of the axilla performed with the patient seated and arm supported.

2. Palpation. This should be performed first standing, then in a reclining position, with the arm on the side being examined placed behind the head. The breast is gently examined with the flat surface of the fingers of her opposite hand. The technique calls for gentle palpation of the breast tissue against the chest wall, usually beginning on the outer half of the breast and systematically covering the entire half of the breast, paying particular attention to the upper outer quadrant where the breast tissue is thickest and where most tumors occur. She should then thoroughly examine the inner half of the breast beginning at the sternum. When the entire breast has been carefully palpated, the woman investigates the second breast in exactly the same manner.

Palpation of the breast should be thorough and unhurried. Every portion of the breast must be deliberately and carefully examined if small lesions are to be detected. If the technique is to have any meaning, the woman must establish a definite pattern and conduct a thorough examination at monthly intervals. The method will be effective only if it is used regularly.

E. Expected findings in elderly women (age >70)

1. Inspection. Because the breasts tend to become pendulous and atrophic with advancing age, identifying areas of skin retraction may require additional maneuvers, particularly asking the patient to lean forward at the waist (Fig. 14-5). Nipple inversion becomes increasingly common with age and may be a relatively normal finding if longstanding.

2. Palpation. The elderly female breast should be relatively free of glandular tissue unless the patient is taking replacement estrogens. In the absence of such hormone therapy, any areas of asymmetric thickening or nodularity—even if not a "dominant mass"—are of concern for malignancy and should be subjected to further evaluation and biopsy. The seated bimanual examination is usually more sensitive for detecting small nodules in pendulous or atrophic breasts than the supine examination.

F. Examination in special situations

1. Augmented breasts. Examining women with breast implants is generally straightforward, recognizing that the breast tissue is characteristically compressed over the surface of the implant. In these patients, seated bimanual examination drawing the breast tissue forward and away from the implant is critical to detecting small masses. Note the presence of any fibrosis or distortion around the implants and any irregularities of the surface of the implant that could represent implant rupture.

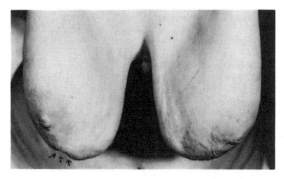

Fig. 14-5. In the patient with atrophic, pendulous breasts, having the patient lean forward at the waist can expose skin retraction (arrows).

   2. The postmastectomy patient. After mastectomy, breast examination focuses on the detection of possible cancer recurrence. Omit bimanual palpation; during the supine examination note the presence of any areas of thickening or nodularity. Always examine the axilla, even if the lymph nodes have been removed. After a thorough axillary dissection, there should be minimal tissue between the chest wall and the skin.

   3. The male patient. Examination of the male is designed to identify gynecomastia or, more rarely, breast cancer. Omit bimanual palpation; during the supine examination note the presence of any tissue beneath the areola, paying particular attention to its shape and consistency and whether there is any fixation to or involvement of the skin. In the normal male, there should be virtually no palpable glandular tissue beneath the nipple.

III. Cardinal Symptoms and Abnormal Findings

A. Inspection and palpation

   1. Symmetry

      a. Increase in size of one breast may indicate development of a cyst, tumor, or infection. At or around puberty, one breast occasionally enlarges significantly more than the other. This juvenile hypertrophy can be a source of concern and embarrassment for the patient.

      b. Decrease in size of one breast may occur with longstanding, neglected cancers.

      c. Congenital absence of one breast (amastia), which may be associated with hypoplasia of the ipsilateral pectoral muscles (Poland's syndrome) is rare.

   2. Skin and nipples

      a. Skin edema *(peau d'orange)* and erythema involving more than one third of the breast is associated with inflammatory breast cancer or severe infections; lesser areas of edema or erythema may be seen with direct tumor invasion, localized infection, or inflammatory conditions.

      b. A visible or palpable cord can be seen in a patient with Mondor's disease.

      c. Retraction of the breast skin is associated with cancer or, rarely, with post-traumatic fat necrosis.

      d. Retraction of the nipple is associated with cancer or periductal mastitis, or it may be a normal congenital finding or occur with age.

      e. Erosion, excoriation, or scaling of the nipple may result from eczema (usually generalized over the body, not restricted only to the nipple), repetitive trauma (such as jogging with loose or irritating clothing), or Paget's disease.

      f. Any nipple discharge should be characterized by its color, consistency, and the presence of blood, whether it is spontaneous or occurs only after stimulation of the nipple, and whether it is unilateral or bilateral.

   3. Consistency and tenderness

      a. Thickened or glandular areas, as well as tender regions, suggest fibrocystic changes in the premenopausal woman or the postmenopausal woman taking replacement estrogen. In the postmenopausal woman not on replacement hormones, such areas should be suspected of malignancy.

      b. Diffuse firmness associated with edema or erythema suggests inflammatory breast cancer or mastitis.

      c. In the male, the presence of glandular tissue is characteristic of gynecomastia.

   4. Regional lymph nodes. Normal supraclavicular nodes are generally not palpable. Normal intramammary or axillary nodes—up to 1 cm in size—can sometimes be felt and will be mobile and rubbery (shotty) in consistency. Lymph nodes larger than 1 cm in size, firm or hard in consistency, fixed to the chest wall, or matted to one another are abnormal.

B. Description of a palpable mass. The main goal of the breast examination is not to definitively diagnose every palpable abnormality, but rather to determine which lesions are of little consequence (e.g., fibrocystic change) and thus may be observed, and which require biopsy to establish or rule out the presence of cancer. In the adult woman, if a dominant mass is detected, it must be considered a cancer until definitively proved otherwise. For any palpable abnormality of the breast, whether a dominant mass or an area of thickening, the following diagnostic points should be accurately described:

1. Location and size of the lesion. Consider the breast as the face of a clock, with the nipple as the central point and 12 o'clock as straight superior. Locate the mass precisely, recording its measured dimensions and the clock position and distance from the nipple (e.g., "2- × 1-cm mass upper inner quadrant left breast, 10 o'clock position, 1 cm from areolar border"). A sketch is often helpful (Fig. 14-6).

2. Number of lesions. Note whether the lesion is solitary or multiple.

3. Consistency and borders of the mass. Consistency of the mass should be described: soft, firm, hard, or cystic. The borders of the mass should be described as well-circumscribed (sharply demarcated from the surrounding tissue) or indistinct. A dominant mass may have indistinct borders yet still be clearly discrete from the surrounding tissue. Although cysts, fibroadenomas, and most benign lesions are well circumscribed, up to 50% of breast cancers can be circumscribed as well.

4. Evidence of fixation. Observe whether the lesion is freely movable or fixed to the skin, underlying pectoralis muscle, or chest wall. (A small deep-seated cancer can become adherent to the pectoralis major, but fixation to the chest wall itself is an ominous sign.) Benign lesions are usually movable; fibroadenomas are often highly mobile. Most breast cancers, however, are also mobile.

5. Breast skin or nipple retraction. Only a very few benign conditions cause breast or nipple retraction. Most breast cancers, however, also do not manifest any signs of fixation to skin or nipple retraction.

6. Presence of tenderness and diffuse nodularity. Malignant lesions are usually not exquisitely tender, but may be sensitive—especially after repeated palpation. The presence of diffuse tenderness or nodularity is consistent with fibrocystic change, but does not eliminate the need for definitive diagnosis of a dominant mass.

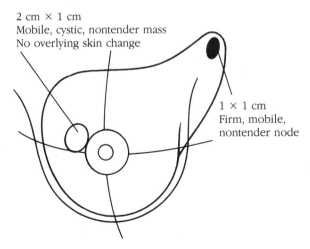

2 cm × 1 cm
Mobile, cystic, nontender mass
No overlying skin change

1 × 1 cm
Firm, mobile,
nontender node

Fig. 14-6. Sample sketch describing the results of the examination of the left breast and axilla in a manner suitable for inclusion in the medical record.

7. Presence or absence of regional lymphadenopathy. No breast examination is complete without noting the status of the regional nodes. Although lymph node enlargement often signals malignant involvement, it can also occur secondary to systemic disease, regional infection, or inflammation, or it may be consequent to a recent breast biopsy (reactive hyperplasia).

8. Palpable thrombosed vein. A palpable cord-like structure, often running vertically in the inferior breast (6 o'clock position), is characteristic of Mondor's disease. It may have some superficial inflammation associated with it.

IV. Common Clinical Disorders

A. Breast cancer. Adenocarcinoma of the breast is the most common malignancy in women in the United States; if detected and treated early, there is an excellent chance for cure. Two histologic types of invasive breast cancer predominate: lobular and ductal carcinoma. Both types are also recognized as noninvasive or *in situ* cancers. Breast cancers are variable in their manifestations and cannot be reliably diagnosed or excluded solely on the basis of physical examination. Remember that even a woman with no identifiable risk factors is still at significant risk of developing breast cancer. Use the American Joint Commission on Cancer (AJCC) staging system (also called the TNM system) to classify all cases of breast cancer (Table 14-1).

1. Typical features of small localized breast cancer (AJCC stage I)
   a. Nontender, dominant mass (or asymmetric thickening in a postmenopausal woman), 2 cm or less in size
   b. Firm or hard consistency, somewhat mobile; possibly well-circumscribed or indistinct borders
   c. No evidence of skin involvement, edema, erythema, chest wall fixation, or axillary or supraclavicular lymphadenopathy

2. Typical features of larger localized or regionally metastatic breast cancer (AJCC stage II)
   a. Nontender, dominant mass (or asymmetric thickening in a postmenopausal woman) 2 to 5 cm in size (or smaller with palpable nodal involvement)
   b. Firm or hard consistency, somewhat mobile; possibly well-circumscribed or indistinct borders
   c. May or may not have palpable axillary node involvement, but no evidence of matted or fixed nodes and no evidence of supraclavicular lymphadenopathy
   d. No evidence of skin involvement, edema, erythema, chest wall fixation

3. Typical features of locally or regionally advanced breast cancer (AJCC stage III)
   a. Nontender, dominant mass (or asymmetric thickening in a postmenopausal woman) >5 cm in size *or* any size tumor with evidence of skin involvement, edema, erythema, *peau d'orange,* or chest wall (*not* pectoralis muscle) fixation
   b. May or may not have palpable axillary node involvement, including evidence of matted or fixed axillary nodes
   c. No evidence of supraclavicular lymphadenopathy

4. Typical features of metastatic breast cancer (AJCC stage IV)
   a. Evidence of supraclavicular lymphadenopathy, *or*
   b. Arm edema or neurologic impairment, *or*
   c. Evidence of cervical lymphadenopathy, *or*
   d. Evidence of visceral or systemic involvement, such as hepatomegaly

5. Diagnostic workup of breast cancer suspected by physical examination
   a. Bilateral mammography. Imaging of both breasts is indicated to rule out the presence of a synchronous contralateral primary. Mammographic features of breast cancer include the following:

Table 14-1. AJCC Staging System for Carcinoma of the Breast

Tumor (T)	Nodes (N)	Metastases (M)
T0: No evidence of a primary	N0: No node metastases	M0: No distant metastases
T1: Tumor <2 cm	N1: Movable nodal metastases	M1: Distant metastases
T2: Tumor 2–5 cm	N2: Fixed nodal metastases	
T3: Tumor >5 cm	N3: Internal mammary node metastases	
T4: Tumor any size with direct extension to chest wall or skin		

Stage I:	Stage II:	Stage III:	Stage IV:
T1N0M0 M1	T0N1M0	T0N2M0	Any T, any N,
	T1N0M0	T1N2M0	
	T2N0M0	T2N2M0	
	T2N1M0	T3N1M0	
	T3N0M0	T3N2M0	
		T4, any N, M0	
		Any T, N3M0	

(1) Presence of a spiculated mass or area of asymmetry or architectural distortion of the breast parenchyma.
(2) Presence of microcalcifications—small clusters of calcifications, 3 to 20 or more in number and each generally under 5 mm in size—alone or with a mass.
(3) Skin edema or nipple or skin retraction in locally advanced cases.
(4) Enlarged lymph nodes seen occasionally but not reliably.
(5) Even with excellent technique, about 10% of palpable breast cancers are not seen on mammography (the percentage is even greater in younger women). Therefore, a negative mammogram in a woman with a dominant mass does *not* exclude the presence of cancer and definitive diagnosis is still required.
   b. Biopsy. A palpable dominant mass is cancer until proved otherwise by a diagnostic breast biopsy. The choice of biopsy technique is described in the next section.
6. Breast biopsy techniques—advantages and disadvantages
   a. Fine-needle aspiration cytology
      (1) Advantages: quick, easy to perform in office setting; requires minimal anesthesia; results available within 48 to 72 hours. If the lesion is a cyst, aspiration will diagnose and treat. If the result is positive for cancer, treatment planning can commence quickly.
      (2) Disadvantages: high false-negative/indeterminate result rate (20% to 30% of all palpable breast cancers have a negative or nondiagnostic aspirate). Therefore, if aspirate is negative, open biopsy is still required. This method has a small but real false-positive rate (0.5% to 1.0% cytology positive for cancer but no cancer present), and it may be difficult to perform hormone receptor analyses.
   b. Core needle biopsy

      (1) Advantages: can be performed in office setting; gives histologic (as opposed to cytologic) result. If result is positive for cancer, treatment planning can commence quickly.

      (2) Disadvantages: more painful than fine-needle aspiration; has a high rate of hematoma formation. The high false-negative rate is due to a sampling error. It may be difficult to perform hormone receptor analyses.

    c. Open biopsy

      (1) Advantages: gives definitive histologic result. It is the optimum technique for performance of hormone receptor analyses. If pathology is benign, no further treatment required.

      (2) Disadvantages: most invasive procedure; may require sedation or even general anesthesia. It also takes the longest to perform and is the *most expensive.*

  7. Metastatic workup. After the diagnosis of cancer is made, a limited workup to assess for the presence of metastatic disease is indicated.

    a. Chest x-ray

    b. Liver function tests (especially alkaline phosphatase)

    c. If alkaline phosphatase is elevated *or* the patient has evidence of stage III or IV cancer on examination *or* the patient has symptoms referable to bone or liver, add bone scan and computed tomography (CT) of liver. Otherwise, these tests are not routinely indicated.

B. Fibroadenoma. Fibroadenoma is the second most common neoplasm of the breast after carcinoma; it occurs most commonly in premenopausal women. Only 2.5% occur in postmenopausal women. They tend to occur and recur more frequently and at an earlier age in black women. Multiple or recurrent fibroadenomas are seen in 13% to 16% of cases.

  1. Clinical features

    a. Nontender or slightly tender dominant mass, usually less than 3 cm in size, often with history of slow enlargement. They are occasionally very large (>3 cm) with history of rapid growth, particularly in adolescents. A fibroadenoma may increase rapidly in size during pregnancy, but there is usually no change in size with menses. It must be differentiated from cystosarcoma phyllodes (phyllodes tumor), an uncommon tumor that presents in a virtually identical fashion and may be either benign or malignant. Cystosarcoma phyllodes is generally larger and more rapidly growing than most fibroadenomas.

    b. Rubbery-firm in consistency, mobile, and oval or round with very well-demarcated margins.

    c. No evidence of skin involvement, edema, erythema, chest wall fixation, or axillary or supraclavicular lymphadenopathy.

  2. Evaluation

    a. Can be safely observed in women younger than 25 years, but most women choose excision. When followed conservatively, 31% and 52% of fibroadenomas diagnosed by fine-needle aspiration were found to regress after 2 and 5 years, respectively. Fibroadenomas are more likely to regress in women younger than 20 years.

    b. Surgical excision is virtually always indicated for women over 35 years to exclude carcinoma.

C. Fibrocystic changes. Lumpiness and diffuse nodular irregularities throughout the breasts have been referred to as fibrocystic disease or benign breast disease. A better name is fibrocystic changes, with the term "disease" restricted to patients with symptoms sufficient to warrant medical or surgical intervention. Fibrocystic changes include cysts, fibrosis, adenosis, and proliferative changes (hyperplasia); some fibrocystic changes can be found within the breast tissue of virtually all women of reproductive age. Most postmenopausal women do not have active fibrocystic changes in the absence of replacement estrogen therapy. Generally, symptomatic or asymptomatic fibrocystic changes do not convey an increased risk for cancer development. Atypical ductal and lobular hyperplasia account collectively for about 5% of cases undergoing biopsy for fibrocystic changes and are associated with an increased breast cancer risk—particularly in the presence of a family history of breast cancer.

1. Clinical features

   a. Patients typically present with complaints of a discrete mass, diffuse lumpiness, or breast pain that may or may not be cyclic. Cyclic breast pain and lumpiness are generally worst in the 2 weeks before menses and least in the week after menses. A mass, if present, may be a nontender or tender dominant mass, an area of thickening, or a nondominant mass not separable from the subjacent breast tissue. Discrete masses of fibrocystic change can mimic carcinoma.

   b. Cysts are usually firm but not hard in consistency, round and mobile with very well-demarcated margins.

   c. No evidence of skin involvement, edema, erythema, chest wall fixation, or axillary or supraclavicular lymphadenopathy is present.

2. Evaluation

   a. The primary goal of the evaluation should be to rule out malignancy, including mammograms for symptomatic patients over 30. Oral contraceptives may be useful. If mastalgia predominates, several medical options and nonhormonal remedies exist. Often, reassurance is the most effective therapy. Some patients experience decreased nodularity and lessened symptoms with a reduction in caffeine intake.

   b. Excisional biopsy may be necessary to exclude carcinoma in a dominant mass (or area of thickening in a postmenopausal woman).

   c. Palpable cysts should be aspirated; if the cyst resolves completely with aspiration and the fluid is not bloody, no further treatment is necessary. If residual mass remains after cyst aspiration or the cyst fluid is bloodtinged or recurs despite aspiration, excisional biopsy is indicated.

D. Mastitis

1. Periductal mastitis. Also called mammary duct ectasia, this is a benign condition most often found in postmenopausal women. It is not associated with an increased risk for carcinoma.

   a. Clinical features. Younger patients are more likely to present with breast pain or a mass, whereas older patients more often present with nipple retraction.

   (1) Nipple retraction (which may mimic a subareolar breast cancer), usually along with a thick, whitish, creamy or purulent nipple discharge.

   (2) Possibly a cause of chronic subareolar infections.

   b. Evaluation. Differentiation from cancer is the main concern in patients with nipple retraction or a subareolar mass.

2. Puerperal (lactation-associated) mastitis. Puerperal mastitis occurs in 1% to 9% of lactating women, with abscess formation in 5% to 11% of cases. It is presumed because of the presence of nipple fissures and milk stasis, which encourages retrograde bacterial infection.

   a. Clinical features. Infections of the breast, both puerperal and nonpuerperal, are most often due to *Staphylococcus aureus* or streptococci. Clinical manifestations of breast infections may range from painful cellulitis to unifocal or multifocal abscesses. If untreated, cellulitis generally progresses to an abscess, especially in the puerperal state. Streptococcal infections are more likely to persist as a diffuse cellulitis, whereas staphylococcal infections present early with suppuration and abscess formation. Lactating women should continue to breast-feed or use a breast pump. Bacteria in the milk does not appear to be pathogenic for the breast-feeding infant.

   b. Prevention. Careful attention to nipple hygiene, including gentle cleaning of the nipple after feeding to remove remaining milk, and antibiotic ointments in case of nipple fissures, can help prevent the development of puerperal mastitis.

3. Acute and chronic abscesses. These may occur spontaneously or in association with one of the types of mastitis previously described. After an acute infection has occurred, there is a high risk of multiple acute and chronic recurrences, owing to the difficulty of eradicating all bacteria from within the network of breast ducts. Any apparent infectious or inflammatory process that does not respond to antibiotics should be suspected of being an inflammatory breast cancer (see **IV.A.3**).

   a. Clinical features. A breast abscess presents as a painful, hot, swollen, and erythematous breast, with or without an underlying fluctuant mass. In contrast to inflammatory breast cancer, it may be associated with an elevated white blood cell count or a fever. Enlarged axillary lymph nodes are frequently encountered, heightening the difficulty in differentiating abscess from cancer.

   b. Exclusion of cancer. Patients with nonpuerperal mastitis and other inflammatory conditions of the breast should undergo a thorough breast examination and mammogram. Any residual mass or mammographic abnormality after treatment or failure to respond appropriately to antibiotics should lead to a biopsy.

E. Mastodynia (mastalgia). This refers to pain in the breast parenchyma without any discrete underlying pathology. Cyclic mastodynia is most often a manifestation of diffuse fibrocystic changes, but may be associated with a discrete lesion such as a cyst.

   1. Clinical evaluation. Most women tolerate the cyclic breast swelling and tenderness associated with menstrual cycles. For those who do not, for whom lifestyle is altered, or for whom the pain becomes constant, an evaluation is indicated. This evaluation should exclude discrete causes of breast pain such as cysts, rule out the presence of an underlying malignancy, and assess the possibility of an extramammary cause of breast pain such as costochondritis. Radiologic studies are done as indicated by age or clinical findings, and abnormal results are managed as appropriate. Mastodynia should not be ascribed to fibrocystic changes until these items have been adequately addressed. In general, cyclic mastodynia is far more responsive to treatment than noncyclic mastodynia. After menopause, most women with mastalgia experience a rapid improvement in symptoms.

   2. Exclusion of cancer. Cyclic mastodynia is not associated with underlying breast cancer, but breast cancer *can* be painful. Any palpable mass should be evaluated and mammograms obtained in women over 30 years of age. Masses suspected of being cystic should be aspirated, since this may result in marked pain relief. Masses suspected of being malignant should be biopsied.

F. Nipple discharge. Elicited nipple discharge is often a normal finding. Management centers around exclusion of breast cancer or prolactinoma; the likelihood of these conditions existing depends to a great degree on the color and bilaterality of the discharge. The most important parts of the clinical history are whether or not the discharge comes from one or multiple ducts, is unilateral or bilateral, is spontaneous, and is associated with a mass.

   1. Galactorrhea. This condition is defined as a white or milky discharge, usually from multiple ducts bilaterally. Differential diagnosis includes the following:

   a. Lactation: may persist months or even years after the cessation of breast-feeding.

   b. Prolactin-secreting pituitary tumors (prolactinoma): associated with elevated serum prolactin. A serum prolactin should be obtained at a time other than that of the breast examination.

   c. Drug intake, especially phenothiazines and oral contraceptives.

   d. Idiopathic causes, including chronic breast stimulation.

   e. Other systemic diseases (uncommon): hypothyroidism, renal failure, and chest trauma, all of which may cause an elevated serum prolactin.

2. Bloody discharge. A discharge may be grossly bloody, serosanguinous, or dark greenish black (guaiac-positive). There are two main causes of bloody discharge.
   a. Cancer. Bloody discharge is the type of nipple discharge most commonly associated with cancer; 70% of cancer cases associated with a nipple discharge had a bloody discharge. Cytology of the discharge (made by smearing the discharge onto a glass slide) may be useful. Mammography should be performed in women over 30 years with a bloody nipple discharge.
   b. Intraductal papilloma. Intraductal papillomas are associated with a unilateral, spontaneous serous (48%), or bloody (52%) discharge, which represents the presenting symptom in 76% of patients and the only complaint in 43%. Twenty-four percent of patients present with a palpable, usually subareolar, mass, and 33% present with both a mass and a discharge. Multiple papillomas are more likely to be associated with subsequent development of carcinoma—possibly because of the coexistent atypical hyperplasia. Ductography (also called galactography), injection of contrast into the discharging breast duct with subsequent mammography, has been demonstrated to identify intraductal lesions such as papillomas, and it may be useful before operative removal by subareolar duct excision.
3. Nonbloody, nonmilky discharge. Other types of nipple discharge are rarely harbingers of serious conditions like underlying cancer. Note that a nonbloody discharge may be dark green or brown in color similar to a bloody discharge. Guaiac test of the discharge can differentiate in these cases. Most nonbloody watery discharges are from fibrocystic changes, whereas most cases of thick, purulent discharge are from periductal mastitis. Mammography should be performed in women over 30 years of age with a nipple discharge.
G. Paget's disease. Ductal carcinoma *in situ* involving the surface of the nipple is usually a manifestation of underlying carcinoma *in situ* deeper within the breast ductal system. Paget's disease is associated with an underlying invasive ductal cancer (as opposed to carcinoma *in situ*) in up to one third of cases.
   1. Clinical features. Paget's disease generally presents as an eczematoid, nonhealing lesion with crusting, scaling, and erythema; it is sometimes accompanied by a bloody discharge. It may spread to involve the entire areolar complex and even the surrounding breast skin.
   2. Diagnostic studies. All nonhealing lesions of the nipple should be biopsied. Scrape cytology may represent an alternative to punch biopsy. Mammography should be performed before biopsy, with the realization that as many as one third of cases may not have a mammographically apparent underlying carcinoma.
H. Cancer in an axillary node without a palpable breast mass. Adenocarcinoma is almost always metastatic breast cancer, even if the breast examination and mammography are negative.
   1. Extensive diagnostic workup to identify other primary tumor sites is not indicated; however, a thorough physical examination—including thyroid, rectal and pelvic examinations—should be performed.
   2. In the absence of positive findings on physical examination, a chest x-ray should be obtained. If the results are negative, the patient should be treated as if she had breast cancer from a known primary site.
   3. It is very important that the axillary node be thoroughly examined histologically, however, prior to carrying out any treatment. This will permit the pathologist to exclude lymphoma or melanoma, both of which can present initially in axillary nodes.
I. Atypical hyperplasia/lobular carcinoma *in situ*. Women with atypical hyperplasia and carcinoma *in situ* of the breast have an increased risk of developing invasive breast cancer. Thus, these conditions can be thought of as "high-risk lesions" or perhaps precursors of invasive breast cancer.

1. Clinical features
    a. Rarely present as a palpable abnormality and rarely symptomatic
    b. May be found incidentally in conjunction with a palpable lesion such as a fibroadenoma or in a woman undergoing breast biopsy for some other reason
    c. Most common associated finding—a mammographic abnormality, usually a cluster of microcalcifications
2. Exclusion of cancer. In all cases, exclusion of a synchronous invasive cancer elsewhere in either breast is a priority, followed by subsequent close clinical follow-up to detect a new invasive or noninvasive cancer early if it occurs. In most cases, this includes annual mammography, twice-yearly examination by a physician, and monthly breast self-examination. Patients with lobular carcinoma *in situ* who are not able to comply with these surveillance requirements should be considered for surgical therapy.

J. Gynecomastia (enlargement of the male breast with a distinct disk of breast tissue palpable immediately beneath the nipple-areolar complex). For most patients, particularly older males with bilateral disease, exclusion of malignancy is all that is required.
    1. Obese patients. Nonspecific breast enlargement from fat deposition must be differentiated from true gynecomastia.
    2. Adolescent males. Asymptomatic gynecomastia is surprisingly common; one study demonstrated a 39% incidence of gynecomastia in boys between ages 11 and 14, declining to 14% by age 16.
    3. Elderly men. Declining serum levels of testosterone in the presence of physiologic estrogen levels may be associated with gynecomastia.
    4. Other causes
        a. Drug-induced. Gynecomastia has been associated with use of a number of drugs, including androgens, estrogens, cimetidine, digoxin, isoniazid, metoclopramide, α-methyldopa, reserpine, spironolactone, and tricyclic antidepressants. It has also been associated with marijuana use. Drug-related gynecomastia is often unilateral or unequal between the two breasts, and discontinuation of the offending drug does not always lead to resolution.
        b. Hyperestrogenemic states. These include Klinefelter's syndrome (XXY chromosomal abnormality), testicular feminization, secondary testicular failure, ectopic estrogen secretion, and hepatic failure.
    5. Clinical features
        a. Begin with a thorough history and systems review aimed at uncovering underlying hormonal, pharmacologic, or pathologic causes.
        b. Physical examination may reveal stigmata of an underlying disorder, such as liver dysfunction, Klinefelter's syndrome, or a testicular tumor. Palpate the breast tissue itself both to verify the presence of gynecomastia and to exclude the possibility of cancer. Benign gynecomastia feels disk-shaped or spherical, firm, and rubbery. The breast tissue is symmetric and centered directly below the nipple. Irregular-shaped masses or those not immediately below the nipple-areolar complex must be considered suspicious for malignancy.
        c. Mammography is feasible in males; it should be used in older men and any patient in whom malignancy is suspected.
        d. Testicular ultrasonography is not used routinely if the testes are normal to palpation.
        e. Liver function tests and a chest radiograph can help to exclude some causes of gynecomastia.
        f. Needle aspiration cytology has proved disappointing in excluding malignancy; equivocal or atypical findings are common in histologically benign cases.

K. Male breast cancer. Only about 0.5% of all cases of breast cancer occur in men; they often present at an older age, about 60 to 65 years, and at a more advanced stage than females because of both a delay in presentation and the smaller amount of breast tissue.

  1. Clinical features
      a. A hard, painless breast lump (most common presentation)
      b. Bloody nipple discharge and skin ulceration (more common than in female patients)
      c. Usually hard, asymmetric, fixed to the skin or chest wall, and frequently associated with axillary adenopathy
  2. Evaluation. Mammography and biopsy can be useful in establishing a diagnosis in questionable cases.

V. Available Technology

  A. Mammography. Up to 50% of cancers detected mammographically are not palpable. Conversely, palpation recognizes 10% to 20% of tumors not detectable mammographically. The low level of radiation exposure associated with mammograms performed using dedicated equipment in certified centers ensures that mammography is safe.
  1. Screening mammography should begin at age 40 according to the guidelines of the American Cancer Society.
  2. Mammography in symptomatic patients may help establish a diagnosis in a woman presenting with a palpable mass or other clinical abnormality (see **IV.A.5.a**). Bilateral mammography should be performed before biopsy in all women over the age of 30 years to detect synchronous, nonpalpable ipsilateral or contralateral disease. *Because of the recognized false-positive rate with mammography, a negative mammogram does not eliminate the need for biopsy of a dominant breast mass.*
  B. Ultrasonography. Ultrasound is a useful adjunct to mammography in the following situations: to distinguish a cystic from a solid mass; to facilitate needle aspiration or core biopsy of nonpalpable lesions; and as a diagnostic tool in women younger than 30 years. Ultrasound does not detect small lesions and calcifications well when compared with mammography and hence has no role in screening for breast cancer.
  C. New technologies
  1. Magnetic resonance imaging (MRI). Interest in MRI of the breast is high. Dedicated breast MRI machines and MRI biopsy localization techniques are being developed. With the use of magnetic contrast agents, diagnosis of nonpalpable breast masses missed by mammography may be possible. MRI also appears very promising for the evaluation of patients with breast implants, particularly for the detection of implant rupture.
  2. Positron emission tomography (PET). PET is unique in that it produces a functional rather than an anatomic view of tissues. PET allows preferential imaging of cells (such as breast cancer cells) that have a high rate of glycolysis. PET may ultimately have a role as a noninvasive method of staging axillary lymph nodes and of detecting metastatic disease. We have found PET to be particularly helpful in distinguishing radiation changes from recurrent disease, particularly in the axilla and the region of the brachial plexus.
  D. The cost figures cited in the table on page 272 are **basic direct costs**. The figures are difficult to obtain and change quickly. They include **only** the cost of the test itself (technician, equipment, time, and materials). No professional costs (interpretation) are included. Costs vary from region to region based on differences in some components such as labor. However, the relative cost ranking should remain similar.

VI. Bibliography

American Joint Commission on Cancer. *Manual for Staging of Cancer,* 4th ed. Philadelphia: JB Lippincott; 1993.

August DA, Sondak VK. Breast. In Greenfield LJ, Mulholland MW, Oldham KT, Zelenock GB (eds). *Surgery: Scientific Principles and Practice,* 2nd ed. Philadelphia: Lippincott–Raven; 1997:1357.

Procedure	Code
Mammography	$$
Ultrasonography	$$
Magnetic resonance imaging (MRI)	$$$$
Positron emission tomography (PET)	$$$$$$

$$ = $50–$100; $$$$ = $200–$500; $$$$$$ = >$1000.

Butler JA, Vargfas HI, Worthen N, Wilson SE. Accuracy of combined clinical mammographic cytologic diagnosis of dominant breast mass. *Arch Surg* 1990;125:893.

Carty NJ, Carter C, Rubin C, et al. Management of fibroadenoma of the breast. *Ann R Coll Surg Engl* 1995;77:127.

Ciatto S, Cariaggi P, Bulgaresi P. The value of routine cytologic examination of breast cyst fluids. *Acta Cytol* 1987;31:301.

Colditz GA, Hankinson SE, Hunter DJ, et al. The use of estrogens and progestins and the risk of breast cancer in postmenopausal women. *N Engl J Med* 1995;332:1589.

Dupont WD, Page DL. Risk factors for breast cancer in women with proliferative breast disease. *N Engl J Med* 1985;312:146.

Early Breast Cancer Trialists' Collaborative Group. Effects of radiotherapy and surgery in early breast cancer. An overview of the randomized trials. *N Engl J Med* 1995;333:1444.

Early Breast Cancer Trialists' Collaborative Group. Systemic treatment of early breast cancer by hormonal, cytotoxic, or immune therapy. 133 randomised trials involving 31,000 recurrences and 24,000 deaths among 75,000 women. *Lancet* 1992;339:1,71.

Fisher B, Anderson S, Redmond CK, et al. Reanalysis and results after 12 years of follow-up in a randomized clinical trial comparing total mastectomy with lumpectomy with or without irradiation in the treatment of breast cancer. *N Engl J Med* 1995;333:1456.

Harris JR, Lippman ME, Morrow M, Hellman S (eds). *Diseases of the Breast.* Philadelphia: Lippincott–Raven, 1996.

Hartley MN, Stewart J, Benson EA. Subareolar dissection for duct ectasia and periareolar sepsis. *Br J Surg* 1991;78:1187.

Hughes LE, Mansel RE, Webster DJT. *Benign Disorders and Diseases of the Breast.* London: Ballire Tindall; 1989.

International Breast Cancer Study Group. Effectiveness of adjuvant chemotherapy in combination with tamoxifen for node-positive postmenopausal breast cancer patients. *J Clin Oncol* 1997;15:1385.

Layfield LJ, Glasgow BJ, Cramer H. Fine needle aspiration in the management of breast masses. *Pathol Annu* 1989;24:23.

National Institutes of Health Consensus Development Panel. National Institutes of Health Consensus Development Conference statement: Breast cancer screening for women ages 40–49, January 21–23, 1997. *J Natl Cancer Inst* 1997;89:1015.

Silverstein MJ (ed). *Ductal Carcinoma In Situ of the Breast.* Baltimore: Williams and Wilkins, 1997.

VII. Key Search Words

The following key words reflect the content of this chapter. They are provided to assist with an on-line search of computer databases, such as MEDLINE, if you wish to pursue the topic of this chapter further.

Breast	Gynecomastia
Breast diseases	Lymph nodes
Breast neoplasms	Mammography
Breast neoplasms, male	Mastitis
Breast self-examination	Nipples
Galactorrhea	Papilloma, intraductal
	Ultrasonography, mammary

15. NERVOUS SYSTEM

Linda M. Selwa

I. Glossary

Anarthria: inability to articulate words (complete voicelessness).

Anosmia: inability to smell.

Aphasia: loss of language functions, that is, either the inability to express thoughts through speech, writing, or signs, or the inability to comprehend spoken or written language (generally caused by dysfunction of cerebral centers mediating expressive or receptive abilities).

Apraxia: inability to use body parts purposefully or to carry out learned skilled movements.

Ataxia: poor regulation of muscular coordination (usually implies cerebellar dysfunction).

Atrophy: diminution in size (wasting) of a muscle.

Autonomic function testing: usually performed in conjunction with electromyographic testing. When indicated, it can quantify sympathetic and parasympathetic responses.

Bulbar palsy: paralysis and atrophy of the muscles of the lips, tongue, mouth, pharynx, or larynx due to degeneration of nerves or nuclei in the brain stem.

Cisternography: nuclear medicine assessment of cerebrospinal fluid (CSF) flow and absorption; useful in normal pressure hydrocephalus and CSF leak.

Clonus: persistent involuntary flexion and extension of a joint stretched in extension or flexion.

Corticography: direct recording of electrographic activity over the cortical surface; useful before cerebral surgery to map brain functions or ictal discharges.

Dysarthria: imperfect articulation of speech.

Dysmetria: inability to control the accuracy of muscular action; a sign of cerebellar dysfunction.

Dysphagia: difficulty swallowing.

Dysphasia: incomplete aphasia.

Dyssynergia: disturbance in coordination of contraction and relaxation in muscle groups usually acting together to produce a single smooth movement; a sign of cerebellar dysfunction.

Extinction (suppression): failure to perceive one of two identical bilateral simultaneous stimuli when sensory perception is otherwise intact. Extinction or suppression may indicate parietal cortex dysfunction.

Fasciculation: visible spontaneous contraction of a group of muscle fibers supplied by a single motor unit.

Functional magnetic resonance imaging (MRI): currently experimental technique for mapping brain regions involved in speech, memory function, motor function, and so on.

Graphesthesia: sense by which figures and numbers written on the skin are recognized.

Homonymous hemianopsia: loss of vision in the nasal half of the visual field in one eye and the temporal half in the other, caused by dysfunction of the cerebral visual pathways.

Horner's syndrome: sympathetic paralysis causing unilateral ptosis of the upper lid, constriction of the pupil, and decreased cephalic sweating.

Intracarotid amobarbital procedure: reversible anesthetization of the distribution of each carotid artery with sodium amobarbital; typically performed to localize language and memory function prior to epilepsy surgery.

Lower motor neurons: peripheral neurons whose cell bodies lie in the ventral gray columns of the spinal cord and whose terminations are in the skeletal muscles.

Nystagmus: involuntary rhythmic oscillations of the eyes.

Optic atrophy: pale appearance of the optic nerve head when the nerve has become demyelinated.

Optic neuritis: inflammation of the optic nerve head resulting in visual disturbances and often acutely causing a swollen appearance of the optic disk similar to papilledema.

Papilledema: edema of the optic disk usually due to increased intracranial pressure.

Paresis (hemi-, para-, quadri-): weakness or partial paralysis.

Plegia: complete paralysis. *Hemiplegia*: paralysis of one side of the body, often caused by cerebral disease. *Paraplegia*: paralysis of the legs and lower part of the body, usually caused by disease or injury of the spinal cord. *Quadriplegia*: paralysis of all four limbs.

Proprioception: perception of movements and position of the body and joints.

Pseudobulbar palsy: weakness of the pharyngeal, laryngeal, or facial muscles, simulating bulbar paralysis but due to supranuclear (upper motor neuron) lesions.

Ptosis: drooping of the upper eyelid.

Quadrantanopsia: blindness in one of the quadrants of the visual field.

Scotoma: blind or partially blind area in the visual field of one or both eyes.

Sensory level: level below which there is a decrease or loss of sensation corresponding to the level of dysfunction of the spinal cord.

Single photon emission tomography/positron emission tomography: useful to image blood flow (SPECT); glucose utilization or neurotransmitter uptake in various degenerative disorders.

Stereognosis: faculty of recognizing objects by the sense of touch.

Upper motor neuron: neuron that conducts impulses from the motor cortex to the motor nuclei of the cranial nerves or to the motor cells in the ventral gray columns of the spinal cord.

II. Techniques of Examination and Normal Findings

A. General considerations

1. Equipment needed
   a. Always required:
      (1) Reflex hammer
      (2) Tuning forks (128 and 256 cps)
      (3) An ophthalmoscope
      (4) A small flashlight
      (5) Tongue blade
      (6) Sharp pin
      (7) Stethoscope
      (8) Wisp of cotton
   b. Often needed:
      (1) An otoscope
      (2) Written materials
      (3) Pen and paper
      (4) Coins
      (5) Snellen's visual acuity card
      (6) A pinhole
      (7) Coffee or strong mint to smell
2. Sequence
   a. Perform a screening examination systematically evaluating mental status, cranial nerves, motor function, coordination, reflexes, sensation and gait.
   b. Expand the section relevant to the patient's complaint as needed.

B. General examination

1. Palpation
   a. Palpate the common carotid arteries in the neck and the temporal arteries in front of the ears. Palpate both radial arteries at the wrist, noting strength of pulse and simultaneousness. Palpate both dorsalis pedis arteries. All these pulses are normally present and equal.
   b. Palpate the ulnar nerves between the olecranon and medial epicondyle and the common peroneal nerves laterally just below the head of the fibula.
2. Auscultation
   a. Listen for a bruit over each eyeball. Ask the patient to close both eyes, place the stethoscope bell over one eyeball firmly, and ask the patient to open the other eye and look steadily at an object.
   b. Listen for a bruit over both carotid arteries high in the neck at the angle of the jaw and in each supraclavicular space. If a bruit is heard in either place, compare blood pressures in the arms.
C. Mental status. Perform a memory examination and some screening of language function in all patients; expand as needed if cognitive functions are a concern of the patient.
   1. Level of consciousness. Assess for lethargy, stupor, or coma by stimulating with voice, visual and tactile stimulation, or even pain, if necessary.
   2. Attention and orientation. Ask the patient to identify the date, time, and place, and their name and situation. Monitor responsiveness to commands; ask the patient to repeat 4 to 7 digits forward and backward. Tests of serial subtraction may also be used to assess attention.
   3. Language function. Conversation can indicate grossly intact fluency and receptive skills when histories are semantically intact and requests for information or performance of the examination are understood. Additional testing is needed if there are any cerebral signs or suspicions.
      a. Fluency/expression. Ask the patient to name objects pointed out by the examiner (thumb, lapel, watch, crystal, colors). Ask him or her to describe the situation or family to assess fluency and semantics.
      b. Comprehension/reception. Ask the patient to perform fairly complex, multi-step commands without demonstration ("Touch your left first finger to your right ear and then close your eyes.") If auditory comprehension is impaired, test reading comprehension of similar or even simpler instructions.
      c. Repetition. Ask the patient to repeat phrases like "no ifs, ands or buts" or other material with high semantic content.
   4. Memory. Ask the patient to recall three items with qualifiers for 5 minutes. These may include a name, place, and object. The patient should always be asked to repeat the items and should be able to recall them without hints at 5 minutes. Ask the patient to list the last several presidents and to discuss a widely understood current event. If family members are present to confirm the information, ask for personal data such as anniversaries, birth dates, or the number of children or grandchildren. One may test for memory of long-past events, such as the date of Pearl Harbor. Tailor your questions to the age, experience, and memory deficits of the individual patient.
   5. Affect. Assess the patient for emotional stability, psychomotor retardation, and sleep or appetite problems.
   6. Abstraction and judgment. Ask patients to describe similarities and differences (e.g., how are an apple and a lemon similar?). Ask what they might do if they found a stamped addressed envelope in the street. Normal patients are able to categorize objects (e.g., fruits, animals) and will say that they would mail the letter.
   7. Construction and visuospatial abilities. When memory or cognition are concerns, ask the patient to draw a clock and include the hands and hour markers. Ask the patient to duplicate a complex drawing. If there is a concern about a subtle neglect syndrome, asking the patient to mark the

midline of a series of horizontal lines scattered across a page can be helpful.

D. Cranial nerves (Fig. 15-1)

   1. Olfactory nerve (I). This is not tested in screening examination, but test if there are concerns about smell or taste. Ask the patient to close the eyes and identify any common, nonirritating odor (e.g., coffee, vanilla, or mint, not alcohol or ammonia). Test each nostril separately. Normally, the patient should be able to identify familiar odors. Loss of the ability to smell can be due to local nasal disorders; when the problem is neurologic, the most common cause is trauma.

   2. Optic nerve (II) (see Chapter 5).

   a. Visual acuity. Test the patient with his or her glasses on, and test each eye separately. Use standardized charts, pocket-sized testing cards, or any available printed material. If the patient cannot read even large print, ask him or her to count your fingers at various distances. Failing that, test the ability to see moving fingers or to distinguish light from dark. To distinguish refractive error from other problems, see whether acuity improves with a pinhole.

   b. Visual fields.

   (1) Check field defects using the confrontation method. Ask the patient to cover one eye, and with the other eye look straight into your eye. Test all four quadrants in each eye by asking the patient to count fingers. Ask about any "blind spots" or test with a small red object for scotomas or desaturation. Normally, the visual fields

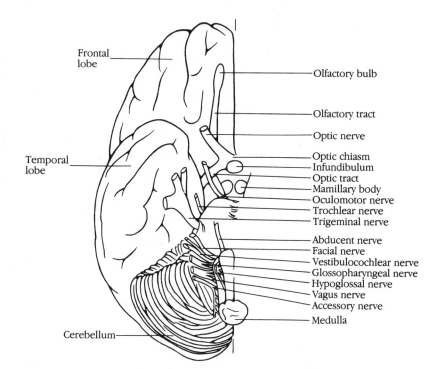

Fig. 15-1. Brain stem with cranial nerves.

are full with no obvious blind spots. Perimetry may be needed to further define small defects.

   (2) Extinction or suppression. Wiggle your finger first in one half of the field, asking the patient, "On which side do you see the finger wiggle?" Next, repeat on the opposite side with a finger from the other hand. Then, move both fingers simultaneously, asking the same question each time. Normally, patients are able to report that both fingers are moving simultaneously.

   c. Fundi. Examine fundi with the ophthalmoscope. The presence of a sharp disk outline and venous pulsations in the disk indicate normal intracranial pressure. Minimal indistinctness along the nasal or medial aspect of the disk may be normal. Examine vessels and check for any hyperpigmentation.

3. Oculomotor nerve (III), trochlear nerve (IV), abducent nerve (VI). These nerves supply the muscles of eye movement and are tested as a unit.

   a. Inspection. Inspect each eye for ptosis, and note any difference between the widths of the palpebral fissures. Assess alignment of the eyes at rest.

   b. Movement. Ask the patient to keep head motionless and follow a small object, such as a fingertip. Move horizontally to the limit of lateral gaze, then move vertically. Return to midposition and test elevation and depression. Pause for a moment at each end point, and inspect for nystagmus and weakness of any eye muscle. Ask about diplopia. Then, bring the object from a distance of about 3 feet to within 1 inch of the patient's nose to test convergence and assess normal pupillary constriction to convergence. Normally, extraocular muscles move the eyes in parallel in all directions. Mild nystagmus may occur at the extreme limit of lateral gaze; no nystagmus is present on upgaze or downgaze even at the extremes.

   c. Pupils. Check pupillary reaction to light by shining light directly into each eye while shielding the other eye. Observe the direct light reflex (constriction in the illuminated eye), and the consensual light reflex (constriction in the shielded eye). Estimate resting diameter and equality of pupils. It is useful to swing a flashlight from one eye to the other to detect any inequality in the amount of light perceived. It is sometimes helpful to evaluate the normal pupillary constriction with convergence.

4. Trigeminal nerve (V).

   a. Sensory. Test the divisions of the trigeminal nerve for sensitivity to light touch, pinprick, and temperature.

   b. Corneal reflex. Test by placing a wisp of cotton on the lateral sclera or cornea while the patient is looking away. Repeat on the other eye. Normally, both eyes blink quickly each time.

   c. Masseter and temporalis muscles. Palpate with the patient clenching jaws. Ask the patient to open the mouth slightly, and tap over the chin to elicit the jaw jerk reflex. If there are cranial nerve concerns, assess deviation of the jaw on opening the mouth and the strength of lateral movement.

5. Facial nerve (VII).

   a. Motor. Ask the patient to smile and show teeth, close eyes against resistance, elevate eyebrows, and contract the platysma. Assess the nasolabial fold bilaterally at rest. Facial movements should be equal bilaterally, but minimal asymmetry may be normal.

   b. Taste. Drop a strong sugar or salt solution on one side of the anterior two thirds of the protruded tongue; ask the patient to report what was tasted. Repeat on other side of tongue.

6. Auditory nerve (VIII). The two divisions are tested separately (see Chapters 6 and 7).

a. Cochlear (hearing). Assess the patient's ability to identify a whispered number at 6 feet. A tuning fork of 256 cycles or more per second may also be applied to the center of the frontal bone (Weber's test). If the patient hears more in one ear than in the other, test air and bone conduction by placing the tuning fork outside the external canal and then over the mastoid process (Rinne test). Normally, hearing should be equal in both ears, and air conduction should be about twice bone conduction.

b. Vestibular (equilibration). Assessed indirectly when evaluating for nystagmus and examining postural stability.

7. Glossopharyngeal nerve (IX), vagus nerve (X). These are largely tested together.

a. Motor function. Note quality of voice and ability to swallow. With head straight forward in the midline, ask the patient to open mouth and say "ah"; observe the position of the soft palate and uvula at rest and with phonation. Normally, the uvula and palate rise in the midline with phonation.

b. Gag reflex. Check by touching each side of the posterior pharyngeal wall with a tongue blade.

c. Taste. If an abnormality of taste is suspected, repeat the taste test on the posterior one-third of the tongue to assess the glossopharyngeal contribution.

8. Spinal accessory nerve (XI).

a. Sternocleidomastoid muscle. Ask the patient to turn head to one side against your hand; palpate the opposite sternocleidomastoid muscle. Repeat contralaterally. Normally, strength is equal bilaterally.

b. Trapezius muscle. Palpate; test strength of "shrug" while you press down on the patient's shoulders with both hands. Strength should be symmetric.

9. Hypoglossal nerve (XII). Ask the patient to protrude tongue in midline; observe any deviation or atrophy. Test for weakness by asking the patient to stick tongue into cheek while you press against the bulging cheek.

E. Motor system

1. Inspection

a. Movement. Look for abnormal movements while the patient is at rest, either large (capable of moving a joint) or small (within the belly of the muscle itself).

b. Muscle bulk. Look for atrophy or hypertrophy. If atrophy is present or progressive disease causing atrophy is suspected, measure and record the circumference of the muscle bilaterally, noting the point at which the measurement is taken. Chronic illness may produce generalized wasting of muscles. Great variation in muscle bulk is found among normal persons, depending on age, sex, and occupation.

2. Strength. It is prudent to briefly assess strength in one muscle in every nerve root distribution. Pay attention to relative weakness in one side compared with the other and in proximal compared with distal groups.

a. Screening examination. Test the strength of the following:

(1) Dorsiflexion and plantar flexion of the feet
(2) Extension and flexion of the knee and hip flexion
(3) Abduction of shoulder, flexion and extension at the elbow
(4) Extension of fingers, abduction of thumb and fingers

b. Grades of strength:

0 = no movement of the muscle
1 (trace) = visible muscular contraction; no joint movement
2 (poor) = minimal movement with gravity eliminated
3 (fair) = full range of motion against gravity
4 (good) = good resistance but not normal
5 (normal) = normal strength against resistance

    c. Normal findings. Significant variation in strength is present among normal persons, depending on age, sex, and occupation. The difference in strength between the nondominant and dominant sides of the body is minimal.

  3. Muscle tone (resistance to passive manipulation). Test by flexing and extending relaxed muscles. Use both fast and slow flexion and extension at the elbows, wrists, and knees. Normally, muscles are somewhat hypotonic at rest. Certain patients cannot maintain muscle relaxation during these manipulations, making the assessment difficult.

F. Cerebellar function. This is tested by assessing the ability to perform skilled and rapid alternating movements in the upper and lower extremities.

  1. Upper extremities. Ask the patient to flip each hand back and forth (supinate and pronate) as rapidly as possible. Finger-to-nose test: ask the patient to touch the index finger of the outstretched arm to the tip of the examiner's finger slowly. Assess rapid fine movements of the fingers, such as touching the tip of the index finger to the thumb. Normally, no wavering, tremor, or misjudging of distance (dysmetria) should occur; performance may be slightly worse with the nondominant hand.

  2. Lower extremities. Ask the patient to tap the foot against the floor as rapidly as possible. Heel-knee-shin test: ask the patient to touch one heel to the opposite knee and run it slowly down the shin to the big toe. Normally, the heel should not fall from the shin. The patient should be able to tap the floor quickly with either foot.

G. Reflexes

  1. Check jaw jerk, biceps, triceps, brachioradialis, finger flexor, patellar, and Achilles reflexes in all patients. The limb should be relaxed and flexed or semiflexed. Strike the tendon or bone directly and smartly with the reflex hammer. To test the biceps reflex, tap your finger, which is placed over the tendon. If the reflex is minimal or apparently absent, ask the patient to "reinforce" by pulling with one hand against the other at the time the tendon is tapped.

    a. Charting reflexes. Label the right and left sides of a human figure, and note the state of the reflex at the appropriate joint.

      0 = absent
      1+ = relatively hypoactive
      2+ = normal
      3+ = relatively hyperactive
      4+ = hyperactive with clonus

    b. Normal findings. Reflexes may be minimal in athletic normal adults or very active in some normal patients. Normal reflexes are always symmetric and are similar in the upper and lower extremities. Grade 0 or 4+ reflexes are abnormal, although nonsustained clonus is sometimes seen at the ankles in normal patients with brisk reflexes.

  2. Pathologic reflexes

    a. Feet. Babinski's reflex: stroke the sole of the foot with a pointed instrument from the heel along the lateral edge of the foot and across the ball of the foot medially. Chaddock's reflex: stroke the lateral edge of the foot from heel to toes just above the sole. Oppenheim's reflex: with the knuckles, press firmly down on the shin from the knee to the ankle. Bing reflex: stimulate the dorsal aspect of the big toe with a pin. With any of these stimuli, no extensor response (dorsiflexion) of the foot or toes should occur after infancy.

    b. Hands. Hoffmann's reflex: quickly extend or flex the last joint of the middle finger, or suspend the limp hand by its middle finger and quickly flip the tip of the finger upward or downward. Normally, little or no flexion response of the thumb and fingers should occur.

    c. Clonus. Quickly flex or extend a joint and maintain stretch.

3. Superficial skin reflexes. These reflexes are normally present in young, relaxed patients, but their absence is common and may be due to a variety of causes.
    a. Abdominal reflex. Using a firm object, stroke over all four quadrants of the abdomen either toward, away from, or at right angles to the umbilicus. Normally, the umbilicus moves toward the stimulus.
    b. Cremasteric reflex (only used in males). Stroke along the internal aspect of the upper thigh. Normally, the testicle on the stimulated side moves upward, owing to involuntary contraction of the cremaster muscle.
H. Sensory examination. This is the most subjective and variable portion of the neurologic examination.
    1. Posterior column sense. Vibratory sense is the most sensitive indicator of posterior column function. Position sense is often not decreased until vibratory sense is markedly diminished or lost.
        a. Vibration. Test with a 128-cps tuning fork placed on a bony prominence in all four extremities (big toe or lateral malleolus on each ankle, first knuckle of each hand). Strike the fork with the same strength, and hold it with the same degree of firmness in each place. Note the duration of vibration perceived.
        b. Joint position sense. With the patient's eyes closed, grasp one toe or finger by the sides and move it up and down; ask the patient to identify the direction of movement in the digit.
    2. Pain and temperature. It is usually not necessary to test both.
        a. Pain. Superficial pain perception is tested with a sharp pin in all four extremities. Develop a standard pattern, such as going laterally to medially and distally to proximally. Test the trunk anteriorly or posteriorly. Map the extent of any loss, going from the area of decreased sensation toward normal. In certain cases (bowel or bladder problems), test the perianal area (buttocks and genitalia). Normally, pain sensation should be felt equally in all areas (assuming equal pressure on the pin).
        b. Temperature. Test temperature sensation with any warm or cool object in the same manner as with the pinprick test (tuning forks are a convenient cold stimulus). Temperature testing assesses the spinothalamic system and should be equal throughout.
    3. Fine sensory modalities. Tests of fine (cortical) sensory modalities are most useful in evaluating parietal cortex function and in the analysis of hysterical sensory loss.
        a. Light touch: test with a wisp of cotton on the hairy surfaces of the trunk and all four extremities, testing one side against the other. Normally, a very light touch can be perceived. (Light touch on nonhairy skin often cannot be perceived.)
        b. Two-point tactile sensation: test with two dull points, one side against the other and upper and lower extremities. Record the threshold at which the patient definitely feels two points. Normally, the threshold on the tip of the index finger is about 3 mm.
        c. Stereognosis: ask the patient to close eyes and identify objects (such as coins or keys) placed in his or her hands by moving them around and feeling them with the fingers. Normally, a person can differentiate among a penny, nickel, quarter, and half-dollar.
        d. Graphesthesia: draw numerals on various parts of the patient's skin, and ask the patient to identify them.
        e. Extinction (suppression): test by double simultaneous stimulation. Ask the patient to close eyes, then touch the patient on the back of the hand. Ask where the touch was. Then touch the identical spot on the other side, and repeat the question. The third time, touch in both places at the same time and with equal pressure. Normally, the patient feels both sides.

I. Gait and station
   1. Walking. Ask the patient to walk normally for some distance. Note posture, size of steps, width of stance, amount and symmetry of arm swing, and balance while walking. Test ability to start and stop on command. Another test of walking balance is tandem walking (walk in a straight line, putting one heel directly in front of the toes of the other foot). Normally, a person should be able to walk in a fairly straight line for 10 or 20 feet with eyes open or closed.
   2. Standing balance. Ask the patient to stand with feet together and eyes open, then with eyes closed. Be ready to catch the patient, since there could be a tendency to fall in this position with eyes closed if proprioception is abnormal (Romberg's sign). Finer tests of balance include standing on one foot and hopping or jumping on one foot. Normally, a person should be able to balance with feet together and eyes closed and to balance and hop on each foot with eyes open and closed.
J. Meningeal signs. Any positive sign indicates the possibility of meningeal irritation.
   1. Nuchal rigidity (stiff neck). Ask the patient to relax, then with both hands flex the neck toward the chest. No resistance or pain should occur.
   2. Brudzinski's sign. This is flexion of the hips when the head is flexed to the chest.
   3. Kernig's sign. Flex the hip on the trunk, allowing the knee to flex at the same time. When the hip is flexed 90 degrees, extend the knee. No resistance, pain, or tendency toward flexion of the neck should be present.
K. Conversion reactions. Recognition of a few common patterns may be helpful in distinguishing organic from functional neurologic impairments:
   1. Patients with feigned visual loss typically present with tunnel vision (visual fields remain just as constricted at farther distances) and navigate their environment normally, whereas it is often difficult for them to perform tasks that normal blind persons have no problem with, such as writing their name. Ask patients suspected of somatasizing to describe the extent of the visual field at different distances from a white wall; ask them to read print (acuity at least 20/100). If a patient claims complete blindness, a mirror moved before him or her may reveal good tracking.
   2. Many patients with hysterical weakness are able to move the limbs fully when recumbent, but are unable to bear weight when standing (astasia abasia). These patients should be tested in both positions.
   3. Factitious gait disorders often result in athletically difficult amounts of swaying and lurching with preserved ability to walk in tandem.
   4. Hysterical movement disorders often vary in location, and patients have many relapses and remissions. These features are unusual in true movement disorders.
   5. Nonepileptic pseudoseizures are very common and often difficult to distinguish historically from epilepsy. The most reliable historical feature for pseudoseizures is a description consisting of long periods of motionless unresponsiveness, which rarely occurs in any seizure type.
L. Expected findings in elderly (age >75)
   1. The ability to smell commonly decreases with advancing age.
   2. Motor power may diminish slightly, but resistance remains symmetric and equal throughout.
   3. Gait examination. It is commonly more difficult for the elderly to perform accurate tandem gait. A mildly stooped and slowed gait may also be normal.
   4. Upgaze is often conjugately and mildly limited in the elderly.
III. **Cardinal Symptoms and Abnormal Findings**
   A. General symptoms
      1. *Numbness* may be due to peripheral nerve or spinal cord (posterior column) involvement, or to sensory pathway interruption in the brain stem, thalamus, or parietal cortex.

2. *Weakness* may result from abnormalities of the muscles, neuromuscular junction, or nerve, or from the corticospinal tract in the spinal cord, brain stem, internal capsule, or motor cortex. Involvement of other central pathways connecting to the main motor system also can produce weakness.

3. *Fainting or loss of consciousness* results from loss of function of the brain (bihemispheric or brain-stem reticular activating system) due to loss of blood supply, inadequate oxygen or glucose, imbalance of nutrients, epilepsy, or cerebral destruction from any cause.

4. *Dizziness* (faintness, vertigo, or imbalance) is caused by dysfunction of the inner ear balance mechanisms or of the vestibular portion of the acoustic nerve or its central connections. Imbalance may result from peripheral nerve, posterior column, cerebellar, or main motor pathway involvement. Syncope can be neurogenic when the autonomic nervous system is damaged.

5. *Pain* may be due to distortion, transection, or irritation of pain endings and pain fibers of peripheral nerves or of the central pain pathways (spinothalamic tracts) in the spinal core, brain stem, or thalamus. Recent data indicate that selective attention to pain is another possible mechanism.

6. *Headache* is caused by distortion of or traction on blood vessels or the meninges or other covering structures of the brain; or by pressure, distortion, traction, or displacement of almost any extracerebral structure in the head including the skull, paranasal sinuses, scalp, and posterior suboccipital muscles of the neck.

7. *Defective memory or thinking* may result from any lesion in almost any area of the brain, although a specific memory defect may result from small lesions in hypothalamic, thalamic, or temporal lobe structures.

B. General examination

1. Palpation

   a. Carotid pulses. When these pulses are absent or markedly decreased, an occlusion is suggested. However, what appears to be a normal carotid artery can be completely or partially occluded.

   b. Temporal arteries. Decreased or absent pulse is presumptive evidence of external carotid occlusion on that side. Retinal artery pressure readings give more reliable information than simple palpation.

   c. The subclavian, brachial, radial, dorsalis pedis, posterior tibial, and femoral pulses, if absent or definitely decreased, give hints of occlusion of the main branches of the aorta and may explain intermittent weakness or numbness.

2. Auscultation

   a. Skull. A bruit may be heard on the side of increased or decreased blood flow through a carotid or vertebral artery. Increased flow may be due to occlusion on the opposite side or to arteriovenous anomaly or tumor on same side. Decreased flow occurs with partial or complete occlusion on the same or opposite sides or can even occur without vascular disease.

   b. Supraclavicular space. A bruit may indicate partial or complete occlusion of the subclavian artery with possible "subclavian steal" syndrome. A decrease in the blood pressure in the affected arm and a delay in the radial pulse on the same side may be present.

C. Mental status. Global abnormalities indicate delirium or dementia, whereas more limited disturbances are often localizing.

1. Level of consciousness, attention, orientation. In dementia, consciousness is generally normal, attention is often good, and orientation is commonly preserved until late in the disease. Delirium, on the other hand, is characterized by a fluctuating level of consciousness with poor attention and orientation and often with hallucinations or affectual changes.

2. Language function. Expressive deficits localize to frontal lobe structures near Broca's area, receptive problems are most prominent in dominant

parietal lesions (Wernicke's area), and deficits in repetition implicate lesions of the arcuate fasciculus, which connects the two areas. Problems with articulation alone can result from lesions in the subcortical regions, thalamus, brain-stem tracts or nuclei, or cerebellum. Dysarthria can usually be classified into ataxic, motor, spastic, dystonic, and hypokinetic types.

3. Memory, abstraction, judgment, and visuospatial skills. Abnormalities can indicate transient (e.g., seizures, transient global amnesia) or permanent (usually associated with cortical degenerative diseases) damage to cerebral structures. Isolated abnormalities in abstraction, affect, or judgment are also frequently seen in patients with psychiatric diseases.

D. Cranial nerves

1. Olfactory nerve (I). The most common neurologic cause of anosmia is trauma. Occasionally, tumors, especially meningiomas of the olfactory groove or sphenoid ridge, can cause anosmia. The ability to smell commonly decreases with advancing age.

2. Optic nerve (II) (see Chapter 5)

   a. Visual acuity. This can be impaired by optic neuritis or ophthalmic artery emboli in addition to the intraocular diseases described in Chapter 5.

   b. Visual fields.

   (1) Homonymous hemianopsia is the most common gross defect of neurologic importance. For example, if the right visual field is lost in both eyes, the left optic tract or visual radiation is diseased somewhere between the optic chiasm and the left visual cortex. The more similar (or congruous) the defect is in both eyes, the more posterior the lesion in the optic radiations is likely to be.

   (2) Homonymous quadrantanopic defect indicates disease involving visual radiations as they pass through the parietal or temporal lobes.

   (3) Upper quadrantanopic defect indicates involvement of the visual radiations in the opposite temporal lobe (Meyer's loop).

   (4) Lower quadrantanopias indicate involvement of the opposite parietal lobe.

   (5) Bitemporal field defects (involvement of the lateral half of the visual field in each eye) indicate a lesion in the center of the optic chiasm interrupting the fibers as they cross from one optic nerve to the opposite tract; this is most commonly caused by a tumor of the pituitary gland.

   c. Fundi. The two most common abnormalities of neurologic concern are the following:

   (1) Swelling or edema of the optic disk (papilledema) first appears as a loss of distinctness of the disk margins, progressing until the margin disappears. The disk may become raised above the surrounding retina, and the edema may spread into the retina. Hemorrhages can be seen in late stages of papilledema.

   (2) Optic atrophy appears as pallor and lack of normal vascularity in the disk.

3. Oculomotor nerve (III), trochlear nerve (IV), abducent nerve (VI)

   a. Movement

   (1) Extraocular muscle paralysis (see Chapter 5)

   (a) Third-nerve paralysis results in a dilated pupil, external deviation of the eyeball, and ptosis of the upper lid.

   (b) Fourth-nerve paralysis is rare and results in weakness of internal rotation of the eyeball and downward and inward gaze. The affected eye is usually hyperopic (higher), and the patient may tilt the head to elevate the eye with the paralyzed superior oblique muscle, bringing the horizontal axes parallel and preventing diplopia.

(c) Sixth-nerve paralysis results in lateral rectus muscle weakness, causing the eye to deviate inward. Sixth-nerve weakness may result from increased intracranial pressure and central herniation syndromes, especially in children.

(2) Nystagmus often gives a clue to the location and type of neurologic disease.

(a) In dissociated nystagmus with lesions of the medial longitudinal fasciculus, the eye on the side to which the gaze is directed has strong horizontal nystagmus in the direction of gaze, and the opposite eye cannot adduct and shows less nystagmus. Multiple sclerosis is the most common cause.

(b) Acute and chronic conditions of the cerebellum, brain stem, and vestibular apparatus cause nystagmus, which is more pronounced on looking toward the side of the lesion. Cerebellar disease can also case spontaneous or gaze-evoked upgaze or downgaze nystagmus.

(c) Cerebral lesions may cause minimal to moderate nystagmus, which is more evident in looking away from the side of the lesion.

b. Pupils

(1) Anisocoria may be caused by sympathetic paralysis (Horner's syndrome), oculomotor nerve weakness, Adie's syndrome, syphilis (Argyll Robertson pupil), diabetes, multiple sclerosis, and trauma or disease of the iris. Mild degrees of anisocoria with normal reactivity to light can be seen in normals.

(2) Bilaterally dilated or constricted pupils may be caused by a variety of drugs, including stimulants such as d-amphetamine, opiates, or eye drops for treatment of glaucoma.

(3) Unilateral dilated pupil often occurs with increased intracranial pressure, when it is a sign of uncal herniation with pressure on the external fascicles of the third nerve. The dilated pupil is usually on the side of the lesion. The Argyll Robertson pupil is irregular and smaller than normal, and it reacts to convergence but not light. In Adie's pupillary abnormality, the pupil is larger than normal and reacts slowly to light. This syndrome is usually found in young women with decreased or absent tendon reflexes.

4. Trigeminal nerve (V)

a. Sensory

(1) The corneal reflex may be diminished unilaterally from either a peripheral or central lesion.

(2) Medullary or upper cervical cord lesions involving the descending tract of the trigeminal nerve can cause loss of pain and temperature sensations exactly to the midline of the face while touch remains intact. It may involve only one division of the nerve, however; therefore, it is important to test all three divisions.

(3) Cerebral infarct may cause some decrease in sensation that does not extend exactly to the midline on the opposite side of the face; there is usually no appreciable weakness of the masseter and pterygoid muscles.

b. Masseter and temporalis muscles. These muscles are most often noticeably weak in muscle and neuromuscular junction disorders, although they are occasionally affected by upper and lower motor neuron lesions. Jaw jerk may be absent in some normal persons.

5. Facial nerve (VII)

a. Movement

(1) Any upper motor neuron lesion results in moderate to marked weakness of the opposite lower facial muscles, including the platysma, orbicularis oris, and sometimes the lower part of the orbicularis oculi. If small, there may be only minimal drooping of the

opposite corner of the mouth at rest and weakness on voluntary movement. Eye closure and frontalis strength may be somewhat affected, although bilateral innervation to these areas usually results in significant sparing.

(2) Lesion of the seventh-nerve nucleus or of the nerve itself (peripheral facial paralysis, lower motor neuron disease, Bell's palsy) causes weakness of all parts of the face on the side of the lesion. The patient will be unable to move the frontalis, orbicularis oculi, or orbicularis oris. Deficient eye closure can lead to corneal abrasions, if not treated.

b. **Taste.** Test for taste on the anterior two thirds of the tongue on the side of the facial weakness when determining the site of the interruption in a peripheral seventh-nerve (Bell's) paralysis.

6. **Auditory nerve (VIII)** (see Chapters 6 and 7)

a. **Conductive deafness.** If air conduction time is lessened while bone conduction time is preserved, the deafness is in the middle ear or external ear.

b. **Perceptive or mixed (sensorineural) deafness.** If both air and bone conduction are reduced, the deafness is caused by nerve damage or is mixed. Central innervation to hearing is bilateral; therefore, a unilateral perceptive deafness indicates a lesion of the cochlear nuclei, the eighth nerve, or the cochlea. Testing the vestibular portion of the eighth nerve may be helpful, since vestibular function will be preserved if deafness is caused by a lesion of the cochlear nuclei but may be lost in lesions of the nerve or cochlea.

7. **Glossopharyngeal nerve (IX) and vagus nerve (X).** The ninth nerve mediates sensory and the tenth nerve provides motor component of palate movement and gag reflex. Unilateral weakness of the palate causes the uvula to deviate toward the intact side during gag testing or phonation. The palate will also be lower on the weak side. Palate weakness alone can be seen in upper or lower motor neuron lesions. If there is marked ipsilateral palate weakness and vocal cord paralysis, the lower motor fibers of the vagal nucleus or nerve are usually involved. If there is no sensory component, the vagus nerve is probably involved after leaving the medulla. Bilateral weakness of the palate can be seen with upper (pseudobulbar) or lower (bulbar) motor neuron disturbances.

8. **Spinal accessory nerve (XI).** Mild unilateral weakness can be seen after upper motor neuron lesions on the same side. Severe unilateral weakness and atrophy of the trapezius and sternocleidomastoid muscles indicates a lesion outside the brain stem, since the nerve has its origin in the upper cervical cord. Bilateral weakness and atrophy of these muscles are often found in primary muscle disease, such as muscular dystrophy.

9. **Hypoglossal nerve (XII)**

a. **Unilateral tongue weakness.** Different sets of muscles control the tongue when it is protruding than those that work when it is resting in the mouth; therefore, the protruded tongue deviates toward the weak side, and the resting tongue toward the strong side. A large acute upper motor neuron lesion may cause temporary unilateral weakness on the opposite side along with a transient dysarthria.

b. **Bilateral tongue weakness.** Check the tongue carefully for continuous fasciculations and atrophy, which may be the earliest sign of lower motor neuron disease affecting the hypoglossal nerve nuclei (i.e., amyotrophic lateral sclerosis). Be careful, tongue movements can be difficult to interpret.

E. Motor system

1. **Inspection.** The presence of fasciculations and atrophy implies rapidly progressive lower motor neuron diseases. Fasciculations may be emphasized in patients or elicited in normals after strong contractions. Atrophy or hypertrophy may assist in the diagnosis of neuromuscular diseases.

2. Abnormal movements
  a. Tremors
    (1) Resting tremor: movements typical of parkinsonism. There are four to five tremors per second; they are usually more evident in hands but also seen in arms, head, face, tongue, and legs. If Parkinson's disease is suspected, look for associated increased tone producing the typical cogwheel rigidity (rhythmic increase and decrease in tone superimposed on passive movements produced by the examiner).
    (2) Kinetic tremor: not present at rest, prominent with sustained posture or fine distal action. This tremor more often involves the head; it can be senile, familial, or essential.
    (3) Intention tremor: usually evident only with carefully directed purposeful movement. This tremor is generally a distal and terminal position tremor common in patients with cerebellar disease and multiple sclerosis.
  b. Chorea: irregular, involuntary spontaneous movements usually involving more than one joint. Movements are purposeless and rapid and can involve any extremity, face, mouth, and tongue. Movements often migrate, with no alteration in tone. Chorea is seen in Huntington's disease, Sydenham's chorea, Wilson's disease, and thyroid disorders.
  c. Athetosis: slow, writhing movements involving mainly the proximal parts of the extremities, trunk, and face. This condition can be seen in cerebral palsy.
  d. Dystonia: slow movements or postures with unopposed action of a fixed set of muscles. Dystonia most often involves face, neck, trunk, and upper extremities in adults and is generally idiopathic. It can be post-traumatic.
3. Strength. If weakness is present, evaluate the distribution of deficits to pinpoint the cause (e.g., cerebral, spinal, nerve root, plexus, neuromuscular junction or muscles). Tests for fatiguability are helpful in myasthenia, and testing in different positions can be helpful in functional disease.
4. Muscle tone
  a. Decreased tone occurs in diseases of the anterior horn cells and peripheral nerves and in uncomplicated diseases of the cerebellum.
  b. Increased tone
    (1) Spasticity occurs in upper motor neuron diseases (pyramidal tract). This common abnormality of tone is classically of the "clasp knife" type, in which tone varies from normal as the joint is rapidly extended or flexed, to a marked increase when full flexion or extension is approached; with continued pressure, the muscle gradually gives way. In general, spasticity is a *rate-dependent* increased resistance to passive manipulation.
    (2) Rigidity occurs in the extrapyramidal group of diseases, such as parkinsonism. It is characterized by increased tone throughout the full range of motion of the joint. Rigidity can produce steady resistance to any superimposed movement (lead pipe) or an intermittent increase in tone (cogwheeling).
    (3) Slow relaxation of muscles occurs in diseases such as myotonia or hypothyroidism. Affected muscles (quadriceps, forearm groups, thenar muscles, or tongue) contract when percussed and then relax at a much slower rate than normal.
F. Cerebellar dysfunction
  1. Disease of one cerebellar hemisphere produces signs (tremor, dysmetria, dysdiachokinesis) ipsilaterally, whereas subcortical and brain-stem lesions can produce contralateral ataxia.
  2. Disease of the cerebellar vermis causes truncal ataxia and proximal tremor; alcohol affects the anterior vermis and gait stability. Other drugs can cause vermian and appendicular (extremity) ataxia and need to be excluded.

3. Sensory loss (especially loss of proprioception), pyramidal tract disease, and marked weakness can interfere with cerebellar testing or give false cerebellar signs.

G. Reflexes. Because abnormalities are difficult to feign, the reflex examination is an objective assessment of neurologic status. Any isolated reflex change requires special attention.

1. Hypoactive or absent reflexes are found in a variety of diseases that interfere with the anterior horn cell, the sensory or motor part of the reflex arc, the motor end plate, or the muscle.

2. Hyperactive or increased reflexes almost invariably represent disease of the upper motor neuron or pyramidal tract, anywhere from the cerebral cortex to just above the appropriate anterior horn cell. The following are reflex arc levels determining level of spinal cord lesions:

Biceps C-5,6
Triceps C-7
Brachioradialis C-6
Finger flexors C-8
Patellar L-3,4
Achilles S-1

3. Pathologic reflexes. Clonus is rarely normal and is an indication of central nervous system disease.

a. Babinski's reflex. A positive response (extension of large toe with fanning of smaller toes) is an unequivocal sign of pyramidal tract disease. This is a reliable sign, which should be tested for in all patients. With extensive disease, the entire leg may withdraw with flexion at the ankle, knee, and hip. If no response occurs, it may be significant if the responses of the two feet differ. Some patients withdraw the leg when the sole is stimulated; using alternative techniques or asking them not to withdraw may help.

b. Hoffmann's reflex. This sign is equivocal and pathologic only when markedly exaggerated or unilaterally present.

4. Superficial skin reflexes. These reflexes are absent in diseases of either the upper or lower motor neurons. Absence of either the upper or lower abdominals may be helpful in determining the "sidedness" of a lesion or the level of a spinal cord lesion (upper: T-7 to 9, lower: T-9 to 11).

H. Sensory responses

1. Posterior column sense. If vibratory sense is decreased or absent in the distal extremities, it is useful to document the most distal joint where it can be felt. "Threshold times" to the end of vibration are less reliable than the absolute presence or absence of vibration at any joint. Motion and position sense should also be tested at progressively higher levels. Some diseases are characterized by marked posterior column sensory loss (e.g., vitamin B_{12} deficiency).

2. Pain, temperature

a. Testing can be carried out with a pin, a broken wooden swab, or the lateral surface of a cold tuning fork. The examination can be somewhat unreliable, owing to variations in pressure by the examiner and the natural variability in different skin areas. Asking the patient to estimate the percentage degree of difference in sensitivity is often helpful, and many examiners disregard small differences of 10%, depending on the setting.

b. Pinprick testing can help to determine the level of a spinal cord lesion. There is often an area of increased response at the level of the lesion, normal responses above the level, and reduced sensitivity below.

c. In patients with bladder or bowel problems, or suspected myelopathies, check the area of the buttocks and genitalia for any sensory loss that might indicate a lesion in the cord, conus medullaris, or cauda equina.

    d. Map the area of sensory loss by testing from the area of loss to the normal exterior zone in all directions. Transfer the information to a sensory chart, and place it in the permanent record (Fig. 15-2).

3. Fine sensory modalities

    a. Parietal cortex disease. If disease is suspected in the parietal cortex, fine sensory tests can help in the evaluation. If a patient demonstrates suppression, the stimulus will be felt only on the side contralateral to the normal parietal lobe.

    b. Hysterical (conversion) sensory loss. Some patients have loss of vibration and light touch but good stereognosis. Others have loss of sensation in an entire extremity, without respecting the boundaries of spinal, nerve root, plexus, or peripheral nerve distributions.

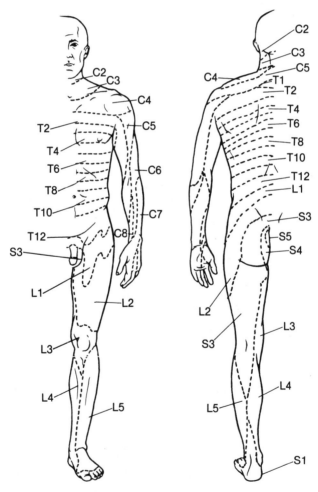

Fig. 15-2. Dermatomes.

I. Gait and station. Describe abnormalities of walking as closely as possible. Note any differences in arm swing, length of stride, or width of stance. Classic gaits include:

1. Foot drop gait: tendency toward dragging of the toes and high lifting of the knees owing to weakness of the dorsiflexors of the feet ("steppage gait").
2. Hemiplegic gait: circumduction of affected leg, weakness of dorsiflexion of the foot, and some tendency toward flexion at the knee on the affected side.
3. Ataxic gait (drunken gait): wide-based lurching walk characteristic of vermian cerebellar dysfunction.
4. Gait of parkinsonism: difficulty initiating gait, small shuffling steps, lack of normal arm swing, flexion of the trunk, tendency to increase speed and decrease the size of steps, and postural instability.
5. Gait of advanced Huntington's disease: a distinctive, dancing gait, with nearly continuous choreiform movements.
6. Scissoring gait: tendency toward internal rotation of both legs, and scraping together of the semiflexed knees as the patient drags the feet forward. This gait is characteristic of lower extremity spasticity.
7. Tabes dorsalis (syphilitic) gait: ataxia, foot slapping, tendency for patient to watch feet while walking, positive Rhomberg sign. (Romberg's sign is positive only when the patient falls with eyes closed, but not with eyes open. This occurs in patients with large fiber sensory dysfunction.)

J. Meningeal signs

1. False-positive signs. These signs can be due to tetanus, extensor rigidity or spasms, parkinsonism, or bony fixation of the neck.
2. False-negative signs. Patients with definite meningitis or subarachnoid hemorrhage occasionally have no signs of meningeal irritation at all, particularly if they are stuporous or comatose.

K. Conversion reactions (hysteria). Making the diagnosis of hysteria in a patient with neurologic complaints is fraught with pitfalls and difficulty. Always examine the patient very carefully for any objective evidence of neurologic illness, even in obviously affectively disturbed persons. Any objective findings (e.g., asymmetric reflexes, extensor plantar responses, and cranial nerve findings) must be evaluated thoroughly in any circumstance. Some typically somatiform complaints or findings can occur in organic neurologic disease, for example:

1. Plexus lesions can cause numbness or weakness or both, which is nondermatomal and involves most of one extremity.
2. A hemisensory defect that splits the midline is found in some lesions of the brain stem and spinal cord.
3. Movement disorders with chorea or athetosis are often masked as volitional behavioral automatisms by embarrassed patients. They will seem less purposeful if elicited while the patient is walking or distracted by another complex task.
4. Any acute significant neurologic impairment or concern can cause severe anxiety or emotional responses.
5. Giving way on strength testing can be found with true weakness, perhaps most commonly in cases of nondominant hemisphere injury in which neglect is prominent.

IV. Common Clinical Disorders

A. Stroke may be due to hemorrhage, arterial ischemia, venous occlusion, or anoxia. Diagnostic studies useful in evaluation include the following:

1. Computed tomography (CT) scans: best for acutely evaluating trauma and hemorrhages
2. Magnetic resonance imaging (MRI) scans: show abnormality earliest
3. Magnetic resonance angiography (MRA): most useful for large or medium vessel stenoses or large aneurysms
4. Carotid duplex studies, transcranial Doppler: best for posterior circulation

5. Transesophageal echocardiogram: to ensure visualization of the left atrium

6. Angiography: definitive evaluation of the intracranial circulation

B. Headache. Classifications are common, classic, or complicated migraine (hemicranial throbbing with nausea, photophobia, scotomata, or neurologic symptoms), tension (continuous dull), cluster (intermittent bouts of unilateral pain with rhinorrhea, lacrimation), icepick, thunderclap, pseudotumor cerebri (young with papilledema), temporal arteritis (often elderly), continuous hemicranial, and trigeminal neuralgia (often stimulus sensitive shooting pain in the trigeminal nerve distribution). Diagnostic tests are more limited than the history diagnostically and include only MRI and CT.

C. Degenerative disorders. These diseases are Alzheimer's disease, Parkinson's disease, Wilson's disease, Huntington's disease and a number of pediatric and genetic disorders.

1. Evaluation typically includes a brain MRI and metabolic serologies as indicated.

2. Formal neuropsychometrics (formal IQ and memory testing) are often helpful in diagnosis.

3. The gene for Huntington's disease (autosomal dominant) has recently been discovered and can be tested directly in the serum of persons at risk after appropriate counseling.

D. Meningitis. This includes viral, bacterial, and opportunistic infections and carcinomatous meningitis. Evaluation includes lumbar puncture and structural imaging to rule out complications (hydrocephalus, radicular encasement).

E. Myelopathy and radicular compression

1. Condition is usually evaluated by imaging the area suggested to be abnormal on physical examination. MRI is simplest and very accurate.

2. Myelography may be useful to assess the degree of block or lower root involvement.

F. Epilepsy: generalized (primary and secondary) and partial

1. Electroencephalography is vital to diagnosis.

2. Brain MRI (preferable) or CT are appropriate in nearly all cases.

G. Neuromuscular diseases: myasthenia, amyotrophic lateral sclerosis, Guillain-Barré syndrome, peripheral neuropathies, myopathies, and dystrophies

1. These diseases are diagnosed by electromyography.

2. Further investigation or confirmation by lumbar puncture, serologies, nerve and muscle biopsies, or imaging studies is sometimes required.

H. Multiple sclerosis. Diagnosis is complex and based on history, examination findings, MRI of brain and spinal cord, evoked potential electrophysiologic studies, and lumbar puncture.

I. Sleep disorders: obstructive sleep apnea, narcolepsy, periodic leg movements/restless legs syndrome, insomnia, phase advance or delay, and parasomnias. Polysomnography and multiple sleep latency tests (electrophysiologic studies of sleep) are required for diagnosis.

V. Available Technology

A. The table lists the various procedures that can be used for the patient with nervous system conditions.

B. The cost figures cited in the table on page 292 are **basic direct costs.** The figures are difficult to obtain and change quickly. They include **only** the cost of the test itself (technician, equipment, time, materials). No professional costs (interpretation) are included. Costs vary from region to region based on differences in some components such as labor. However, the relative cost ranking should remain similar.

Procedure	Indication
Computed tomography (CT)	Stroke Trauma Hemorrhage
Magnetic resonance imaging (MRI)	Stroke Degenerative diseases Myelopathy/radicular compression Demyelinating diseases
Magnetic resonance angiography (MRA)	Large/medium vessel stenoses Large aneurysms, arteriovenous malformations
Carotid duplex studies	Evaluate anterior cranial circulation
Transcranial doppler	Evaluate posterior cranial circulation
Transesophageal echocardiogram	Visualize left atrium
Angiography	Evaluate intracranial circulation
Neuropsychometrics (IQ/memory testing)	Degenerative diseases Cognitive concerns
Genetic testing	Huntington's disease
Lumbar puncture	Meningitis Neuromuscular diseases Demyelinating diseases
Myelography	Myelopathy/radicular compression (assess degree of block or lower root involvement)
Electroencephalography	Epilepsy Degenerative disorders
Electromyography	Neuromuscular diseases
Evoked potential electrophysiologic studies	Demyelinating diseases
Polysomnography/multiple sleep latency tests	Sleep disorders Excessive daytime somnolence Parasomnias
Intracarotid amobarbital procedure	Language and memory function Localization for proposed cortical resections
Corticography	Localization of epileptogenic zones in epilepsy
Single photon emission tomography/positron emission tomography	Degenerative diseases Localization of ictal focus
Functional MRI	Neuromuscular disease Autonomic system dysfunction
Autonomic function testing	Neuromuscular disease Autonomic system dysfunction
Cisternography	Cerebrospinal fluid leak Normal pressure hydrocephalus

Procedure	Code
Computed tomography (CT)	$$$
Magnetic resonance imaging (MRI)	$$$$
Magnetic resonance angiography (MRA)	$$$$$
Carotid duplex studies	$$
Transcranial Doppler	$$
Transesophageal echocardiography	$$$
Angiography	$$$$$
Neuropsychometrics (IQ/memory testing)	$$
Genetic testing	*
Lumbar puncture	$$$
Myelography	$$$$
Electroencephalography	$$$
Electromyography	$$$$
Evoked potential electrophysiologic studies	$$$
Polysomnography/multiple sleep latency tests	$$$$
Intracarotid amobarbital procedure	$$$$$
Corticography	$$$$$$
Single photon emission tomography/positron emission tomography	$$$$$$
Functional MRI	*
Autonomic function testing	$$$
Cisternography	$$$$$

$$ = $50–$100; $$$ = $100–$200; $$$$ = $200–$500; $$$$$ = $500–$1000; $$$$$$ = >$1000; * = highly variable or not available.

VI. Bibliography

Brazis P, Masdeu J, Biller J. *Localization in Clinical Neurology*, 2nd ed. Boston: Little, Brown; 1990.

Burde R, Savino P, Trobe J. *Clinical Decision-Making in Neuro-ophthalmology*. St. Louis: Mosby-Year Book; 1985.

DeJong R. *The Neurologic Examination*, 4th ed. Hagerstown, MD: Harper & Row; 1979.

Gelb D. *Introduction to Clinical Neurology*. Boston: Butterworth Heinemann; 1995.

Gilman S, Winans S. *Manter and Gatz's Essentials of Clinical Neuroanatomy and Neurophysiology*, 8th ed. Philadelphia: FA Davis; 1994.

Mayo Clinic and Mayo Foundation. *Clinical Examinations in Neurology*, 6th ed. St. Louis: Mosby-Year Book; 1991.

Pryse-Phillips W. *Companion to Clinical Neurology*. Boston: Little, Brown; 1995.

Weintraub MI. Malingering and conversion reactions. *Neurol Clin* 1995;13(2): 255–266,321–340.

VII. Key Search Words

The following key words reflect the content of this chapter. They are provided to assist with an on-line search of computer databases, such as MEDLINE, if you wish to pursue the topic of this chapter further.

Neurologic examination
Reflex
Diagnosis, neurologic
Cranial nerves

16. MUSCULOSKELETAL SYSTEM

Mark A. McQuillan

I. Glossary

Abduction: motion of a part away from the midline.

Active range of motion: limits of motion through which a joint may be moved by those muscles which cross the joint.

Adduction: motion of a part toward the midline.

Ankylosis: complete loss of motion of a joint.

Arthritis: inflammation of a joint.

Bursa: potential space often filled with fluid between two soft tissue layers that move upon each other.

Calcific tendinitis of the shoulder: inflammatory condition of a tendon about the shoulder, one stage of which is the deposition of crystals containing calcium within the structure of the tendon.

Capsule: the fibrous tissue sheath about a joint.

Carpal tunnel: the potential space on the volar (anterior) aspect of the wrist, the floor of which is formed by the carpal bones, the roof by the transverse carpal ligaments. Within the carpal tunnel travel the deep and superficial flexors of the fingers, the long flexor to the thumb, and the median nerve.

Cavus foot: foot deformity in which a very high arch is present.

Club foot (talipes equinovarus): foot deformity consisting of varus of the heel, equinus of the ankle, and adduction and supination of the forefoot.

Contracture: shortening of soft tissues about a joint, which limits normal motion of the joint.

Contralateral: on the opposite side.

Crepitation: grating or cracking sensation produced by motion.

Eversion: position achieved by turning a part away from the midline of the body.

Fatigue: physical or mental exhaustion, increased discomfort and decreased efficiency. Fatigue is a subjective experience that can mean exhaustion, loss of strength, stamina or endurance, breathlessness, or loss of ambition (consider depression).

Inversion: position achieved by turning a part toward the midline of the body.

Joint effusion: excessive fluid within a joint.

Kyphosis: angular curvature of the spine, the convexity of which is posterior.

Meniscus: fibrocartilaginous structure found between the articular surfaces of certain joints (e.g., knee).

Pain: a sensation of hurting or strong discomfort or distress, more or less localized; noxious stimuli with aversive emotional component; also any departure from normal sensory comfort.

Paresthesia: sensation of burning, crawling, or tingling.

Passive range of motion: limits of motion through which a joint may be moved without use of the muscles that cross the joint.

Pes planus: foot deformity in which the arch is flattened.

Pronation: position of the forearm achieved by turning the palm down; position of the foot achieved by turning the sole down.

Pseudoarthrosis: lack of bony continuity after the process of bone repair has ceased.

Pseudoclaudication: pain, tension, and weakness with exertion that resolves with rest. It is not related to circulation and involves buttocks and proximal thighs. Pseudoclaudication suggests spinal stenosis.

Rotator cuff: common insertion of the subscapularis, supraspinatus, infraspinatus, and teres minor muscles into the proximal humerus (shoulder).

Spondylolisthesis: forward displacement of a vertebra on the vertebra below as a result of bilateral defects in the vertebral arch.

Subluxation: lack of a completely normal relationship between the articular surfaces of two bones that make up a joint, such that abnormal motion may occur. However, the articular surfaces are still in contact (i.e., not dislocated).

Supination: position of the forearm achieved by turning the palm up; position of the foot achieved by turning the sole up.

Supine: position of lying on the back, face upward.

Synovitis: inflammation of the lining of a joint.

Tendinitis: inflammation of a tendon.

Thoracic outlet: anatomic region between the base of the neck and the axilla through which pass the brachial plexus and subclavian vessels.

Valgus: angulation of a part of an extremity away from the midline.

Varus: angulation of a part of an extremity toward the midline.

Special tests used in physical examination:

Adson's maneuver (Fig. 16-1): used to test for thoracic outlet syndrome. With patient in sitting position, hands resting on thighs, palpate both radial pulses as the patient rapidly inspires, holds breath, hyperextends neck, and turns head toward affected side. Transiently depressed or obliterated radial

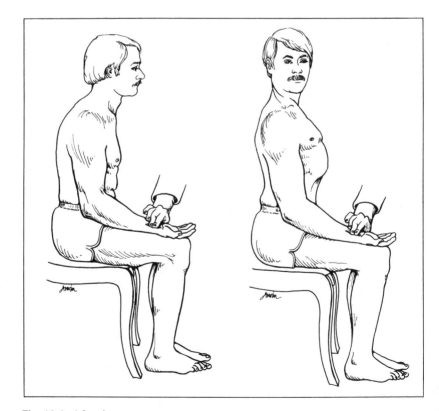

Fig. 16-1. Adson's maneuver.

pulse on that side indicates temporary occlusion of the subclavian artery. Intensification of pain and paresthesia in the arm, tenderness to palpation over the brachial plexus, and neurologic changes in arm and hand (particularly a decrease in ability to appreciate light touch over fourth and fifth fingers) indicate compression of brachial plexus in supraclavicular fossa. These signs may be intensified as the shoulder is abducted and externally rotated.

Compression test: used to detect degenerative, prolapsed, or herniated intervertebral disks. Vertically compress the extended cervical spine by pressing on the head. Increase in symptoms upon vertical compression of extended cervical spine with head tilted to side indicates degenerative changes in the facet joints or uncovertebral articulations (joints of Luschka).

Cozen's test (Fig. 16-2): used to test for epicondylitis (tennis elbow). Dorsiflexion of the wrist against resistance causes pain in the area of the lateral epicondyle.

Drawer sign: used to test the integrity of the cruciate ligaments. With the knee flexed, the examiner alternately forcefully pushes or pulls the proximal tibia and watches for forward or backward motion relative to the femoral condyles. The latter indicates posterior cruciate laxity, and the former suggests pathology in the anterior cruciate.

Fabere sign (for flexion, abduction, and external rotation): used to detect sacroiliac disease. In the supine position the leg is flexed, abducted and externally rotated with the heel placed on the knee. A positive test results when downward pressure on the flexed knee produces pain in the ipsilateral sacroiliac region.

Finkelstein's test (Fig. 16-3): used to diagnose de Quervain's tendinitis. Move the wrist rapidly into ulnar deviation as the patient holds the thumb flexed in the palm. Pain in the region of the radial styloid (anatomic snuff box) is a positive test.

Gower's maneuver: used to detect proximal muscle weakness of the lower extremities. Ask the patient to rise from a seated position without using the hands and arms to help. Inability to stand without an assist from the arms is a positive result.

Lachman's test: used to detect anterior cruciate ligament tears. With the patient supine, the examiner grasps the distal femur and proximal tibia and

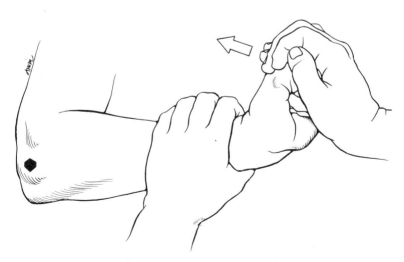

Fig. 16-2. Cozen's test.

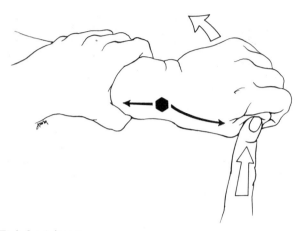

Fig. 16-3. Finkelstein's test.

flexes the knee to 15 to 20 degrees; anterior force is applied to the tibia. Excessive anterior translation of the tibia is a positive test result.

Lasègue's sign: used to detect radiculopathy and herniated disk. Ask the seated patient to extend the knee fully. Pain in the sciatic distribution, or compensation by leaning back toward recumbency, is a positive result.

Lhermitte's sign: used to detect irritation of spinal dura either by tumor or protruded cervical disk. With patient sitting and knees in full extension, ask patient to flex neck and hips simultaneously. Sharp pain that radiates down spine and into upper or lower extremities is a positive result.

McMurray's test (Fig. 16-4): used to detect tears in the anterior portions of either meniscus. Flex the patient's knee fully while supine, steadying the knee with one hand. Slowly extend the knee while holding the tibia in internal rotation. A palpable snap with momentary discomfort as the knee is extended suggests a tear in that portion of the lateral meniscus that was between the femoral condyle and the tibial plateau when the snap occurred. Repeat with tibia held in external rotation to test the posterior aspect of the medial meniscus. (This test does not confirm tears involving the anterior third of either meniscus.)

Patrick's test (also known as fabere sign; see previous text).

Schöber test: used to detect arthritis of the lumbar spine. A perpendicular line is drawn from the midpoint between the posterior iliac spines and an arbitrary point 10 cm above. The distraction of the line joining these two points is measured on anterior flexion. In a normal individual, this 10-cm line distracts to a total of 16 to 22 cm. A patient with degenerative or inflammatory arthritis involving the lumbar spine may have only 1 to 2 cm of distraction.

Spurling's test: used to detect cervical radiculopathy. Axial pressure is applied to the head with the head rotated toward the painful shoulder. Cervical nerve root irritation is revealed by increased shoulder pain or radicular symptoms.

Straight-leg raising test (Fig. 16-5): used to detect sciatic nerve or nerve root irritation. Flex the patient's hip with knee in full extension by raising the foot. A sharp pain traveling from the lower back or buttock down the posterior aspect of the leg indicates a positive result.

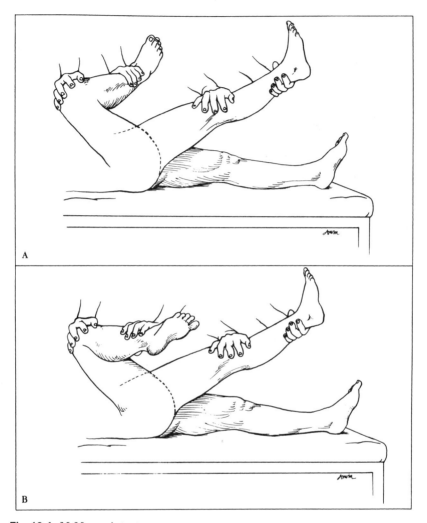

Fig. 16-4. McMurray's test.

Thomas' test (Fig. 16-6): used to detect flexion contractures of the hip. In the supine position, the patient flexes both legs to the chest, then reextends one leg. Lack of full extension indicates hip disease.

Tinel's sign (Fig. 16-7): used to detect a partial lesion or beginning regeneration of a nerve. Percuss over the site of a nerve. A tingling sensation in the distal end of a limb is a positive result.

Trendelenburg's sign (Fig. 16-8): used to evaluate the strength of the gluteus medius muscle. Stand behind the patient and observe dimples over the iliac spines. Ask the patient to stand on one leg. If the pelvis on the unsupported side does not elevate, the test result is positive and suggests ipsilateral weakness of the gluteus medius.

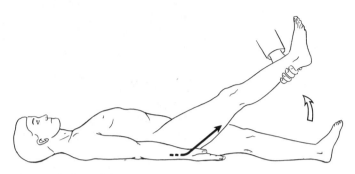

Fig. 16-5. Straight-leg raising test.

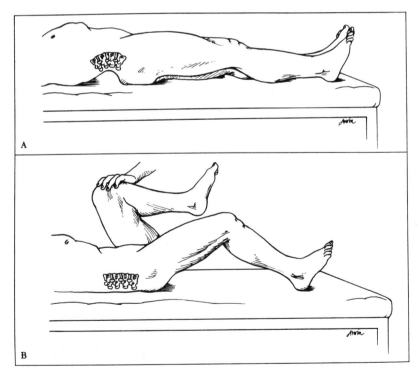

Fig. 16-6. Thomas' test. **(A)** With the patient supine, a flexion contracture of the hip may be masked by lordosis of the lumbar spine. **(B)** When the lumbar lordosis is eliminated by maximally flexing the left hip, the angle that the right thigh makes with the examining table designates the degree of flexion contracture in the right hip.

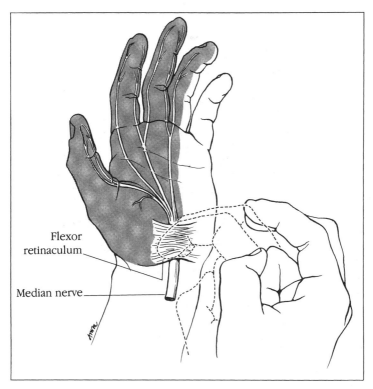

Flexor retinaculum

Median nerve

Fig. 16-7. Tinel's sign. Strike the median nerve in the wrist as it passes through the carpal tunnel. A tingling sensation radiating from the wrist to the hand is a positive test result.

II. Techniques of Examination
A. Setting. This chapter covers examination of adults and does not include the method of measuring and recording joint motion.

1. Acute problems. The physician's approach must be modified to accommodate patients in acute, severe distress. Examination differs in acutely injured patients. (For example, active and passive ranges of motion of the cervical spine would not be determined in an acutely injured patient until the mechanical stability of the cervical spine had been shown by x-ray; see Chapter 17.)

2. The elderly patient with chronic limitations or debilitating illness may often seem unaware of diminished range of motion (active or passive).

3. The small child or infant with musculoskeletal difficulties provides the most information during careful inspection and observation of the gait, movement, stance, and posture exhibited during normal play activities.

4. Sports injuries. An injured athlete in "the heat of battle" may be at once extremely anxious, fearful of permanent injury, reluctant to leave the competitive arena, and difficult to evaluate underneath heavy equipment. Proper immobilization with or without removing headgear and protective padding is a special challenge.

5. Posture and gait.

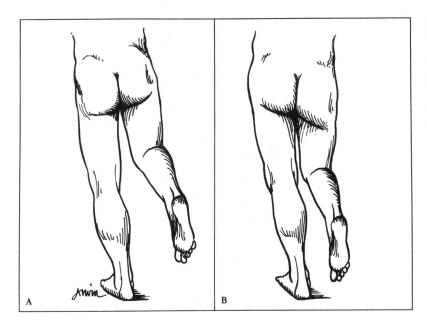

Fig. 16-8. Trendelenburg's sign. **(A)** Normal. The right side of the pelvis rises when weight is borne on the left leg. **(B)** Positive Trendelenburg's sign of the left hip. The right side of the pelvis falls when weight is borne on the left leg.

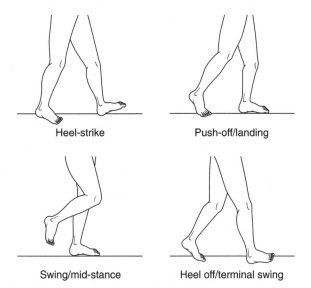

Heel-strike

Push-off/landing

Swing/mid-stance

Heel off/terminal swing

Fig. 16-9. Normal gait. (Adapted from Doherty M, Hazleman BL, Hutton CW, et al. *Rheumatology Examination and Injection Techniques.* Philadelphia: WB Saunders; 1992:14.)

    a. Inspection of the patient's gait reveals much about the musculoskeletal system. Have the patient walk several steps away from you, then toward you. Observe as the patient walks; note any grimacing, awkwardness, or change in rhythm. The phases of the normal gait are demonstrated in Figure 16-9 (Doherty, 1992).

    b. Abnormalities of gait may arise from the following:

      (1) Mechanical or structural abnormalities.

      (2) Pain. There are various *types* of antalgic gaits such as those arising from problems in the low back, hip, knee, or foot. *Causes* of antalgic gait are summarized in Table 16-1.

      (3) Muscular disorders.

      (4) Neurologic disorders.

      (5) Psychiatric disorders.

B. Goals and key questions

  1. The goal of the musculoskeletal examination is to differentiate among the five major causes of musculoskeletal complaints.

    a. Infection

    b. Crystalline disease

    c. Inflammation

    d. Degenerative disease

    e. Neoplasm

  2. Key questions to answer in the examination may include the following:

    a. Is the patient safe:

      (1) To move?

      (2) To travel?

Table 16-1. Some Causes of Antalgic Gait

BONE DISEASE
  Fracture
  Infection (osteomyelitis)
  Tumor
  Avascular necrosis (if in childhood, often called by eponym)
    Femoral head (Perthes' disease, Legg-Calvé disease)
    Tibial tubercle (Osgood-Schlatter disease)
    Tarsal navicular (Köhler's bone disease)

MUSCLE DISEASE
  Traumatic rupture, contusion
  Cramp secondary to fatigue, strain, malposition
  Inflammatory myositis

VASCULAR DISEASE
  Claudication of arterial insufficiency
  Thrombophlebitis

JOINT DISEASE
  Traumatic arthritis
  Infectious arthritis
  Immune arthritis (rheumatoid, lupus, vasculitis of other sorts)
  Crystalline arthritis (gout, pseudogout)
  Hermarthrosis (hemophilia, scurvy)

NEUROLOGIC DISEASE
  Lumbar spine disease with nerve root irritation or compression
  Pelvic masses involving sacral roots

OTHER
  Foot trauma (including blisters, ingrown toenails)
  Foreign bodies of the foot
  Corns, bunions

        (3) To exercise? (bracing, splinting, spine board, removal of football helmet)

        (4) To compete?

    b. Is the patient infected (gonococcemia, bacterial endocarditis, osteomyelitis, septic arthritis)?

    c. Does the patient have acute vascular occlusion? (Arterial or venous thromboembolic events may present as joint pain or painful limb.)

    d. Is objective inflammation present? (Distinguish between arthralgia and arthritis.)

    e. Is the problem worsening?

        (1) Gradual—rheumatoid arthritis, pannus

        (2) Sudden—hematoma

        (3) Dramatic, excruciating—malignant tumor, crystalline disease

C. General examination techniques. The minimal screening rheumatologic examination is an attempt to balance brevity and thoroughness with reasonable sensitivity for detection of musculoskeletal abnormalities. The examiner inspects the joints at rest, and during specified movements the patient is instructed to perform. The exact sequence of the inspection and its overall duration will be developed by each examiner individually. A suggested guideline is to begin with the hands and proceed to the upper extremities, progressing proximally. The head and neck are examined next, then the lower extremities from proximal to distal. Finally, the low back and gait are evaluated. The overall survey may be accomplished in many cases within 2 to 3 minutes.

  1. Inspection

    a. At rest

      (1) Swelling

      (2) Contours

      (3) Atrophy/muscle bulk

      (4) Redness/erythema

      (5) Deformity

      (6) Posture

      (7) Guarding

      (8) Nodules, rashes, miscellaneous

    b. With motion

      (1) Active range of motion. The patient demonstrates active range of motion by mimicking the examiner. The patient provides the power; the examiner observes the ease and limits of motion. Facial expression may reveal painful maneuvers. Have the patient rapidly perform the following:

        (a) Fingers: fist formation, finger flexion with palms up and open, finger extension

        (b) Wrists: dorsiflexion and palmar flexion

        (c) Elbows: flexion, extension, supination, pronation

        (d) Shoulders: elevation and back scratch

        (e) Neck: flexion, extension, lateral bending, lateral rotation

        (f) Hips: cross legs over knees—flexion, extension, internal rotation, external rotation

        (g) Knees: flexion, extension

        (h) Ankles: plantar flexion, dorsiflexion, inversion, eversion

        (i) Toes: flexion, extension

      (2) Passive range of motion. If pain is present with active motion but not present with passive movement, the pathology is likely to be in the muscles, tendons, or ligaments. If pain persists with passive movement, abnormalities of the bony structures or synovium are present.

  2. Percussion (used little in the musculoskeletal examination)

    a. Spinous processes

    b. Tinel's sign

3. Palpation. Gentle, light palpation is sufficient to reveal problem areas while conveying concern and goes a long way toward building rapport.

    a. Passive range of motion: to determine pain, tenderness, and the limits and ease of motion.

    b. Heat: to detect heat or warmth. Use the dorsum of the hand that is more sensitive to subtle temperature differences. Large joints have less vascular supply than neighboring large muscle groups (knee versus gastrocnemius complex). Thus, similar temperatures at the knee and calf suggest pathology of the knee.

    c. Effusions: soft tissue swelling (STS).

    d. Joint line tenderness: synovitis.

4. Auscultation (used little in the musculoskeletal examination)

    a. Temporomandibular joint: for crepitus

    b. de Quervain's tenosynovitis: for rubs

    c. Achilles tendon: for tendon rubs (scleroderma)

D. Examination of a muscle

    1. Muscle fibers

        a. Inspect the muscle for gross hypertrophy or atrophy and for fasciculations (isolated contractions of a portion of the fibers).

        b. Measure circumference of an extremity at a given point above and below the patella or olecranon; compare with the opposite side.

        c. Test muscle strength (Table 16-2).

        d. Palpate the muscle; note consistency and presence of tenderness over muscle or its tendon.

        e. Areas of muscle spasm can be easily palpated, are tender to palpation, and often are accentuated because the joint they span is moved passively.

    2. Nerves. Test deep tendon reflex. (Spinal segments and peripheral nerves that generally innervate major muscle groups of the extremities are listed in Table 16-3.)

E. Regional examinations

    1. Temporomandibular joint

        a. Test range of motion. Have the patient open and close the mouth and move the jaw from side to side.

        b. Inspect for asymmetry or deformity.

        c. Percuss for pain.

        d. Palpate for crepitus, snapping.

        e. Auscultation. Listen for crepitus.

    2. Cervical spine

        a. Determine range of motion.

            (1) Active range of motion (flexion, extension, lateral bending, rotation). Ask the patient to touch chin to chest, then to look up at ceiling. Also, touch chin to shoulders; touch ear to shoulders.

            (2) Passive range of motion (Fig. 16-10).

Table 16-2. Testing for Muscle Strength

100%	5	Normal	Complete range of motion against gravity with full resistance
75	4	Good	Complete range of motion against gravity with some resistance
50	3	Fair	Complete range of motion against gravity
25	2	Poor	Complete range of motion with gravity eliminated
10	1	Trace	Evidence of slight contractility No joint motion
0	0	0	No evidence of contractility

Table 16-3. Innervation of the Muscles of the Extremities

Upper Limb Muscles	Nerve	C2	C3	C4	C5	C6	C7	C8	T1
Sternocleidomastoid; trapezius	Spinal accessory	X	X	X					
Diaphragm	Phrenic		X	X	X				
Deltoid	Axillary					X			
Supraspinatus	Suprascapular				X	X			
Infraspinatus	Suprascapular				X	X			
Teres minor	Axillary				X	X			
Subscapularis; teres major	Subscapular				X	X			
Serratus anterior	Long thoracic				X	X	X		
Rhomboideus	Dorsal scapular			X	X				
Clavicular pectoralis major	Lateral and medial pectoral				X	X	X		
Biceps; brachialis	Musculocutaneous				X	X			
Brachioradialis	Radial				X	X			
Latissimus dorsi	Thoracodorsal					X	X	X	
Sternal pectoralis major	Lateral and medial pectoral					X	X	X	X
Flexor carpi radialis; pronator teres	Median					X	X		
Extensor carpi radialis, longus and brevis; extensor digitorum communis; extensor indicis proprius; extensor carpi ulnaris; extensor pollicis, longus and brevis; abductor pollicus longus; triceps	Radial					X	X	X	
Flexor digitorum sublimis	Median						X	X	X
Flexor digitorum profundus	Volar interosseous; ulnar							X	X
Flexor carpi ulnaris	Ulnar						X	X	X
Pronator quadratus	Volar interosseous						X	X	X

Muscle	Nerve	L1	L2	L3	L4	L5	S1	S2	S4	S5
Interossei	Ulnar								X	X
Lumbricals; flexor pollicis brevis	Median; ulnar								X	X
Adductor pollicis; opponens digiti minimi	Ulnar								X	X
Biceps tendon reflex	Musculocutaneous						X			
Brachioradialis reflex	Radial						X			
Triceps tendon reflex	Radial							X		

Lower Limb Muscles	Nerve	L1	L2	L3	L4	L5	S1	S2	S4	S5
Hip flexion	Iliopsoas; sartorius; rectus femoris; tensor fasciae latae — Lumbar plexus; femoral; superior gluteal; obturator		X	X	X	X	X			
Hip adduction	Adductor magnus; adductor brevis; adductor longus — Obturator		X	X	X					
Knee extension	Quadriceps femoris — Femoral		X	X	X					
Hip abduction	Gluteus medias; gluteus minimus; tensor fascia femoris — Superior gluteal				X	X	X			
Foot inversion & dorsiflexion	Tibialis anterior — Peroneal				X	X				
Toe extension	Extensor digitorum, longus and brevis — Peroneal				X	X	X			
Great toe extension	Extensor hallucis, longus and brevis — Peroneal				X	X	X			
Foot eversion	Peroneus, longus and brevis — Peroneal				X	X	X			
Foot inversion & plantar flexion	Tibialis posterior — Tibial					X	X			
Toe flexion	Flexor digitorum, longus and brevis — Tibial					X	X	X		

Table 16-3. *Continued*

Lower Limb Muscles	Nerve	L 1	L 2	L 3	L 4	L 5	S 1	S 2	S 4	S 5
Great toe flexion	Flexor hallucis longus	Tibial				X	X			
Hip extension	Gluteus maximus	Inferior gluteal				X	X	X		
Knee flexion	Biceps femoris; semimembranosus; semitendinosus	Peroneal; tibial				X	X	X		
Foot plantar flexion	Gastrocnemius; soleus	Tibial				X	X	X		
	Cremasteric reflex	Genital-femoral	X	X							
	Patellar tendon reflex	Femoral			X	X					
	Achilles tendon reflex	Tibial						X			
	Anal reflex	Pudendal							X	X	X

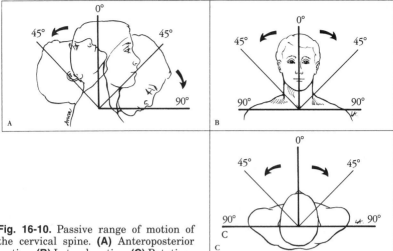

Fig. 16-10. Passive range of motion of the cervical spine. **(A)** Anteroposterior motion. **(B)** Lateral motion. **(C)** Rotation.

  b. Inspection
     (1) Look for gross deformities, visible muscle spasm.
     (2) Normal findings include normal cervical lordosis.
  c. Percussion—spinous processes
  d. Palpation
     (1) Spinous processes. Palpate for general alignment and tenderness.
     (2) Cervical muscles. Palpate for tenderness and muscle spasm.
     (3) Spinal dura. Assess by performing Lhermitte's test.
     (4) Thoracic outlet. Measure circumference of upper and lower arms, compare with opposite side. Test muscle strength, sensory modalities, and deep tendon reflexes in upper extremity.
3. Thoracic spine
  a. Inspect for kyphosis. Observe symmetry of ribs during flexion, extension, and lateral bending. Observe inspiration and chest circumference.
  b. Palpate spinous processes for general alignment and tenderness.
4. Lumbar spine
  a. Test range of lumbar motion in flexion, extension, lateral bending, and rotation. Have the patient touch toes, bend backward and look up, bend to the sides, and twist shoulders to the sides.
  b. Inspect contour (e.g., posture, list, tilt) with patient standing.
  c. Palpate.
     (1) Palpate paraspinal muscles for tenderness and spasm.
     (2) Palpate spinous processes, noting general alignment and tenderness. Differentiate bony tenderness from tenderness of the paraspinous muscles or costovertebral angle.
     (3) Measure leg length from anterior superior spine to medial malleolus.
     (4) Test for radiculopathy. Test deep tendon reflexes at the knee and ankle, and test sensory modalities of light touch, pain, and position sense. Perform straight-leg raising test.
     (5) Perform abdominal, hernia, and rectal examinations to check for sphincter tone and pelvic pathology.

      (6) Evaluate the distal lower extremity pulses.

      (7) Test muscle power of the dorsiflexors and plantar flexors of the foot and ankle by having the patient support the body weight on the toes and on the heels.

   d. Normal findings. Lumbar lordosis is normally present.

5. Sacroiliac joints

   a. Provocative testing of the sacroiliac joints is of questionable sensitivity and specificity.

   b. Use Schöber's maneuver to detect arthritic changes.

   c. Imaging techniques are the best diagnostic tools: plain films, bone scan, computed tomography (CT), magnetic resonance imaging (MRI).

6. Shoulder

   a. Determine active range of motion; ask the patient to perform full overhead elevation and back scratch (internal rotation).

   b. Inspect shoulder anteriorly and posteriorly, look for general contour and muscle atrophy. The deltoid muscle covers the shoulder anteriorly, laterally, posteriorly; the infraspinatus muscle originates on the posterior border of the scapula below the scapular spine. The rotator cuff represents the insertion of the subscapularis, supraspinatus, infraspinatus, and teres minor muscles into the proximal humerus.

   c. Palpate the bony landmarks around the shoulder carefully for points of tenderness.

7. Elbow

   a. Determine active range of motion; ask the patient to flex and extend the elbows and to pronate and supinate the hands.

   b. Inspect general contour; look for loss of full extension.

   c. Palpate the bony landmarks: olecranon, radial head, and epicondyles.

   d. Test the active and passive ranges of motion of the elbow in flexion, extension, supination, pronation. Compare with the opposite side.

   e. Palpate the head of the radius and the tissue just anterior to it for points of tenderness as the forearm is supinated and pronated.

   f. Palpate the extensor surface of the forearm for nodules, often found with rheumatoid arthritis.

8. Wrist

   a. Inspect contour; note any fullness about the joint.

   b. Palpate the bony and tendinous structures for tenderness and nodularity.

   c. Percuss over the median nerve at the wrist to detect nerve compression (Tinel's sign).

   d. Auscultation; listen for audible rub (de Quervain's tenosynovitis).

9. Hand

   a. Ask the patient to perform:

      (1) Full fist formation

      (2) Full extension

      (3) Spread fingers against resistance

      (4) Phalen's sign for carpel tunnel (Tinel's sign is nonspecific)

   b. Inspect carefully for interosseous muscle atrophy on the dorsum of the hand.

   c. Palpate for presence of nodules or fibrous bands.

10. Hip

   a. Determine active range of motion. Ask the patient to flex and extend the hip while supine and lying in lateral decubitus position; cross ankle over knee.

   b. Inspect range of motion in flexion, extension, abduction, adduction, and rotation; compare with opposite side.

   c. Palpate the hip anteriorly for points of tenderness. The femoral head is about 1 inch distal and 1 inch lateral to the point at which the femoral artery crosses the inguinal ligament. Palpate the greater trochanter laterally and the ischial tuberosity posteriorly.

d. Determine the strength of the flexor, extensor, abductor, and adductor muscle groups by having the patient move the thigh against the resistance of your hand.

11. Knee

a. Determine active range of motion. Have the patient flex and extend the knee fully.

b. Inspect the knee for joint swelling and gross deformity; inspect the thigh for atrophy of the quadriceps muscle group.

c. Test for effusion.

(1) Ballottement: press the patella against the femur with the knee in full extension.

(2) Bulge sign: place fingers on lateral and medial sides of the patella; move back and forth while feeling for a fluid wave on the other side.

d. Palpate about the joint line, about the circumference of the patella, over the attachments of the medial and lateral collateral ligaments, over the anserine bursa (on the medial posterior aspect of the proximal tibia about 1 inch distal to the joint line), and in the popliteal fossa.

e. Assess the integrity of the ligaments.

(1) Medial collateral ligament. Test integrity by attempting to force the knee into valgus (knock-knee) deformity with the knee in full extension. If more than 5 to 10 degrees of deformity can be produced, ligament instability is suspected.

(2) Lateral collateral ligament. Test by attempting to force the knee into varus (bowleg) deformity with the knee in full extension. If more than 5 to 10 degrees of deformity can be produced, ligament instability is suspected.

(3) Cruciate ligaments. Test with the patient sitting with knees flexed to 90 degrees. If the tibia can be pulled anteriorly from under the femur (positive "drawer" sign), laxity of the anterior cruciate ligament is present. If the tibia can be pushed posteriorly under the femur, laxity of the posterior cruciate ligament is present.

(4) Lachman's test for anterior cruciate ligament tears.

f. Normal findings: full extension and at least 120 degrees of flexion from full extension are normally present.

12. Ankle

a. Determine active range of motion. Ask the patient to dorsiflex, plantar flex, invert, and evert the foot.

b. Inspect for gross deformity or swelling.

c. Palpate for tenderness or fullness within the joint.

d. Test the active and passive motions of the ankle joint.

e. Test the stability of the joint, particularly in inversion and eversion.

f. Determine the strength of the muscles crossing the ankle joint by having the patient support body weight on the ball of the foot (stand "on tiptoe") and then walk on the heels. Look for asymmetry.

g. Normal findings: at least 30 degrees of plantar flexion and 15 degrees of dorsiflexion are normally present.

13. Foot

a. Inspection

(1) Look for obvious deformities and swelling.

(2) Look at shoes for abnormal wear pattern.

(3) Observe heel from the rear; look for straight alignment with leg.

(4) Inspect toes for deformities and calluses.

(5) Inspect sole of the foot for calluses over the metatarsal heads.

b. Palpation

(1) Assess the foot tissues by palpating the skin, noting the presence or absence of hair on the dorsum of the toes.
(2) Palpate the dorsalis pedis and posterior tibial pulses.
(3) Test individual muscles by having the patient perform appropriate movements against the resistance of your hand.
(4) Palpate for points of tenderness indicating inflammation of bursae or joints.
(5) Assess the stability of the midfoot and hindfoot. Test inversion and eversion of the foot by rocking the heel medially and laterally while stabilizing the lower leg, rotating the foot by supinating, and pronating the metatarsals as a unit while stabilizing the heel and flexing and extending the toes.

c. Normal findings: the axis of the heel is normally a continuation of the long axis of the lower leg when observed from the rear.

F. Examination of the elderly (age >65)

  1. History. It is often helpful to seek additional information from the patient's family, companion, attendant, or personal care assistant. Ask whether the patient's hobbies, activity level, gait, or motion recently changed.
  a. Inspection
  b. Observation
  c. Activities of daily living
  d. Stairs
  e. Toileting
  f. Gower's maneuver (important clue to proximal muscle weakness, myositis)

  2. Observation during the history and examination is very useful.
  a. Climbing onto examination table
  b. Lying down and sitting up again
  c. Rising from chair

  3. Important abnormalities
  a. Pain
  b. Stiffness/pseudoparkinsonism
  c. Weakness
  d. Lameness
  e. Deformity
  f. Pseudoclaudication (important clue to spinal stenosis)
  g. Pseudophlebitis
  h. Depression/pseudodementia/global impairment

III. Cardinal Symptoms

A. Constitutional symptoms. These symptoms are important but nonspecific clues to possible systemic illness.
  1. Fatigue
  2. Weight loss
  3. Fever
  4. Adenopathy

B. Stiffness
  1. Morning stiffness. Inflammatory conditions are often accompanied by morning stiffness of longer than 20 minutes.
  2. Gelling (need to limber up after brief immobility).

C. Pain. Note its characteristics (location, onset, quality, duration, timing, severity, radiation) and its relation to the patient's activity. Describe in the patient's terms. Note any factors that exacerbate or ameliorate the pain, any accompanying symptoms, and the results of previous treatments.
  1. Rest pain
  2. Pain with motion
    a. Active—musculotendinous problem
    b. Passive—bone or synovium problem
  3. Pain worsened by immobility

4. Pain worsened by activity
5. Night pain causing awakening
6. Referred pain: perceived by the patient in an anatomic location removed from the site of the lesion
   a. Hip. Pain from a hip disorder is often first noted in the anterior and lateral aspect of the thigh.
   b. Shoulder. Pain from a shoulder lesion may be felt at the insertion of the deltoid muscle on the lateral aspect of the proximal portion of humerus.
   c. Lower cervical spine. Pain is often referred to the interscapular region of the back, along the vertebral aspect of the scapula, or to the tips of the shoulders and the lateral aspects of the arms.
7. Specific types of pain
   a. Bone erosion (tumor or aneurysm): deep, constant, boring pain. This pain is often more noticeable and intense at night; it may not be relieved by rest or position.
   b. Degenerative arthritis, muscle disorders: aching pain, often accentuated by activity and lessened by rest. It may be increased by certain positions or motions. Degenerative changes of the cervical or lumbar spine often cause subjective paresthesias that do not follow a dermatome distribution (described as a "sandy" feeling or as if the part were "going to sleep").
   c. Fracture, infection of bone: severe, throbbing pain. This pain is increased by any motion of the part.
   d. Acute nerve compression: sharp, severe pain, radiating along the distribution of the nerve. It is often associated with weakness of muscles supplied by the nerve and sensory changes over the area supplied by it.
8. Lower lumbosacral spine: distinguish among back, buttock, hip, and groin pain.

IV. **Abnormal Findings**
   A. Temporomandibular joint: crepitus, subluxation
   B. Cervical spine
      1. Absence of normal cervical lordosis, abnormal shortness of neck due to congenital malformations of cervical vertebrae.
      2. Spinous processes. Decreased motion is associated with points of tenderness commonly seen in tumors and infections of the cervical vertebrae and in degenerative, prolapsed, herniated cervical intervertebral disks.
      3. Muscle spasm.
      4. Intervertebral disks, facet joints. Intensified discomfort with the compression test indicates degenerative, prolapsed, or herniated intervertebral disks. Increase in symptoms with head tilted to side indicates degenerative changes in the facet joints or uncovertebral articulations (joints of Luschka).
      5. Spinal dura. Positive Lhermitte's test result suggests irritation of spinal dura either by tumor or protruded cervical disk.
      6. Thoracic outlet.
         a. Disappearance of the radial pulse during the Adson's test signifies temporary occlusion of the subclavian artery.
         b. Intensification of pain and paresthesia in the arm during the Adson's test, tenderness to palpation over the brachial plexus, neurologic changes in arm and hand (particularly a decrease in ability to appreciate light touch over fourth and fifth fingers) indicate compression of the brachial plexus in the supraclavicular fossa. These signs may be intensified as the shoulder is abducted and externally rotated.
   C. Thoracic spine
      1. Kyphosis
      2. Scoliosis

D. Lumbar spine
 1. The absence of lumbar lordosis suggests spinal abnormality.
 2. Tenderness of the paraspinous muscles or costovertebral angle suggests renal pathology.
 3. Tenderness to palpation over lumbar spinous processes associated with limited motion of the spine may indicate tumor, infection, disk lesions, osteoarthritis, or spondylolisthesis.
 4. Sharp pain traveling from the lower back or buttock down the posterior aspect of the leg during the straight-leg raising test indicates irritation of the sciatic nerve or its roots of origin within the spine.
 5. Lasègue's sign versus straight-leg raising. Results should be concordant if there is radiculopathy or herniated disk disease. Discordant results indicate a need for further evaluation. Ascertain the exact location of the pain; hamstring tightness may confound the results. Malingering is another possible cause.
 6. Pseudoclaudication suggests spinal stenosis.
E. Sacroiliac joints
 1. Positive Schöber's maneuver suggests sacroiliitis.
 2. All other physical examination maneuvers for sacroiliitis have been shown to be unreliable; ascertainment of sacroiliac involvement is dependent on Schöber's maneuver or sacroiliac films.
F. Shoulder
 1. Muscle atrophy/weakness
    a. Deltoid. Visible atrophy follows disuse, injury to axillary nerve, and diseases of nervous system (e.g., poliomyelitis).
    b. Infraspinatus. Visible atrophy results from nerve injury, diseases of the nervous system, tears of the insertion of the muscle into the rotator cuff, and calcific tendinitis of the rotator cuff at its insertion site.
    c. Anterior serratus muscle. Weakness often follows injury to the long thoracic nerve of Bell in the neck or in the axilla. (Determine function by having the patient push with both hands against a wall. The medial border of the scapula is normally held firmly against the chest wall; if displaced posteriorly ["wings"], weakness of the muscle is present.)
 2. Tenderness
    a. Diffuse tenderness over the entire shoulder suggests adhesive capsulitis (frozen shoulder) or synovitis of the joint.
    b. Tenderness over a segment of the rotator cuff indicates rotator cuff tear or calcific tendinitis.
    c. Tenderness over the long head of the biceps tendon as it lies in the bicipital groove between the greater and lesser tuberosities of the humerus suggests biceps tendonitis. This diagnosis is strengthened if shoulder pain is accentuated when the forearm is flexed and supinated against resistance.
 3. Range of motion. If passive motion is normal but active motion is limited, rotator cuff tear or muscle weakness is indicated. If active and passive motions are both limited to an equal degree, contractures, arthritis, or mechanical block (e.g., calcific tendinitis) are suggested.
G. Elbow
 1. Tenderness. Tenderness lateral or anterior to the radial head may indicate lateral epicondylitis (tennis elbow); tenderness increases as the patient pronates the forearm and extends the wrist against resistance.
 2. Palpable effusion or synovitis is present within the joint.
 3. Ulnar neuropathy. Localized tenderness suggests irritation of the nerve, which often follows fractures about the elbow. It is associated with pain and paresthesia in the fourth and fifth fingers and weakness of the hand muscles supplied by the ulnar nerve (adductor pollicis, third and fourth lumbricals, and interossei).
 4. Nodules (rheumatoid arthritis).

H. Wrist
1. Tenderness over the anatomic snuffbox on the lateral aspect of the wrist may indicate abnormality of the navicular or greater multangular bones.
2. de Quervain's disease. Tenderness over the lateral aspect of the distal radius suggests inflammation of the tendon sheaths of the extensor pollicis brevis and the abductor pollicis longus, confirmed when a tender nodule can be felt within one or both of the tendons over the lateral aspect of the distal radius and when a positive Finkelstein's test is noted.
3. Median nerve. Phalen's sign: compression at the wrist causes tenderness over the nerve, loss of normal sensation in the portion of the hand supplied by this nerve (flexor surfaces of thumb, index and middle fingers, lateral half of ring finger) and weakness of thumb muscles supplied by the nerve. Percussion over the nerve at the wrist will produce pain radiating distally into the hand (positive Tinel's sign).

I. Hand
1. Nerve injury, tendon rupture, muscle fibrosis, joint contracture, arthritis
2. Interosseous muscle atrophy on the dorsum of the hand
3. Dupuytren's contracture: nodules within the fourth or fifth flexor tendon in the palm associated with firm fibrous bands which limit extension of the fingers
4. Trigger finger: palpable click as the finger is flexed or extended (the nodule snaps into or out of the tendon sleeve through which it passes); may be associated with a palpable nodule or diffuse swelling within a flexor tendon overlying a metacarpal-phalangeal joint.

J. Gait. Abnormalities of gait may be caused by leg-length inequality, muscle weakness, habit patterns, fusion, contractures, pain-producing lesions of hip, knee, ankle, or foot.
1. Trendelenburg gait (see Fig. 16-8). When weight-bearing, the pelvis on the side opposite the involved hip falls rather than rises, indicating weakness of the abductor muscles due to intrinsic muscle disease, lack of normal innervation of the muscle, or unstable hip joint.
2. Antalgic (anti-pain) gait. The patient leans over the involved hip as weight is borne through it, moving the center of gravity toward the hip joint. This decreases the force exerted on the hip, which decreases discomfort.

K. Hip
1. Inflamed bursae may account for hip pain.
2. Flexion contracture. If the hip flexes during the Thomas' test (see Fig. 16-6), flexion contracture is present; the angle that the involved thigh makes with the flat surface indicates the degree of contracture.
3. Trochanteric bursitis.

L. Knee
1. Joint swelling and gross deformity.
2. Atrophy of the quadriceps muscle group.
3. Effusion.
4. Tenderness about the patella suggests osteoarthritis or chondromalacia. Confirm chondromalacia with the patellar inhibition test: firmly press the patella against the underlying femur and move the patella medially, laterally, proximally, and distally. Crepitation and pain confirm the diagnosis.
5. Tenderness over the medial or lateral collateral ligament suggests a tear of the ligament or an inflamed bursa between the ligament and the bone.
6. Tenderness over the anserine bursa or in the popliteal fossa suggests symptomatic bursitis in these regions.
7. Palpable crepitation within the knee joint during flexion and extension suggests a mechanical incongruity, which may be the result of arthritic

changes, a tear of the medial or lateral meniscus, or a loose fragment of cartilage or bone within the joint.

8. Mechanical block (locking of the joint during flexion or extension) signifies a block within the joint, most commonly a torn meniscus or bone fragment. When the knee cannot be fully extended passively, a mechanical block or a contracture of the posterior capsule is suggested.

9. Torn meniscus is suggested by a positive McMurray's sign (see Fig. 16-4).

10. Ligament instability.

M. Ankle

1. Tenderness just anterior to the Achilles tendon at its insertion into the calcaneus suggests an inflamed bursa, often noted in the patient with rheumatoid arthritis or Reiter's syndrome.

2. Tenderness over the posterior tibial tendon or peroneal tendons at the point of constriction posterior to the malleolus is an indication of tenosynovitis, similar to de Quervain's disease of the wrist. Passive motion of the foot intensifies the discomfort; a palpable nodule may be present within the tendon.

3. If tilting of the talus can be demonstrated as the ankle is forced into eversion, instability of the medial collateral ligament is present.

N. Foot

1. Deformities and swelling.

2. If the heel is tilted toward the midline when observed from the rear, the heel is in varus (often associated with clubfoot and cavus foot). If the heel is tilted away from the midline, the heel is in valgus (often associated with flat foot).

3. Bunion. A swelling may be seen over the medial aspect of the metatarsophalangeal joint of the great toe, which may be associated with a medial deviation of more than 15 degrees when compared with the lateral four metatarsals (metatarsus primus varus) or with lateral deviation of the great toe (hallux valgus).

4. Toes.

   a. Clawtoe. Proximal phalanx is hyperextended; proximal interphalangeal joint acutely flexed.

   b. Hammertoe. Proximal interphalangeal is joint acutely flexed; metacarpophalangeal joint in neutral position.

5. Circulatory problems.

6. Inflammation of bursae or joints.

   a. Diffuse tenderness over the calcaneus itself is often associated with early rheumatoid arthritis or Reiter's syndrome.

   b. Inflammation in any of the joints of the foot may be caused by septic arthritis, rheumatoid arthritis, osteoarthritis, or gout.

   c. Tenderness to palpation over the metatarsal heads on the ball of the foot indicates metatarsalgia; tenderness between the metatarsal heads on the dorsum of the foot suggests interdigital neuroma (strengthened if a sensory abnormality can be demonstrated on the opposing surfaces of the contiguous toes supplied by the involved interdigital nerve, and if medial to lateral compression of the forefoot induces metatarsal pain, which radiates into the involved toes).

7. Morton's neuroma (painful nerve nodule usually between the third and fourth toes).

8. Peripheral neuropathy.

V. Available Technology

A. The table on the following page lists the methods available for diagnosing musculoskeletal conditions.

Procedure	Indication
X-ray (plain films)	Demonstrate bony fractures, osteophytes, erosions
Arthrocentesis	Joint infection Crystalline diseases Hemarthrosis
Doppler arterial wave analysis (noninvasive vascular studies)	Exclude acute vascular occlusion
Bone scan	Inflammation Infection Necrosis
Ultrasonography	Soft tissue injuries (e.g., rotator cuff tears)
Magnetic resonance imaging (MRI)	Avascular necrosis of hip Spinal cord disease Neoplasm
Computed tomography (CT)	Infection Neoplasm Disk disease Avascular necrosis
Electromyography (invasive test)	Radiculopathy Myopathy Neuropathy
Arthrography (invasive radiologic contrast imaging)	Capsular tears (shoulder/knee joints) Tendon rupture (partial or complete)
Myelography (invasive test)	Spinal cord imaging
Arthroscopy (invasive internal joint visualization)	Mechanical and pathologic joint derangement; leads to directed therapeutic interventions
Synovial biopsy (invasive test, most often done as part of arthroscopy)	Obscure chronic arthritis, especially fungal
Compartment pressures (invasive test)	Compartment syndrome
Intraosseous pressures (invasive test)	Avascular necrosis
Arthroplasty (joint revision or replacement surgery)	Osteoarthritis Rheumatoid arthritis Avascular necrosis

B. The cost figures cited in the table on the following page are **basic direct costs.** The figures are difficult to obtain and change quickly. They include **only** the cost of the test itself (technician, equipment, time, and materials). No professional costs (interpretation) are included. Costs vary from region to region based on differences in some components such as labor. However, the relative cost ranking should remain similar.

Procedure	Code
X-ray (plain films)	$$
Arthrocentesis	$$
Doppler arterial wave analysis	$$
Bone scan	$$$$
Ultrasonography	$$
Magnetic resonance imaging (MRI)	$$$$
Computed tomography (CT)	$$$
Electromyography	$$
Arthrography	$$$
Myelography	$$$
Arthroscopy	$$$$
Synovial biopsy	$$$$
Compartment pressures	*
Intraosseous pressures	*
Arthroplasty	*

$$ = $50–$100; $$$ = $100–$200; $$$$ = $200–$500; * = highly variable or not available.

VI. Bibliography

Birrer RB, ed. *Sports Medicine for the Primary Care Physician*, 2nd ed. Ann Arbor, MI: CRC Press; 1994.

Doherty M, Hazleman BL, Hutton CW, et al. *Rheumatology Examination and Injection Techniques*. Philadelphia: WB Saunders; 1992.

Hoppenfeld S. *Physical Examination of the Spine and Extremities*. Norwalk, CT: Appleton-Century-Crofts; 1976.

Kelley WN, Harris ED, Ruddy SR, Sledge CB, eds. *Textbook of Rheumatology*, 4th ed. Philadelphia: WB Saunders; 1993.

McCarty DJ, Koopman WJ. *Arthritis and Allied Conditions*, 12th ed. Philadelphia: Lea & Febiger; 1993.

Paget S, Pellici P, Beary JF III. *Manual of Rheumatology and Outpatient Orthopedic Disorders,* 3rd ed. Boston: Little, Brown; 1993.

Polley HF, Hunder GG. *Rheumatologic Interviewing and Physical Examination of the Joints*, 2nd ed. Philadelphia: WB Saunders; 1978.

Schrier RW. *Geriatric Medicine*. Philadelphia: WB Saunders; 1990.

VII. Key Search Words

The following key words reflect the content of this chapter. They are provided to assist with an on-line search of computer databases, such as MEDLINE, if you wish to pursue the topic of this chapter further.

A. Title words: musculoskeletal physical diagnosis
B. Subject words:
    1. Physical examination + (joint)
    2. Diagnosis + _____
C. Second subject words:
    1. Joint deformities, acquired
    2. Joint diseases
D. Third subject words:
    1. _____ joint +
    2. Eponymous + _____

17. THE ACUTELY INJURED PATIENT

Christopher J. Andershock
William G. Barsan

I. Glossary
The medical terms used for emergency medicine are generally the same as those used in other situations. For that reason, no glossary is included in this chapter.

II. Initial Assessment and Management

  A. General considerations

    1. Acutely injured patients are generally younger members of the population without significant underlying disease. Prompt appropriate treatment can make a significant difference in both initial recovery and long-term morbidity.

    2. It is often difficult to obtain a detailed or even cursory history; physical findings must be relied on for diagnosis and directing initial treatment.

    3. In the United States, over 57 million people were accidentally injured in 1985. Trauma is among the leading causes of death in people ages 1 to 44, with over 150,000 deaths annually, and is responsible for over one third of all hospital admissions. The long-term effects (e.g., individual loss, pain, suffering, incapacitation, disability) are difficult to quantify.

    4. Aims of management of the acutely injured patient:

      a. Rapid, safe, and reliable assessment of the patient's condition

      b. Resuscitation and stabilization on a priority basis

  B. Treatment priorities based on the injuries sustained, the patient's clinical stability, and the injury mechanism (resuscitation ongoing)

    1. Rapid primary evaluation, called the *primary survey*

    2. Resuscitation and stabilization; initial clinical management is highly prioritized

      a. Establish and protect the patency of the airway, ensuring adequate ventilation.

      b. Treat shock and obvious external hemorrhage.

      c. Assess potential for cerebral herniation and cervical spine injuries.

      d. Assess/treat neurologic status.

      e. Assess/treat cardiac, thoracic, and abdominal injuries.

      f. Assess/treat musculoskeletal and soft tissue injuries.

    3. Secondary, more detailed assessment

    4. Constant reevaluation

  C. Primary survey. Management of life-threatening conditions is begun during this rapid, initial evaluation of high-priority systems. Priorities for pediatric patients are the same as for adults, although the quantities of blood, fluids, medications, degree of heat loss, and injury patterns may differ. The sequence of the primary survey can be remembered by the mnemonic, ABCDE:

    Airway management with cervical spine control
    Breathing and ventilation
    Circulation and control of obvious hemorrhage
    Disability and neurologic status
    Exposure and environmental control

    1. Airway management/breathing and ventilation. These are carried out simultaneously.

      a. Airway assessment

        (1) Open the airway and observe the rate and quality of respirations.

        (a) If no there is no cervical spine injury, use the head-tilt, chin-lift method.

        (b) If cervical spine must be immobilized, use the jaw-thrust method.

    (2) Assess airway for obstruction.

        (a) Remove with suction: blood, emesis, dislodged teeth, and other foreign bodies.

        (b) Posterior retraction of the tongue (in an unconscious patient): place an oral or nasal pharyngeal airway to hold the airway open.

        (c) Neck trauma: difficult to assess and manage, often requiring emergency airway control and possibly a surgical airway. Causes include displaced anatomic structures, edema, hematoma, direct compression, and tracheal transection.

b. Breathing and ventilation assessment

    (1) Assess the quality and rate of the patient's respirations.

    (2) Inspect the chest for signs of compromise, such as labored or accelerated respirations, penetrating wounds, obvious flail chest segments, distended neck veins, and tracheal deviation.

    (3) Palpate for rib fractures or subcutaneous emphysema.

    (4) Auscultate to ensure bilateral adequacy and symmetry of air exchange.

c. Airway management

    (1) Provide supplemental oxygen to all trauma patients. If the patient shows signs of compromise or inadequate respirations, assist breathing with high-flow oxygen through a bag-valve-mask system with an oxygen reservoir.

    (2) Determine need for intubation. Conditions mandating intubation include airway obstruction, inadequate ventilation, and inability of unconscious patient to protect the airway. If in doubt, early intubation is recommended.

        (a) Nasal or oral airway. Choose the method based on the skill of the examiner, since recent studies show no significant difference in terms of patient safety.

        (b) Surgical airway. This is indicated when oral and nasal approaches have failed or when significant intraoral hemorrhage or massive supraglottic edema is present.

            (i) Cricothyrotomy. Place either a cuffed endotracheal or tracheal tube through the cricothyroid membrane directly into the trachea.

            (ii) Percutaneous transtracheal ventilation (most commonly used in children). Introduce a large-bore needle through the cricothyroid membrane and ventilate with high-flow oxygen through the needle. This temporary measure will provide adequate ventilation for about 30 minutes.

2. Circulation and control of hemorrhage. The most serious abnormality of the circulatory system is circulatory shock, which must be recognized quickly and treated to prevent serious sequelae, including death.

  a. Signs and symptoms of shock. Shock is often difficult to recognize, unless the patient has decompensated. The body has many compensatory mechanisms that mask shock—especially if one relies on single indicators such as pulse or blood pressure. This is particularly perilous in pediatric trauma. Elderly patients who have underlying cardiac disease or who are on medications such as β-blockers may not have an elevated heart rate. A narrowed pulse pressure with tachycardia signifies significant blood loss and involvement of compensatory mechanisms.

    (1) Decompensated shock. Inadequate perfusion of the skin, kidneys, and central nervous system is usually easy to recognize, causing ashen or cyanotic skin, decreased urine output, and mental status changes.

(2) Early shock.

   (a) During the physical examination, pay specific attention to pulse rate, respiratory rate, pulse pressure, state of skin perfusion, and peripheral circulation. Vital signs are a valuable tool in gauging the severity of shock, although in young otherwise healthy adults compensatory mechanisms permit a 30% to 40% blood loss (2000 mL) before hypotension, tachycardia, tachypnea, and mental status changes occur. The most common abnormalities are tachycardia (Table 17-1) and tachypnea. The earliest signs of shock are tachycardia and peripheral vasoconstriction. An acutely injured patient who presents with tachycardia and cool or cyanotic extremities should be considered as being in shock.

   (b) Laboratory tests of immediate benefit in the acute phase of shock include arterial pH and bicarbonate levels, which can be used to assess the quality of the patient's resuscitation.

b. Causes of shock. As a general rule, shock does not result from isolated head injuries.

   (1) *Hypovolemia.* Loss of blood is the most common cause of shock. Because an individual can lose up to 30% of circulating blood volume with good compensation, the patient who presents with signs and symptoms of shock has suffered significant blood loss. Such a patient must be managed aggressively and therapeutic interventions instituted quickly to optimize the chances for a good outcome.

   (a) Obvious *external hemorrhage* can be controlled by direct pressure. Small vessels can be clamped or ligated under direct visualization to control active bleeding. Blind clamping in a wound is contraindicated.

   (b) If no obvious source of external hemorrhage exists, look for blood loss in other areas *(internal hemorrhage)*.

   (i) Thoracic cavity. A massive hemothorax can account for up to 2000 mL of blood loss. On physical examination, auscultation will display decreased breath sounds on the affected side, and the trachea may be deviated away from the site of bleeding.

   (ii) Abdominal cavity. The abdomen can contain an exsanguinating hemorrhage. In an unconscious patient, the only sign may be a rigid abdomen; in a conscious patient, blood irritates the peritoneum and causes rebound tenderness and localizing peritoneal signs.

   (iii) Retroperitoneal space. Pelvic fracture or kidney laceration can cause significant hemorrhage into the retroperitoneal space.

   (iv) Soft tissue. Soft tissue injuries associated with a femur fracture can contain a hematoma of up to 1 L of blood; bilateral femur fractures could be the sole source of shock.

Table 17-1. Criteria for Tachycardia

Infant	Heart rate >160
Preschool-age child	Heart rate >140
School age through puberty	Heart rate >120
Adult	Heart rate >100

  (2) *Cardiogenic shock.* This can be caused by direct myocardial contusion, tamponade, air embolism, pulmonary embolus, or myocardial infarction. On physical examination, tamponade is suggested by tachycardia, muffled heart sounds, engorged neck veins, and hypotension resistant to fluid therapy.

  (3) *Tension pneumothorax.* In the patient with acute respiratory distress, subcutaneous emphysema, ipsilateral loss of breath sounds, or tracheal shift are suggestive of tension pneumothorax. Emergent treatment with either a chest tube or needle decompression based on clinical grounds is warranted.

  (4) *Neurogenic shock.*

  (5) *Septic shock.*

 c. Treatment of shock. Treatment is aimed at identifying and treating the underlying cause. Current advanced trauma life support (ATLS) guidelines for treating shock are as follows:

  (1) Secure airway; ensure adequate ventilation.

  (2) Obtain two large-bore peripheral intravenous sites for fluid replacement.

   (a) Fluid resuscitation in adult: 2-L bolus of isotonic crystalloid solution (normal saline or Ringer's lactated solution)

   (b) Fluid resuscitation in child: 20 mL/kg bolus

  (3) Place a urinary catheter to monitor urine output (adequate output in an adult: 0.5 to 1.0 mL/kg/hr or 30 to 50 mL/hr).

  (4) Monitor hemodynamic response (urine output and acid-base balance most commonly); base therapeutic decisions on the response.

3. Disability and neurologic status. The most critical area to assess is level of consciousness by means of a rapid neurologic examination.

 a. Level of consciousness. Assess by carrying out the following:

  (1) Check pupillary size, reactivity, and obvious asymmetry.

  (2) Use a mnemonic, AVPU, in which the patient is judged to be **a**lert, responsive to **v**ocal stimuli, responsive to **p**ainful stimuli, or **u**nresponsive.

  (3) Another method is the Glasgow Coma Scale, which is easy to perform and predictive of patient outcome. This assessment is often performed as part of the secondary survey.

 b. Change in level of consciousness. Change may be an ominous sign, and its cause should be considered traumatic until another etiology is found. Changes in level of consciousness can be caused by head injury, inadequate oxygenation, ventilation, or hypotension. The assessment may be complicated by drugs or alcohol.

 c. Posturing. The presence of posturing is a sign of impending herniation, which may require urgent craniotomy.

4. Exposure and environmental control.

 a. Exposure. The patient should be completely undressed to facilitate the physical examination and continued management.

 b. Environmental control. Traumatically injured patients are often hypothermic and should be placed in a warm environment with warm blankets covering the parts of the body not being examined. Warm intravenous fluids should be used during resuscitation.

D. Secondary survey. After the primary survey has been completed and resuscitation has begun, a formal secondary survey can be done. Before beginning, reassess the airway, breathing, circulation and vital signs. Special procedures are performed during the time of the secondary survey, including portable radiologic studies and a diagnostic peritoneal lavage (DPL), if needed.

 1. History. Talk to prehospital personnel and any family member who accompanied the patient. Allergies, current medications, past medical history, the last meal, and any events related to the injury are ascertained at this time.

2. Physical examination. A complete examination is performed, including a detailed inspection of the entire body from head to toe. A consistent, systematic approach, either organ-based or region-based, is recommended. Vital signs should be reassessed frequently during the examination.

   a. Head.

      (1) Palpate entire scalp and head for lacerations, contusions, and evidence of fracture.

      (2) Examine ears for hemotympanum.

      (3) Recheck eyes for visual acuity, pupillary size, retinal hemorrhages, penetrating injury, presence of contact lenses or lens dislocation.

      (4) Palpate the temporomandibular joints and all facial bones.

   b. Cervical spine and neck. If any maxillofacial or head injuries discovered, assume that an unstable cervical spine injury exists until proven otherwise.

      (1) Inspect for obvious deformities, bruises, lacerations, or the distended neck veins.

      (2) Palpate for bony tenderness, step-off fractures, or subcutaneous emphysema.

   c. Chest. Significant chest injury is usually manifested by pain and shortness of breath.

      (1) Inspect the chest for contusions or hematomas of the chest wall. Injuries such as open pneumothorax or flail chest should be identified at this point.

      (2) Palpate ribs and clavicle. Place sternal pressure to evaluate for fracture of the sternum, costochondral separation, or subcutaneous emphysema.

      (3) Auscultate both anteriorly and posteriorly.

      (4) A single-view, portable chest x-ray study can confirm the presence of a suspected hemothorax or pneumothorax. A widened mediastinum or loss of distinct mediastinal structures is suggestive of vascular injury including aortic disruption.

   d. Abdomen. Abdominal injuries must be identified and treated aggressively; specific diagnosis is not as important as identifying that an injury exists and that surgery may be necessary. An initial normal examination does not rule out significant intra-abdominal injury. Repeated examinations must be done to assess for progression of subclinical injury, preferably by the same examiner.

      (1) Inspect the gross appearance of the abdomen, looking for distended or scaphoid appearance, obvious signs of hematoma, or penetrating injuries.

      (2) Auscultate all four quadrants, listening for bowel sounds, bruits, and breath sounds in the upper quadrants.

      (3) Palpate for tenderness, rigidity, or rebound tenderness.

   e. Perineum, rectum, genitalia.

      (1) Inspect the entire area looking for contusions, hematomas, lacerations, or urethral bleeding.

      (2) Perform a rectal examination to determine the presence of blood in the bowel lumen, a high-riding prostate in men, the potential for open pelvic fractures, rectal wall integrity, and sphincter tone.

      (3) Perform a vaginal examination in women to assess for the presence of blood in the vaginal vault, vaginal lacerations, and open pelvic fractures.

   f. Musculoskeletal system.

      (1) Inspect all four extremities for obvious deformity or contusion.

      (2) Palpate all long bones for tenderness, crepitation, and abnormal movements. Palpate the hip and pubic symphysis for abnormal movement. Obtain peripheral pulses to help identify the presence of vascular injuries.

(3) Ascertain the stability of all joints. In the conscious patient, active motion of the muscle tendon units can determine stability; in the unconscious patient, abnormal joint movement with passive motion is suggestive for joint disruption.

g. Neurologic status. In the acutely injured patient, complete spinal immobilization is required until spinal injury is excluded. Any evidence of paralysis or paresis suggests a major injury, either to the spinal cord or the peripheral nervous system.

(1) Assessment. Mental status changes should not, initially, be attributed to drugs or alcohol.

(a) Level of consciousness. The Glasgow Coma Scale (see Table 17-2) is a prognostic, standardized examination, scored by assessing eye-opening, motor response, and verbal response. For triage purposes, the following results are useful:

<8 = severe head injury
8 to 12 = moderate head injury
>12 = mild head injury

(b) Pupil size and reactivity. Shine a light directly onto the pupils; look for symmetry, dilation, and full extraocular eye movements. Loss of light reflex in an unconscious patient may be associated with intracranial hemorrhage on the ipsilateral side, especially if there is a fixed, dilated pupil. Unequal, nonreactive pupils are a cardinal sign of impending herniation.

(c) Motor examination.

(i) Conscious patient. Evaluate strength, tone, and reflexes in all extremities. Look for abnormal posturing or lack of movement. Paraparesis or quadriparesis suggests a cervical or thoracic spine fracture with cord injury. Hemiparesis can be caused by brain-stem herniation, severe brain contusion, or brain hemorrhage.

(ii) Unconscious patient. The motor examination is limited to response to painful stimuli; no response is an ominous sign.

(2) Reassessment. Serial neurologic examinations, preferably by the same examiner, are critical if there is any question of head injury. Any changes must be addressed and aggressively treated.

Table 17-2. Glasgow Coma Scale

	Response	Points
Eye opening	Spontaneous	4
	To verbal command	3
	To pain	2
	No response	1
Best motor response	Obeys command	6
	Purposeful movement to pain	5
	Withdrawal to pain	4
	Decorticate posturing	3
	Decerebrate posturing	2
	No response	1
Best verbal response	Oriented	5
	Confused	4
	Inappropriate words	3
	Incomprehensible	2
	No response	1

E. Monitoring. The patient must be frequently reassessed and continuously monitored. Changes must be quickly addressed as they arise.
  1. Indwelling urinary catheter
  2. Cardiac monitor
  3. Continuous pulse oximetry
  4. Frequent vital signs (every 10 to 15 minutes)
F. Radiologic examination. X-ray examinations can be performed during the time of the secondary survey.
  1. Traditional three-view radiologic examination: portable x-rays of the chest, pelvis, and a cross-table lateral of the cervical spine. (Before obtaining the chest and pelvis films, it may be helpful to place a nasogastric tube in the stomach on low continuous wall suction.)
  2. Further radiologic studies, as needed for each individual patient.
III. **Mechanism of Injury.** Understanding the biomechanics of various types of trauma allows prediction of injury patterns, which in turn allows the physician to anticipate certain complications.
  A. Blunt trauma
    1. Biomechanical vectors
      a. Shear strain. Changes in speed (acceleration or deceleration) cause transection or laceration of mobile organs and tissues as they pull against their points of attachment.
      b. Tensile strain. Direct compression causes injury to tissue and, depending on the site, damage to underlying structures and organs.
    2. Motor vehicle collisions (cause of most acute injuries)
      a. Frontal impact. The force and energy are modified by use of restraints, type of vehicle involved, and whether the vehicle struck a stationary or moving object.
        (1) Down and under dashboard. Lower extremities absorb the energy of impact, causing dislocated knees, fractured femurs, and posterior dislocation of hips.
        (2) Up and over steering wheel. More diverse and potentially life-threatening injuries may be sustained when chest and abdomen strike the steering wheel, causing injuries to anterior chest wall, lungs, heart, and compression injuries of the liver or intestines. The head striking the windshield may cause spinal cord injuries, and closed head injuries.
      b. Rear impact. Forward acceleration can cause acute hyperextension of the neck, resulting in cervical spine injury.
      c. Lateral impact. When one car strikes another car in the passenger compartment, lateral crushing injuries to the torso, pelvis, and spine may occur. These injuries may be worse if the occupant is restrained. Secondary injuries may be caused by the person striking other passengers or objects inside the vehicle.
      d. Rollover. Impact may occur at several angles; many injuries are possible.
    3. Pedestrian/motor vehicle collisions
      a. Adults. Leg injuries occur during initial impact; if the victim falls over the hood, pelvic, abdominal and thoracic injuries can occur. Head injuries can occur as the body strikes the ground.
      b. Children. The initial impact on children is higher, and pelvic injuries can result. Children are more likely to be dragged under the vehicle, causing unpredictable injuries.
    4. Falls. The height of the fall determines magnitude of injury, and the surface on which the victim lands modifies the injuries. Multiple injuries may occur in any type of fall.
      a. Feet first: bilateral calcaneal fractures, compression fractures of the lumbar and thoracic spine
      b. Forward, arms extended: Colles' wrist fractures, hip dislocations, pelvic fractures

    c. Head first: brain and cervical spine injuries

B. Penetrating trauma

    1. Low-energy missiles. Knives, screwdrivers, and similar objects produce damage primarily by sharp cutting edges. The extent of injury cannot be determined by examination of the entrance wound alone.

    2. Gunshot wounds.

        a. Low- and medium-velocity weapons (most handguns, some rifles) cause injury to tissue in the path of the projectile. The injury is generally three to six times the area of the bullet's frontal surface.

        b. High-velocity weapons create a wide area of injury often contaminated by clothing, bacteria, and debris pulled into the wound. The entrance and exit wounds are evaluated to assess the number of projectiles, path, and organs at risk.

IV. Anatomic Considerations

A. Head injury. Traumatic brain injuries (TBIs) are often associated with other major trauma. The main priority is stabilization of the patient and management of life-threatening chest and abdominal injuries; management of TBIs must wait. However, hypotension and hypoxia must be zealously avoided to prevent secondary brain injury, and reversible causes of coma (hypoglycemia, narcotic overdose) and the potential for cervical spine injury must be recognized.

    1. Concussion: transient episode of neuronal dysfunction after blunt trauma with a rapid return of normal neurologic activity; no anatomic brain damage. Management is by observation and nonopiate analgesics. Any worsening of signs and symptoms warrants an aggressive workup. Many patients complain of persistent symptoms weeks or even years after the injury.

    2. Contusion: a bruise of the brain, which may be accompanied by bleeding into the injured area. Bleeding causes decreased level of consciousness (drowsiness) and focal neurologic deficits depending on the area of brain injured. Significant edema may develop, requiring monitoring of intracranial pressure.

    3. Skull fracture: not always associated with significant traumatic brain injury. Severe TBI can occur without skull fracture.

        a. Linear nondepressed. This usually requires no treatment.

        b. Across arterial grooves or suture lines. Assess for vascular injury; monitor for epidural or subdural hematoma.

        c. Depressed. If the fragment is depressed more than the thickness of the skull, surgery may be required to minimize sequelae such as seizures.

        d. Open (direct communication between scalp and cranial contents). Early surgery is needed. Diagnosis is made when brain is visible or cerebrospinal fluid (CSF) is leaking from the wound.

        e. Basilar. Basal skull fractures often are not apparent on routine skull radiographs. CSF leaking from ears or nose is diagnostic; Battle's sign (ecchymosis in mastoid region) and hemotympanum are suggestive of basal skull fracture. Treatment is supportive. CSF leak, if present, requires neurosurgical evaluation.

        f. Cribriform plate. Raccoon eyes are associated with this fracture. Oral insertion of a gastric tube is recommended.

    4. Hemorrhage: classified according to anatomic location. Bleeding within the cranial vault has potentially catastrophic consequences.

        a. Epidural hematoma. This injury carries a 25% to 50% mortality rate. Eighty percent of epidural hematomas occur within 12 hours of injury, and 5% to 10% have no demonstrable fracture.

            (1) Cause. Most are due to a tear in a dural artery, commonly the middle meningeal artery; less often a tear in a dural sinus is the cause.

            (2) Diagnosis. Classic presentation is loss of consciousness, followed by a return to full consciousness lasting minutes to hours, then a second depression of consciousness. Physical examination shows a decreased level of consciousness, contralateral hemiparesis, ipsilateral pupillary dilatation. Computed tomography (CT) scan will show the biconvex hyperdensity of the hematoma.

(3) Treatment. Emergent surgical evacuation of the epidural hematoma is required; secondary brain injury, including herniation, can occur rapidly without this treatment.

b. Subdural hematoma. Rupture of the bridging veins between the cerebral cortex and the dura, and laceration of the brain or cortical arteries results in bleeding into the subdural space. The underlying brain injury is often severe. Subdural hematoma is six times more common than epidural hematoma.

(1) Acute. Presentation is focal findings and deteriorating level of consciousness within 24 hours of injury. Many patients require surgery; the mortality rate is 60% to 80% without early intervention and 30% or less if surgery occurs within 4 hours of injury.

(2) Subacute. This injury becomes symptomatic in 2 to 14 days; mortality rate is 12% to 25%, which markedly decreases with operative evacuation.

(3) Chronic. Symptomatic (altered level of consciousness, personality change) after 14 days is often seen in elderly patients and alcoholics who may be unable to recall a fall or suspected TBI. Overall mortality rate is 3% to 15%.

5. Diffuse axonal injury. Widely scattered microscopic damage throughout the brain is caused by diffuse shearing injury and results in increased intracranial pressure secondary to cerebral edema. It is characterized by prolonged coma lasting days to weeks. The patient often displays decorticate or decerebrate posturing. Autonomic dysfunction (high fever, hypertension, diaphoresis) may be present. Forty-four percent of comatose head-injured patients have this injury, which carries an overall mortality rate of 33% to 50%.

6. Penetrating injuries

a. Impalement. Leave object in place for neurosurgical removal. Obtain skull films to determine angle and depth of impaling object.

b. Missile wounds. Very high mortality rate is associated with this wound, especially with Glasgow Coma Scale results of less than 6, with through-and-through wounds, and with wounds that cross the midline. A bullet that does not penetrate may still cause TBI from concussive force.

B. Thoracic trauma. Delays in diagnosis and treatment are a common cause of preventable death.

1. Chest wall. Injuries may cause mechanical breathing problems. Underlying lung or vascular injuries may be present.

a. Rib fracture.

(1) Treat simple rib fractures by pain management.

(2) Flail chest (fracture of three or more adjacent ribs in two locations) is diagnosed by observing paradoxical motion of the chest wall with respirations. This causes decreased ventilation and decreased venous return. The injury can be stabilized by turning the patient onto the injured side; supplemental oxygen or continuous positive airway pressure (CPAP) may be all that is needed for treatment. More aggressive treatment is required if the patient is in shock, has three or more associated injuries, previous pulmonary disease, fracture of eight or more ribs, age greater than 65, or O_2 saturation <60% on 100% oxygen.

b. Sternal fracture. This often-missed injury is caused by anterior blunt chest trauma. Point tenderness and pain suggest the diagnosis. Significant underlying injuries (myocardial contusion, cardiac rupture, tamponade, pulmonary injury) must be sought; provide pain control and aggressive pulmonary toilet as needed.

2. Lung.
   a. Pneumothorax: air in the pleural space.
      (1) *Simple pneumothorax* involves collapse of the lung, no communication with atmosphere, and no shift of mediastinal structures. This may result from a ruptured alveolus or a small laceration in the pulmonary parenchyma from either blunt or penetrating trauma. Highly variable symptoms and signs may occur: shortness of breath and chest pain are most common, cyanosis and tachycardia may occur, decreased or absent breath sounds and hyperresonance may be over the involved side, and subcutaneous emphysema may be present. Treat with tube thoracostomy with low continuous suction to evacuate the air and allow reexpansion of the lung.
      (2) *Open pneumothorax* involves a chest wall defect causing equilibration of intrathoracic and atmospheric pressure. This creates a large functional dead space and loss of ventilation due to collapse of the lung. Emergency treatment includes covering the defect with a clean dressing; this eliminates the major physiologic abnormality. Do not occlude the defect, which could convert the injury into a tension pneumothorax. Definitive treatment is endotracheal intubation and tube thoracostomy before surgery.
      (3) *Tension pneumothorax* can be caused by the same injuries that cause a simple pneumothorax, but the injury acts like a one-way valve—air can enter, but not exit. Air accumulates, resulting in positive intrathoracic pressure. This causes collapse of the lung, shift of the mediastinum toward the opposite side, compression of the other lung and great vessels resulting in severe respiratory disturbance, and decreased venous return. Hypoxia, acidosis, and shock occur rapidly. Cardinal signs are hypotension, tachycardia, jugular venous distention, and absent breath sounds on the involved side. To treat, immediately decompress with a large-bore needle inserted into the second intercostal space in the midclavicular line; follow by inserting a chest tube.
   b. Hemothorax: blood in the pleural space caused most commonly by hemorrhage from lung parenchyma or by disruption of intercostal and internal mammary arteries, resulting from blunt or penetrating trauma. Breath sounds are diminished or absent; neck veins may be distended. With loss of >1000 mL, signs include restlessness, anxiety, pallor, tachycardia, and hypotension. To treat, restore circulating blood volume, control the airway, and evacuate accumulated blood with a chest tube.
   c. Traumatic diaphragmatic hernia: rupture of the diaphragm, most often the left hemidiaphragm, resulting in herniation of abdominal contents into the thoracic cavity. If caused by penetrating trauma, the tear is usually less than 2 cm; in blunt trauma the tear can be up to 15 cm. Small tears may go undiagnosed for years. The varied signs and symptoms include tachypnea, hypotension, absence of breath sounds or presence of bowel sounds in the chest. Treat with operative repair.
   d. Pulmonary contusion: lung parenchymal damage with edema and hemorrhage, but without laceration; commonly seen with rib fractures, flail chest, and sternal fractures. Signs of pulmonary contusion include dyspnea, tachypnea, cyanosis, tachycardia, hypotension, chest wall bruising, and hemoptysis (in about 50%). Diagnosis is based on increased work of breathing and hypoxia. Chest x-ray is useful, since 70% show signs of infiltrate or contusion within 1 hour of injury. Treat with vigorous pulmonary toilet and supplemental oxygen. Large contusions may require intubation and mechanical ventilation.
   e. Pulmonary laceration: direct parenchymal damage causing hemorrhage; most often caused by penetrating injury but may be from frac-

tured rib or avulsion of pleural adhesion. This injury is usually not life-threatening. Treat with observation; place a chest tube, if needed.

f. Subcutaneous emphysema: air in subcutaneous tissue. It is important to identify and treat the underlying cause. It is commonly associated with pneumothorax, ruptured bronchus, and ruptured esophagus. If heard over the chest wall, it is usually indicative of pneumothorax; over the supraclavicular area, pneumomediastinum.

g. Tracheobronchial tree injuries: relatively rare but extremely lethal and can occur with either blunt or penetrating trauma. Patients who reach the hospital complain of dyspnea, cough, and hemoptysis; subcutaneous emphysema is nearly always present. Consider these injuries if chest tube placement fails to reexpand the pneumothorax and massive air leak continues. Surgical repair is needed.

3. Mediastinal structures

a. Thoracic aortic injuries are caused by excessive force causing tearing; the tearing may involve some or all layers. Associated injuries are very common.

(1) Clinical findings are often meager. They include retrosternal or interscapular pain, dyspnea (from tracheal compression and deviation), stridor or hoarseness (from esophageal or laryngeal nerve compression), dysphagia, ischemic pain of the extremities, lower extremity pulse deficit, lower extremity paralysis, palpable sternal fracture, scapular or multiple rib fractures of the left chest, or hypertension (secondary to stretching of the sympathetic fibers at the aortic isthmus).

(2) Rapid diagnosis and early surgical repair are necessary.

b. Pericardial tamponade is compression of the heart caused by hemorrhage into the pericardial space. This injury can result from either blunt or penetrating trauma and may be immediately life-threatening.

(1) Findings classically include Beck's triad (distant heart sounds, hypotension, and jugular venous distention); tachycardia and pulsus paradoxus (i.e., systolic blood pressure drop >10 torr during inspiration) are often present. Electrical alternans by electrocardiogram (EKG) is highly specific for tamponade. Suspect tamponade in patients with penetrating injury who are tachycardic and hypotensive despite resuscitation and who show no evidence of hemorrhage into the chest, abdomen, or pelvis.

(2) If tamponade is suspected, perform a thoracotomy or pericardial window immediately. Pericardiocentesis may be performed for diagnosis and treatment. Advance a large-bore spinal needle placed on a 30-mL syringe into the pericardial space (identified by return of blood); removal of 20 to 30 mL of blood may result in dramatic improvement. If unsuccessful, immediate thoracotomy is indicated.

C. Abdominal trauma

1. Assessment of abdominal injuries may be difficult. Most are caused by blunt trauma.

a. History. It may not be possible to obtain an adequate history from the patient; witnesses may supply some useful information. Time and mode of injury are important.

b. Important clinical signs:

(1) Hypotension—most often due to hemorrhage from solid organs

(2) Ecchymosis, abdominal wall—suspect intraperitoneal injury

(3) Ecchymosis, flank or periumbilical—suspect retroperitoneal injury

(4) Tenderness, local or generalized—suspect intra-abdominal visceral injury

(5) Blood or subcutaneous emphysema on rectal examination—rare, but highly correlated with abdominal injury

  c. Treatment. Surgical intervention is required for hemorrhage control and hollow viscus injury. These patients must be identified quickly. Because the clinical examination is often equivocal, laboratory testing (radiographs, ultrasonography, CT, diagnostic peritoneal lavage) is essential.

2. Penetrating trauma. Concurrent abdominal and chest injuries often occur.

  a. Stab wounds. Initial clinical assessment is difficult and often inaccurate. Assess hemodynamic status, and examine the patient repeatedly. Surgery is indicated if any of the following are present: hemodynamic instability, signs of intraperitoneal injury or implement *in situ*. If otherwise stable, further diagnostic studies (local wound exploration, diagnostic peritoneal lavage, CT) can be undertaken.

  b. Gunshot wounds. Assess the extent and number of injuries and the patient's hemodynamic stability. Immediate laparotomy is indicated for unstable patients and those with obvious peritoneal penetration. Further diagnostic testing and observation are helpful in those with obviously superficial injuries or when peritoneal penetration is not certain.

3. Blunt abdominal trauma. Initial presentation is often deceptive. Pain and tenderness are the most reliable signs of injury in the alert patient. In those with an altered sensorium, physical signs are unreliable.

  a. Spleen. The spleen is the intra-abdominal organ most often injured by blunt trauma. Physical signs are variable. Left upper quadrant pain may be present; referred pain to the left shoulder (Kehr's sign) is common. Most spleen injuries have prompt, significant bleeding; others are subject to rupture after hours or days. Splenectomy has been the classic approach; however, aggressive attempts to save the spleen are now common, particularly in children, to avoid the complications of postsplenectomy sepsis.

  b. Liver. Because of its size and weight, the liver is prone to damage from blunt trauma, including subcapsular hematoma, parenchymal contusion, venous or arterial damage, and disruption of the biliary duct system. Findings include right upper quadrant tenderness, guarding, rebound tenderness, and hypoactive bowel sounds.

  c. Retroperitoneal structures. Injuries to the duodenum, pancreas, and kidneys are difficult to detect on physical examination. Duodenal injury is almost always associated with other injuries, most often those of the liver.

  d. Vasculature. Major abdominal vascular injuries due to blunt trauma are rare. If aortic injury does occur, it is associated with a high mortality rate. Hypotension is the most common sign of injury to the inferior vena cava.

D. Spine and spinal cord trauma. Remember that manipulation, movement, and inadequate immobilization can cause or worsen a spinal injury. Disposition of the patient must be determined promptly. If a neurologic deficit is present, the patient should be seen by a neurosurgeon, although the role of surgery in spinal injuries is limited.

1. Spinal column injuries. Mechanically unstable fractures may present without neurologic deficits. Mechanically stable fractures may result in spinal cord damage from fracture fragments, vascular compromise, or soft tissue damage.

  a. Physical examination. Carefully palpate the entire spine, using logroll precautions. Assess for pain, tenderness, and step-off fractures. Local tenderness is usually present; palpable deformity is occasionally present. Prominence of spinous processes, edema, ecchymosis, pain with attempted motion, and muscle spasm are variably present. Tracheal deviation or dysphagia suggest retropharyngeal hematoma with associated cervical spine injury.

    b. Causes. Specific injury patterns can be predicted from the mechanism of injury. All can produce unstable injuries.

      (1) Flexion

      (2) Flexion/rotation

      (3) Extension; more often associated with unstable fractures

      (4) Vertical compression

    c. Management. Total spine immobilization must be maintained until fracture can be ruled out by clinical examination or radiographic studies. If an unstable fracture is identified, immobilization must continue until the fracture can be stabilized.

2. Spinal cord injuries. Suspect these injuries in patients with impaired consciousness, neck or back pain, facial or head trauma, localized spinal tenderness, focal neurologic deficit, or unexplained hypotension. Associated injuries are often difficult to detect in patients with known spinal cord injury. Diagnostic peritoneal lavage or CT is usually needed to assess the abdomen. Pressure sores can develop in as little as 1 hour in spinal cord–injured patients on a backboard.

    a. Causes. Injuries occur with either penetrating or blunt trauma. Blunt trauma can cause disruption of the vertebral column and transection of the spinal cord, displaced bony fragments, and herniated disks. Primary vascular damage can cause an epidural hematoma or disruption of vertebral and spinal arteries. Forced hyperextension in patients with degenerative joint disease of the cervical spine can result in high cord injury.

    b. Secondary injury. Decreased spinal cord blood flow may cause secondary injury, believed to be initiated by free radical formation from peroxidation reactions. High-dose steroids are now used to prevent these injuries.

    c. Assessment.

      (1) Determine whether the injury is complete or incomplete.

        (a) Complete cord lesion is indicated by total loss of motor and sensory function distal to the injury. If condition lasts longer than 24 hours, 99% will not have functional recovery. This injury can be mimicked by spinal shock.

        (b) Incomplete cord lesion is indicated by any evidence of cord function (sensory or motor) distal to the injury, and thus the chance of some functional recovery is present.

          (i) Central cord syndrome: occurs in hyperextension injuries to patients with arthritic necks. Deficit is greater in upper extremities than in lower extremities.

          (ii) Brown-Séquard syndrome: penetrating trauma causing hemisection of the cord. It results in ipsilateral motor paralysis with contralateral sensory hypesthesia.

          (iii) Anterior cord syndrome: caused by cervical flexion injuries, herniated disks, or bone fragments. Paralysis and hypalgesia occur below the lesion with preserved position, touch, and vibration senses.

          (iv) Treat with high-dose steroids: initial bolus of 30 mg/kg methylprednisolone, followed by continuous infusion of 5.4 mg/kg per hour for 24 hours.

      (2) Examine for motor strength, sensory disturbances, reflex changes, and autonomic dysfunction (loss of bladder and rectal control, priapism).

      (3) Perform the neurologic examination. Three spinal cord tracts can be tested.

        (a) Corticospinal tract. Located in the posterolateral aspect of the cord, this tract controls motor function on same side of body. Test by voluntary muscle contraction.

        (b) Spinothalamic tract. Located on the anterolateral aspect of the cord, this tract transmits pain and temperature from the contralateral side. Test by pinch or pinprick.

        (c) Posterior columns. These provide ipsilateral proprioception. Test by position sense of the fingers or toes, or tuning fork vibration.

    d. Management. Stabilize the patient.

        (1) Carry out *complete spinal immobilization.*

        (2) *Airway management* is crucial in cervical spine injury and must be secured in a restless, agitated, or violent patient.

        (3) Use maintenance fluids for *circulatory support* unless treating hypotension.

  3. Spinal shock. This can be suspected when there is loss of neurologic function and autonomic control below the level of the lesion. It is caused by a concussive injury. Examination shows flaccid paralysis, no sensation, and loss of deep tendon reflexes and bladder tone; signs include bradycardia, hypotension, hypothermia, and ileus. This condition usually resolves within 24 hours.

  4. Neurogenic hypotension. This is usually secondary to spinal shock; it is caused by impairment of descending sympathetic pathways. Neurogenic hypotension is a diagnosis of exclusion; other causes of shock must be aggressively ruled out. Patients usually respond to Trendelenburg positioning, fluid resuscitation, and, rarely, vasopressors.

E. Genitourinary trauma. Suspect this in patients with injuries of the back, abdomen, genitalia, flank, pelvis, or perineum. Localized abrasions, lacerations, or contusions may point to underlying injury; flank, abdomen, or back tenderness and hematuria are often present.

  1. Renal injuries. Hematuria is characteristic and is very sensitive but not specific.

    a. Diagnostic studies are needed for definitive diagnosis in penetrating trauma and are useful in blunt trauma when definite indications are present. Three studies are used routinely: intravenous pyelogram, CT, and angiography.

    b. Management. At least 85% of renal injuries do not require surgery. Absolute indications for surgery include severely shattered kidneys, renal pedicle injuries, and penetrating abdominal wounds. The goal is to preserve tissue and function without increasing morbidity or mortality.

  2. Bladder injuries. Most injuries are caused by blunt trauma to a distended bladder; pelvic fracture is associated in 10% to 15%. There is a high incidence of associated severe injury.

    a. Type.

        (1) Intraperitoneal rupture usually involves injury to the dome of the bladder, which is often extensive, requires early operative repair, and is associated with other intra-abdominal injuries.

        (2) Extraperitoneal bladder injuries involve extravasation into the retroperitoneum alone. It is usually managed without surgery.

    b. Clinical symptoms include suprapubic tenderness, urgency with inability to void, and (if intraperitoneal) the development of fever, abdominal distention, nausea, and vomiting. Diagnosis of bladder injuries is made by radiographic studies, particularly cystogram.

    c. Management. Bladder contusions and extraperitoneal ruptures are usually managed conservatively with a suprapubic cystostomy or indwelling urethral catheter. To avoid infection, patients with extraperitoneal ruptures should receive antibiotics for the duration of the catheter placement. Intraperitoneal rupture requires surgical repair and suprapubic drainage.

  3. Ureter injuries. Traumatic injuries are rare, usually caused by penetrating trauma, and often missed. Definitive diagnosis is by intravenous pyelogram; treatment is surgical repair. Late diagnosis is associated with a high incidence of nephroureterectomy.

4. Urethral injuries. These are uncommon and occur almost entirely in males. Untreated severe injuries have significant morbidity.
    a. Anterior injuries (below the urogenital diaphragm). These are usually caused by straddle injuries or falls and rarely by penetrating trauma.
        (1) Findings include considerable perineal pain, blood at the meatus, and good urinary stream with voiding. Anterior injury is associated with significant morbidity if there is concomitant injury to Buck's fascia.
        (2) Treatment. If a catheter can be threaded into the bladder, surgery is not needed. If not, suprapubic urinary diversion for 2 to 3 weeks is necessary.
    b. Posterior disruption. Pelvic fracture is usually present; complete transection is common.
        (1) Findings include blood at the meatus, inability to void, perineal bruising, and a boggy, high-riding prostate. Diagnose with retrograde urethrogram.
        (2) Treatment. Insert a suprapubic catheter for urinary diversion; repair can be delayed, sometimes for months.
        (3) Complications can be significant, including urethral stricture, incontinence, and impotence.
F. Musculoskeletal trauma. Rarely life-threatening, these injuries usually involve bone, muscle, nerve, and soft tissue. Limb-threatening injuries include devitalization of an extremity, compartment syndromes, open fractures, and major joint dislocations.
    1. History. Determine the mechanism of injury and the environment (exposure, toxins, foreign bodies). Ascertain preinjury status (alcohol, drugs, preexisting conditions), and obtain a description of the findings at the accident site.
    2. Physical examination. Assess color and perfusion; look for open wounds, obvious deformities, swelling, discoloration. Assess tenderness, sensation, pulses, and crepitation. Check active voluntary motion to confirm intact muscle-tendon units. Use passive movement to identify motion that should not exist. Test pelvic stability with gentle anteroposterior pressure; any motion is abnormal and suggests significant disruption.
    3. Specific injuries.
        a. Traumatic amputation. Wound care and hemostasis are the highest priority. Place a bulky dressing with direct pressure as needed to control hemorrhage. Do not blindly clamp arterial bleeding sites. Replantation must be done early. Transport the cooled (*not* frozen) amputated part with the patient. If cooled, the amputated tissue remains viable for up to 18 hours after injury.
        b. Open wounds. Assume that any skin wound near a fracture or joint communicates with a skeletal injury. Do not probe open wounds—probing increases risk of infection and provides little information. Minor wounds can be cleaned and closed. Larger wounds may require surgical closure. Closure of open extremity wounds is not urgent. Treat wounds that communicate with skeletal injuries more aggressively; they have a high risk for osteomyelitis and nonunion of the fracture. Debridement, open reduction, and internal fixation are required, usually within 6 hours.
        c. Compartment syndrome. Swelling in a muscle compartment causes interstitial pressure to exceed capillary perfusion pressure; this develops over several hours or days. The resulting ischemia can cause paralysis, necrosis, and Volkmann's ischemic contractures. Compartment syndrome is associated with crush injuries, closed or open fractures, and reperfusion of a previously ischemic extremity. Findings include pain with passive motion, paresthesias, weakness or paralysis,

and tense edema. If elevated intracompartmental pressures are present, fasciotomy is performed.

  d. Dislocations (painful injuries with obvious deformities involving a joint). Knee, hip, shoulder, and elbow dislocations have potential for compromise, although actual incidence of serious arterial injury is only 1% to 2%. Findings include local pain, obvious deformity, instability, and impaired motion; tenderness, ecchymosis, paresthesias, and decreased or absent distal pulses may be present. Immediate reduction is required if neurovascular compromise is present. Conscious sedation or general anesthesia may be needed to overcome muscle spasm and pain.

 G. Pelvic fractures. These are caused by high-energy impact and are often associated with abdominal, central nervous system, and genitourinary injuries.

  1. Signs and symptoms include significant pain, abnormal pelvic motion, and inability to void.

  2. Diagnosis is usually made by plain radiographs.

  3. Management includes intravenous fluid resuscitation to replace blood loss. If multiple fractures are present, external fixation or open reduction may be needed to stop hemorrhage.

V. Available Technology for Trauma Diagnosis

 A. The table lists the methods available for diagnosis of the acutely injured patient.

Procedure	Indication
Chest x-ray	Chest trauma Difficulty breathing Unconscious patient
Flat-plate abdomen	Abdominal pain Pelvic pain/instability Hip dislocation Unconscious patient
Abdominal ultrasonography	Suspected retroperitoneal injury Abdominal trauma Pregnancy
Diagnostic peritoneal lavage	Unstable/unconscious patient with suspected intra-abdominal injury
Computed tomography (CT)	Head injury Suspected abdominal, retroperitoneal, or pelvic injuries Confirmation/evaluation of spinal injuries
Magnetic resonance imaging (MRI)	Limited usefulness emergently Evaluation of suspected spinal cord injury
Intravenous pyelogram	Screening exam for renal injury Largely replaced by CT scanning
Angiography	Suspected aortic disruption Penetrating injury involving major vascular structures Crush injuries/partial amputations
Cystogram	Pelvic fractures Suspected bladder injury
Retrograde urethrogram	Pelvic fracture with abnormal prostate exam Suspected urethral injury
Intracompartmental pressure measurement	Suspected compartment syndrome

B. The cost figures cited in this table are **basic direct costs.** The figures are difficult to obtain and change quickly. They include **only** the cost of the test itself (technician, equipment, time, and materials). No professional costs (interpretation) are included. Costs vary from region to region based on differences in some components such as labor. However, the relative cost ranking should remain similar.

Procedure	Code
Chest x-ray	$
Abdominal x-ray	$
Abdominal ultrasonography	$$
Diagnostic peritoneal lavage	$$$$
Computed tomography (CT)—head	$$$$
CT—abdomen	$$$$
Magnetic resonance imaging (MRI)	$$$$$
Intravenous pyelogram	$$$$
Angiography	$$$$$
Cystogram	$$$$
Retrograde urethrogram	$$$$
Intracompartmental pressure measurement	*

$ = $0–$50; $$ = $50–$100; $$$ = $100–$200; $$$$ = $200–$500; $$$$$ = $500–$1000; * = highly variable or not available.

VI. Bibliography

American College of Surgeons Committee on Trauma. *Advanced Trauma Life Support Reference Manual.* Chicago: American College of Surgeons; 1993.

Greenfield LJ, Mulholland MW, Oldham KT, Zelenock GB (eds). *Surgery: Scientific Principles and Practice.* Philadelphia: JB Lippincott; 1993.

Rosen P, Barkin R, Braen C, et al. *Emergency Medicine: Concepts & Clinical Practice,* 3rd ed. St. Louis: Mosby-Year Book; 1992.

VII. Key Search Words

The following key words reflect the content of this chapter. They are provided to assist with an on-line search of computer databases, such as MEDLINE, if you wish to pursue the topic of this chapter further.

Glasgow Coma Scale
Head injuries
Multiple trauma
Shock, hemorrhagic
Surgery, operative
Wounds and injuries

18. PEDIATRIC EXAMINATION

Ronald D. Holmes

I. **Glossary**. The medical terms used for pediatric conditions are generally the same as those used for adults. For that reason, no glossary is included in this chapter.

II. **Techniques of Examination**. The approach to the pediatric physical examination varies with the age of the patient and can conveniently be divided into three parts: (1) the newborn and young infant; (2) the toddler and young child; and (3) the older child and adolescent. The approach to the older child and adolescent is very similar to that for an adult. However, examination of newborns, infants, and young children is more variable, and the technique of the examination and expected "normal" findings may be age-specific.

  A. The approach to the physical examination of the infant and young child must be flexible and often varies according to the age of the child. It is not typically done by means of the accustomed head-to-toe, organ-to-organ approach used in the adult.

  B. Begin with a general observation of the infant's or child's interaction with the parents and the examiner. Observe behavior, facial expression, posture, muscle tone, and coordination. Failure of newborns or young infants to make eye contact may be a sign of serious illness.

  C. Make as many observations as possible before touching the child.

  D. Initially focus on aspects of the examination that are most relevant to the clinical problem. Delay the most objectionable parts of the examination until last. Listening to the chest and palpating the abdomen are best done before the child cries. Children often do not like the throat and ear examination, since restraint is often necessary.

  E. Interact and communicate with the child and parent during the examination to help the child relax and to prevent unnecessary worry by the older child or parent.

  F. Respect the child's sense of modesty and level of understanding. It is important to gain the child's cooperation with a friendly attitude, casual play, simple explanations of what will happen, and considerable patience.

  G. In the very ill child or premature infant, performing the examination in several brief stages may be necessary. It is very important to keep the child warm and to warm your hands and instruments during the examination.

  H. Children constantly grow and develop, and "normality" can only be evaluated by assessing certain characteristics and measurements over time. It is important to refer to growth charts and age-appropriate blood pressure graphs and to become familiar with Tanner staging of secondary sexual characteristics to assess normal growth and development.

III. **Normal Findings**. The pediatric examination is almost never completed in the systematic fashion that follows, and the examiner must take every opportunity to look at *what* he or she can *whenever* possible.

  A. Measurements
    1. Height, weight, and head circumference
      a. Rate of growth is of great value in estimating the state of nutrition, general health, and some aspects of endocrine balances and maturation. Failure to gain normal increments in weight or height, and actual loss of weight, are often the first recognized signs of disease.
      b. Head size is relatively larger in children than in adults. Head circumference measurements are directly related to intracranial vol-

ume. Careful, frequent measurements to determine the rate of growth are important, especially when hydrocephalus or microcephalus is suspected. More than 85% of children with a circumference of more than 2 SD above or below the mean are mentally retarded or have other neurologic abnormalities.

c. Measurements must be compared with standards for age using appropriate growth charts. Measurements should be recorded in standard units and as percentile rank. Disproportionate measurements of height, weight, and head circumference may indicate serious illness.

d. Measure the head circumference by passing a tape measure over the occipital protuberance and just above the supraorbital ridges.

e. Infants appear rotund because of abundant subcutaneous fat. Toddlers age 2 to 3 years become more linear and lean.

2. Temperature
   a. Temperature is usually obtained rectally until age 3 years or older.
   b. Temperatures a degree or more above the adult average (98.6° F /37° C) are normal in infants and young children.

3. Pulse and respiratory rate
   a. These rates should be obtained when the child is quiet. Both are sensitive to fever and increase about 15% to 20% with each degree of rise in temperature (° C). Respiratory rate and depth of breathing may increase with respiratory disease, heart disease, or metabolic disease.
   b. Normal rates are more rapid in younger children and decrease with age.

4. Blood pressure
   a. Blood pressures are measured routinely in all children over 3 years of age by the auscultation method. Measuring blood pressure in younger children and infants is more difficult and is generally done using Doppler flow techniques.
   b. A quiet subject, and a cuff of the proper width (covering about ⅓–⅔ of upper arm) are necessary for accurate readings.
   c. Normal findings vary according to age (Figs. 18-1 through 18-5).

B. Skin and subcutaneous tissues reflect the general state of hydration and nutrition.
   1. Examination
      a. The condition of the skin and subcutaneous tissue reflect the general state of nutrition and hydration.
      b. A thorough inspection should be completed to detect any abnormalities and to recognize normal variations that may cause the child or parent to worry.
      c. The examination should include an assessment of tissue turgor. Tissue turgor is determined by picking up a fold of abdominal skin between the thumb and index finger and then releasing it. Normally, the skin rapidly returns to the former position. Skin that remains creased and raised is an indication of dehydration or undernutrition.
      d. Turgor is a manifestation of capillary refill. Capillary refill can also be assessed by lightly compressing the nail bed until it blanches and then observing the time (usually <2 seconds) before the pink returns.

C. Head
   1. Examination
      a. Observe shape of head, head control, and movement. Examine the face for shape and symmetry.
      b. Palpate the bones, fontanelles, and sutures in newborns and young infants.
   2. Findings in newborn
      a. Molding. Distortion of shape with overlapping of the large flat bones often occurs as the head passes through the birth canal. A few days to a few weeks may pass before normal anatomic relationships are reestablished.

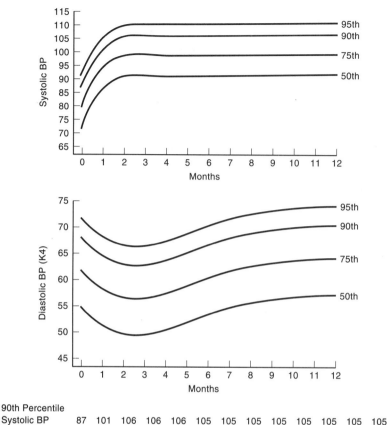

90th Percentile													
Systolic BP	87	101	106	106	106	105	105	105	105	105	105	105	105
Diastolic BP	68	65	63	63	63	65	66	67	68	68	69	69	69
Height cm	51	59	63	66	68	70	72	73	74	76	77	78	80
Weight kg	4	4	5	5	6	7	8	9	9	10	10	11	11

Fig. 18-1. Age-specific percentiles of blood pressure measurements in boys—birth to 12 months of age; Korotkoff phase IV (K4) used for diastolic blood pressure. (Adapted from Report on the Second Task Force on Blood Pressure Control in Children—1987. *Pediatrics* 1987;79:1–25 [Fig. 21-1].)

    b. Caput succedaneum. Soft tissue molding of the scalp at the time of birth may cause a soft, poorly outlined swelling from edema that pits on pressure and may overlie suture lines.

    c. Asymmetry of the head. This may occur in normal infants who always lie in the same position, because bones at this time are very soft.

    d. Head control and movement are indicators of neuromuscular development. By 2 months, the baby can raise the head from a prone position and hold it relatively steady when supported in an erect position. By 4 months, head control is good with no unsteadiness.

    e. Fontanelles. The posterior fontanelle normally closes to palpation within a few weeks; the anterior fontanelle varies in size throughout early infancy but is usually only a slight depression by the time the

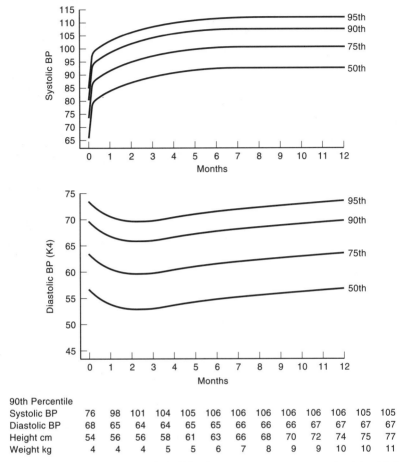

Fig. 18-2. Age-specific percentiles of blood pressure measurements in girls—birth to 12 months of age; Korotkoff phase IV (K4) used for diastolic blood pressure. (Adapted from Report on the Second Task Force on Blood Pressure Control in Children—1987. *Pediatrics* 1987;79:1–25 [Fig. 21-2].)

90th Percentile												
Systolic BP	76	98	101	104	105	106	106	106	106	106	106	105	105
Diastolic BP	68	65	64	64	65	65	66	66	66	67	67	67	67
Height cm	54	56	56	58	61	63	66	68	70	72	74	75	77
Weight kg	4	4	4	5	5	6	7	8	9	9	10	10	11

child is 12 to 18 months. Until they close, some arterial pulsation is transmitted through the fontanelles.

D. Eyes

    1. Examination

        a. The eyes of older children are examined as in an adult. In infants and younger children, the goals are to observe extraocular movements for strabismus and to visualize the red reflex with the ophthalmoscope to exclude corneal or retinal abnormalities.

        b. Participation in a game or following a toy moved by the examiner may help ascertain ocular movements and pupillary responses. By 2½ to 3 years, visual testing with a Snellen's E or other chart can be accomplished.

        c. Assessment of visual acuity in younger children is subjective and typically based on observation by the parent and examiner.

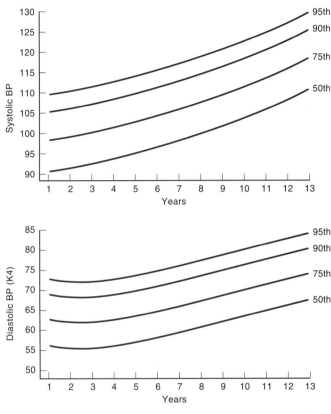

90th Percentile													
Systolic BP	105	106	107	108	109	111	112	114	115	117	119	121	124
Diastolic BP	69	68	68	69	69	70	71	73	74	75	76	77	79
Height cm	80	91	100	108	115	122	129	135	141	147	153	159	165
Weight kg	11	14	16	18	22	25	29	34	39	44	50	55	62

Fig. 18-3. Age-specific percentiles of blood pressure measurements in boys—1 to 13 years of age; Korotkoff phase IV (K4) used for diastolic blood pressure. (Adapted from Report on the Second Task Force on Blood Pressure Control in Children—1987. *Pediatrics* 1987;79:1–25 [Fig. 21-3].)

    2. Findings
        a. Complete eye coordination may not develop until near the end of the first year.
        b. Evaluate carefully for strabismus to prevent amblyopia.
  E. Ear, nose, mouth, and pharynx
    1. Examination
        a. Delay ear, nose, and throat evaluation until the end of the physical examination, since restraint may be needed (Fig. 18-6).
        b. Hearing assessment in children less than 5 years is often subjective.
        c. Formal auditory testing should be considered for infants at increased risk for hearing loss, such as family history of hearing loss, congenital infections, meningitis, and previous treatment with ototoxic antibiotics.

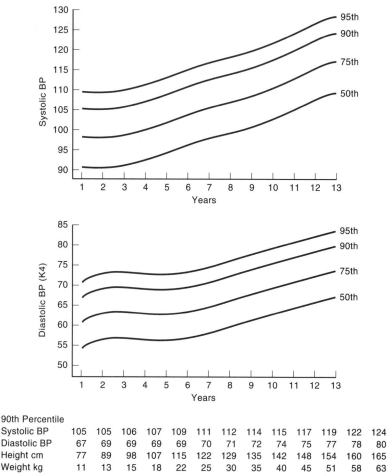

90th Percentile													
Systolic BP	105	105	106	107	109	111	112	114	115	117	119	122	124
Diastolic BP	67	69	69	69	69	70	71	72	74	75	77	78	80
Height cm	77	89	98	107	115	122	129	135	142	148	154	160	165
Weight kg	11	13	15	18	22	25	30	35	40	45	51	58	63

Fig. 18-4. Age-specific percentiles of blood pressure measurements in girls—1 to 13 years of age; Korotkoff phase IV (K4) used for diastolic blood pressure. (Adapted from Report on the Second Task Force on Blood Pressure Control in Children—1987. *Pediatrics* 1987;79:1–25 [Fig. 21-4].)

    d. Examination should include inspection of the auricle, periauricular tissues, and external auditory canal and visualization of the tympanic membrane. This includes assessment of the mobility of the tympanic membrane.

    e. Familiarity with the technique of pneumatic otoscopy is required to properly examine the ear and tympanic membrane. Otitis media is commonly seen in asymptomatic infants and children.

    f. Examination of the tympanic membrane may be stressful for children and parents, and patients may have to be restrained during pneumatic otoscopy.

       (1) Most patients can be examined sitting in the parent's lap (Figs. 18-7 and 18-8).

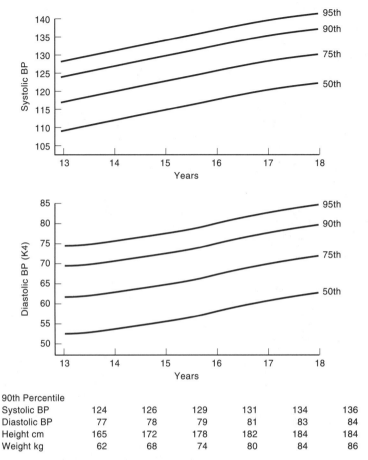

Fig. 18-5. Age-specific percentiles of blood pressure measurements in boys—13 to 18 years of age; Korotkoff phase IV (K4) used for diastolic blood pressure. (Adapted from Report on the Second Task Force on Blood Pressure Control in Children—1987. *Pediatrics* 1987;79:1–25 [Fig. 21-5].)

    (2) The pinna must be manipulated to straighten out the external canal (Fig. 18-9).

    (3) The otoscope speculum is advanced toward the anterosuperior quadrant of the tympanic membrane to see the bony landmarks, and membrane mobility is tested.

  g. Direct visualization of the nasal passage is usually avoided unless specific signs are present, such as unilateral nasal discharge and mouth breathing.

  h. The mouth and oral pharynx are examined last and should be omitted if the child is asymptomatic and if previous examinations have not shown anatomic anomalies.

2. Toddlers and young children

  a. Cerumen may occlude the auditory canal and may be removed by curettage or lavage. The procedure should be performed carefully

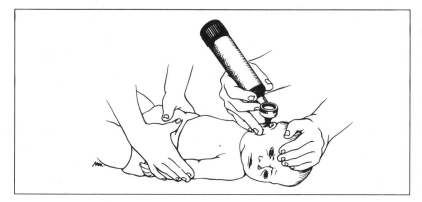

Fig. 18-6. Examination of the ear. Note that the examiner's hand, holding the otoscope, rests on the child's head so that any sudden movement will be transmitted to both the hand and the instrument, minimizing trauma to the external canal.

      and gently and attempted only after the child has been immobilized to prevent trauma.

    b. Tonsils and adenoids are often large and cryptic; enlarged tonsils do not necessarily indicate chronic infection.

F. Lymph nodes and glands
  1. Examination
    a. The distribution of lymph glands is similar to that in adults, but they are more prominent up to the time of puberty.
    b. The thyroid gland should be palpated in older children (>9 years) and the size defined by digital manipulation of each lobe.
  2. Findings
    a. Nodes are easily palpable as shotty, small, bean-sized nodules.
    b. Nodes usually undergo considerable hypertrophy in response to infections throughout childhood. Nodes are often <1 cm in diameter, but cervical enlargement to 2 cm may persist for several weeks after upper respiratory infection.

G. Chest and lungs
  1. Examination
    a. Examine the child as you would an adult.
    b. Because the chest wall is thin, evaluation of underlying structures is often easier than in the adult.
  2. Inspection
    a. The chest of the infant and young child has a relatively greater anteroposterior diameter than that of the adult.
    b. Small nodular breast hypertrophy is found in most newborns and may be associated with small amounts of milk-like secretions for a few days. Some breast hypertrophy may be found transiently in adolescent boys. Obese children may have apparent breast hypertrophy due to adipose tissue.
  3. Auscultation
    a. Breath sounds in young children are normally loud, harsh, and somewhat bronchial in character. Rhonchi transmitted from the trachea or large bronchi can confuse the listener. Their character, position, and differentiation may be facilitated by holding the stethoscope 1 or 2 inches from the infant's mouth or nose and comparing these sounds with those heard over the chest.

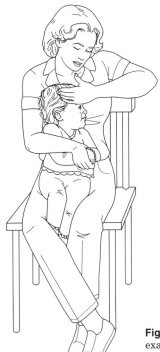

Fig. 18-7. Mother assisting in restraining a child for examination of the ear. (Adapted from Bluestone CD, Klein JO. *Otitis Media in Infants and Children,* 2nd ed. Philadelphia: WB Saunders; 1995 [Fig. 21-1B].)

    b. In the infant, even slight changes in position, such as turning the head, may influence the relative positions of the intrathoracic structures and therefore the intensity of breath sounds or the degree of resonance.

    c. Respiration is controlled by the diaphragm with little or no intercostal movement until the child is about 6 years of age.

  4. Percussion. Percussion note over the lung fields is more resonant in the child, and even approaches being tympanic in quality.

H. Cardiovascular system

  1. Examination

    a. Inspect and palpate the precordium to assess cardiac size.

    b. Focus auscultation on rate, rhythm, heart sounds, and murmurs.

    c. Palpate the brachial and femoral pulses to detect coarctation of the aorta. Other pulses are not routinely palpated.

  2. Findings

    a. The heart fills more of the thoracic cavity in children than in adults, and the apex is one or two intercostal spaces higher than that in the adult.

    b. Sinus arrhythmia is a physiologic finding and is prominent throughout infancy and childhood; in fact, its absence is suggestive of cardiac abnormality.

    c. Heart sounds are of a higher pitch and shorter duration with greater intensity than later in life. The pulmonary second sound is regularly louder than the aortic until adolescence.

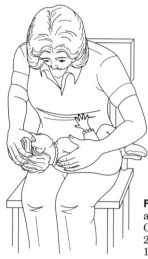

Fig. 18-8. Mother using lap position of infant for examination of the infant's ear. (Adapted from Bluestone CD, Klein JO. *Otitis Media in Infants and Children,* 2nd ed. Philadelphia: WB Saunders; 1995 [Fig. 21-1C].)

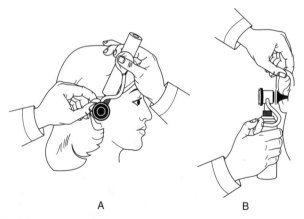

A   B

Fig. 18-9. Positioning of otoscope to enhance visualization and to minimize the chance that head movement will result in trauma to the ear canal. Both of the otoscopist's hands can be used **(A)**, or when the child is cooperative, a finger touching the child's neck is sufficient **(B)**. (Adapted from (Adapted from Bluestone CD, Klein JO. *Otitis Media in Infants and Children,* 2nd ed. Philadelphia: WB Saunders; 1995 [Fig. 21-2]).

  d. Functional murmurs are common during childhood. Between ages 6 to 9 ears, over 50% of children have obvious murmurs. As adolescence is approached, parasternal murmurs become less frequent and pulmonic murmurs more prevalent. These usually are grade 2 intensity or less, well localized, and blowing or vibratory in character. Change in position may change intensity or cause disappearance (Table 18-1).

e. A venous hum is a continuous purring sound common in childhood and is best heard above or below the clavicles. It is accentuated in the upright position and can be confused with the murmur of patent ductus arteriosus.

I. Abdomen

1. Examination

a. Examine as in adult.

b. Because of crying, repeated attempts may be needed.

c. Distraction with conversation or a toy may be helpful. To encourage relaxation, palpation is sometimes done with the child in a prone position; in the infant, examination during feeding can be helpful.

2. Findings

a. Infants and preschool children often have a protuberant abdomen that is accentuated by lumbar lordosis.

b. Umbilical hernias are common and usually resolve without treatment by age 5 years.

c. The liver edge is palpable by using light palpation. The spleen tip may be palpable during deep inspiration.

J. External genitalia and secondary sexual characteristics

1. Examination

a. Genitalia

(1) The penis and scrotum should be inspected and palpated.

(2) The external genitalia of girls are examined by spreading the labia, thumbs placed on the labia majora and moving the thumbs

Table 18-1. Description of Innocent Murmurs

Murmur	Position	Quality	Timing, Duration, and State
SYSTOLIC			1 ... 2 3
Still's	Apex LLSB	Musical, low pitch	
Basal	ULSB URSB	Blowing, high pitch	
Carotid	Neck	Blowing, high pitch	
PPPS	Axillae, ULSB, Back	Blowing, high pitch	
CONTINUOUS			
Mammary souffle	Lactating breasts	Hum Low pitch	Continuous
Venous hum	Infra-clavicular Bilateral or unilateral (R >L)	Low pitch sometimes snoring quality	Continuous

LLSB = lower left sternal border; ULSB = upper left sternal border; URSB = upper right sternal border; 1 and 2 = first and second heart sounds; R = right; L = left; PPPS = physiologic peripheral pulmonic stenosis.

From Rudolf, AM, and Hoffman, JIE. *Pediatrics*. 18th ed. Norwalk, CT: Appleton and Lange; 1987.

laterally and posteriorly to expose the clitoris, labia minora, and vaginal introitus.

(3) Examination should be avoided or limited when the child is embarrassed or frightened and previous examinations have been normal.

b. Sexual development

(1) Time of onset of puberty varies greatly.

(2) Sexual development should be described using the Tanner stage criteria.

2. Findings

a. The foreskin does not retract over the glans penis (phimosis) at birth.

b. The testicles may be present in the scrotum and normally retract into the inguinal canal during the examination.

c. Hymenal tags may protrude and are normally seen around the introitus.

d. Adhesions of the labia minora are common.

e. The size of male genitalia must be evaluated in relation to age, not body size. The penis and scrotum often appear disproportionately small in obese boys.

K. Rectum

1. Examination

a. The anus and perineum must be examined.

b. Digital examination must be done with adequate lubrication and slow, steady pressure with the finger until it passes the sphincter.

c. Use the little (fifth) finger in infants and young children or a nasal speculum in infants.

2. Findings

a. Although anal fissures are not normal, they are very common.

b. The tone of the anal sphincter is difficult to estimate and may seem "tight" as a normal response to digital examination.

L. Musculoskeletal system

1. Examination

a. Examine as in an adult.

b. Ambulation is not present in the early months of life; therefore, it is important to look carefully for lack of motion, weakness, or distortion of normal relationships.

c. Arms and legs are comparatively short early in life, and the span of outstretched arms is less than the standing height until about age 10 years in boys and 14 in girls.

d. The most important part of the examination in young infants is to examine the hips to exclude subluxation or dislocation of the femoral head (Ortolani and Barlow maneuvers (Fig. 18-10).

e. Examination of the spine for scoliosis is critical in older children.

2. Findings

a. Infants appear rotund due to abundant subcutaneous fat; toddlers age 2 to 3 years become more linear and lean.

b. Some degree of lordosis and "pot belly" is normal until mid-childhood.

c. Tibial bowing and adduction of the foot resulting from *in utero* positioning are common and normal if the foot can be passively straightened with ease.

d. Some infants have "in-toeing" during the first 2 years.

M. Nervous system

1. Examination

a. In addition to the usual examination, an evaluation of behavior and expected responses to stimuli is useful. For example, give a 9-month-old infant three blocks. Does he or she grasp firmly? Reach accurately? Transfer from hand to hand? Use fingers in grasping?

b. Proper examination requires knowledge of normal development.

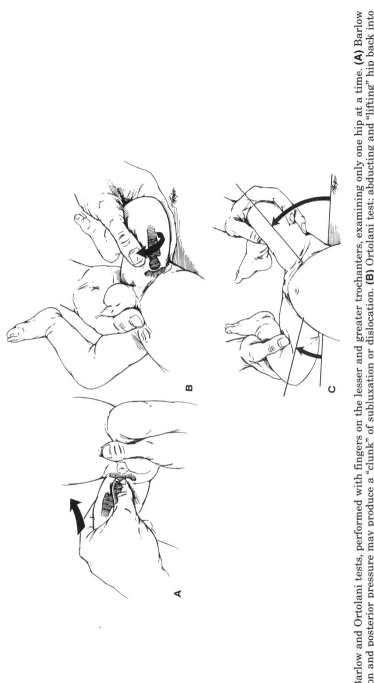

Fig. 18-10. Barlow and Ortolani tests, performed with fingers on the lesser and greater trochanters, examining only one hip at a time. **(A)** Barlow test: adduction and posterior pressure may produce a "clunk" of subluxation or dislocation. **(B)** Ortolani test: abducting and "lifting" hip back into place. **(C)** In children older than age 3 to 6 months, Barlow and Ortolani tests are often negative despite diminished laxity. The most important finding in this age group may be limitation of abduction. (From Oski FA, DeAngelis CD, Feigin RE, Warshaw JB. *Principles and Practice of Pediatrics*. Philadelphia: JB Lippincott, 1994:1019.)

2. Findings
   a. Reflex behavior is important in estimating neurologic integrity.
   b. Tonicity and activity are normally equal bilaterally, and decreased in premature newborns.
   c. The full-term infant lies in flexed position with hands fisted and resists being straightened.
   d. When supported with one hand under the abdomen in a horizontal position, the baby raises the head and legs toward the plane of the body (Landau reflex). Normally easily elicited, this reflex may be absent in a premature infant.
   e. A full-term infant firmly grasps an object placed in its palm and can be lifted up until most or all of its weight is supported (grasp reflex). The reflex is less strong in premature infants and may be absent in an infant of less than 36 weeks' gestation.
   f. Sucking (reflex) is vigorous by 38 weeks' gestation.
   g. When one cheek is stroked, the infant turns his or her head toward the side stroked, and the lips prepare for sucking (rooting reflex).
   h. A sudden change in position or a loud noise causes the infant to tense muscles, spread arms wide, and extend legs (Moro's reflex). This reflex normally disappears by 2 months of age; persistence beyond that indicates neurologic abnormality.
   i. Blinking, sneezing, gagging, and coughing can be elicited with appropriate stimuli in all but the smallest premature infants.
   j. When stimulated, plantar flexion of the great toe is present in most infants and may persist throughout much of the first year (Babinski's reflex). This reflex disappears when the child begins to walk.
   k. Deep tendon reflexes are present at birth.

IV. **Special Concerns: Examination of the Newborn and Adolescent**
   A. Examination of the newborn infant
      1. Determine the Apgar score at 1 minute and 5 minutes (Table 18-2). These scores are a general indication of the viability of the infant; scores of 6 or less indicate actual or potential problems.
      2. Perform a limited examination immediately, including a search for major defects.
      3. Perform a complete examination within the first several hours of life, including auscultation of heart and lungs, palpation of abdomen (best done while infant is quiet or asleep).
         a. Ensure airway patency, if necessary, by passing a soft catheter through the nose, pharynx, and esophagus into the stomach.
         b. Inspect and palpate the oral cavity.

Table 18-2. Apgar Score for the Newborn

Signs	Score		
	0	1	2
Heart rate	Absent	<100	>100
Respiratory effort	Absent	Weak	Good
Muscle tone	Limp	Some flexion	Well-flexed extremities
Response to stimulus to feet	None	Some motion	Motion and crying
Color	Pale or blue	Acrocyanosis	Completely pink

The score is computed at 1 and 5 minutes following delivery by assigning 0, 1, or 2 to each item. A total score of 10 indicates optimum. A total score of 0 indicates a moribund infant.
Source: From V Apgar, DA Holaday, LS James, IM Weisbrot, and C Berrien. Evaluation of the newborn infant: Second report. *JAMA* 168:1985, 1958. Copyright 1958, American Medical Association.

  c. Examine the umbilicus to determine the number of blood vessels; normally, two arteries and one vein are present.

  d. Examine the genitalia for anomalies.

  e. Evaluate the central nervous system by observing spontaneous alertness and activity, strength and character of cry, response to stimuli, vigor of sucking and feeding, and postural tone.

  f. Measure the length, weight, and head circumference and plot them on the growth chart.

4. Estimate the gestational age and correlate it with the birth weight. Not all infants weighing <2500 g are premature; some are full-term but malnourished from maternal disease or poor placental function (Fig. 18-11).

  a. Before 36 weeks' gestation, the following are seen:

   (1) One or two transverse creases on the sole of the foot

   (2) Breast nodule <3 mm in diameter

   (3) No cartilage in the ear lobe

   (4) Testes seldom descended into the scrotum, which has few or no rugae

   (5) Decreased muscle tone, flaccid posture, hands open

  b. By 40 weeks' gestation, the following are seen:

   (1) Many creases on the sole of the foot

   (2) Breast nodule >4 mm in diameter

   (3) Cartilage in the earlobe

   (4) Testes descended into the scrotum, which is covered with rugae

   (5) Increased muscle tone and posture of predominantly flexed extremities

5. Common skin findings

  a. Skin. In premature and newborn infants, the skin appears thin, almost transparent, red, and wrinkled.

  b. Vernix caseosa. The soft, moist, white, or clay-colored material is the covering on all newborn infants.

  c. Flaky desquamation. This occurs shortly after birth; the degree varies with individuals.

  d. Nevus vasculosus. Small, flat, red patches that blanch under pressure may be present over occiput, forehead, and upper eyelids.

  e. Milia. Very small, white-to-yellow, discrete, raised lesions are seen normally in groups, especially over the face. They are caused by plugging of the sebaceous glands.

  f. Miliaria. Red "prickly heat" rash is caused by heat in summer or in overdressed infants.

  g. Acrocyanosis. Blotchy blue appearance of the hands and feet is normal in early infancy but not a constant finding.

  h. Mongolian spots. Bluish, irregular-shaped, flat areas that vary greatly in size are sometimes present over sacral and buttock areas.

  i. Physiologic jaundice. This is present to a mild degree in many infants starting after the first day of life and usually disappearing by the 8th or 10th day.

B. Adolescent examination

  1. Explain the objectives of the examination in a gentle and sensitive manner, and provide an appropriate examination gown and the opportunity to disrobe in private.

  2. Ask the patient whether the parent should remain in the room during the examination.

  3. Develop rapport and define the limits, if any, of confidentiality and under what circumstances the findings during the interview and examination will be discussed with the parent.

  4. Teach the adolescent about his or her body.

  5. Answer questions promptly without an authoritarian or patronizing attitude.

Physical Maturity

	-1 / -2	0	1	2	3	4	5
Skin	Sticky, friable, transparent	Gelatinous, red, translucent	Smooth pink, visible veins	Superficial peeling and/or rash, few veins	Cracking, pale areas, rare veins	Parchment, deep cracking, no vessels	Leathery, cracked, wrinkled
Lanugo	None	Sparse	Abundant	Thinning	Bald areas	Mostly bald	
Plantar surface	Heal-toe 40–50 mm –1; <40 mm –2	>50 mm, no crease	Faint red marks	Anterior transverse crease only	Creases anterior 2/3	Creases over entire sole	
Breast	Imperceptible	Barely perceptible	Flat areola, no bud	Stippled areola 1–2 mm bud	Raised areola 3–4 mm bud	Full areola 5–10 mm bud	
Eye/ear	Lids fused: loosely–1 tightly–2	Lids open, pinna flat, stays folded	Slightly curved pinna; soft; slow recoil	Well-curved pinna; soft but ready recoil	Formed and firm instant recoil	Thick cartilage, ear stiff	
Genitals (male)	Scrotum flat, smooth	Scrotum empty, faint rugae	Testes in upper canal, rare rugae	Testes descending, few rugae	Testes down, good rugae	Testes pendulous, deep rugae	
Genitals (female)	Clitoris prominent, labia flat	Prominent clitoris, small labia minora	Prominent clitoris, enlarging minora	Majora and minora equally prominent	Majora large, minora small	Majora cover clitoris and minora	

Maturity rating

Score	Weeks
-10	20
-5	22
0	24
5	26
10	28
15	30
20	32
25	34
30	36
35	38
40	40
45	42
50	44

Fig. 18-11. Expanded NBS includes extremely premature infants and has been refined to improve accuracy in more mature infants. Adapted from Ballard JL et al. New Ballard score, expanded to include extremely premature infants. *J Pediatr.* 1991;119:417–423. (Fig 1).

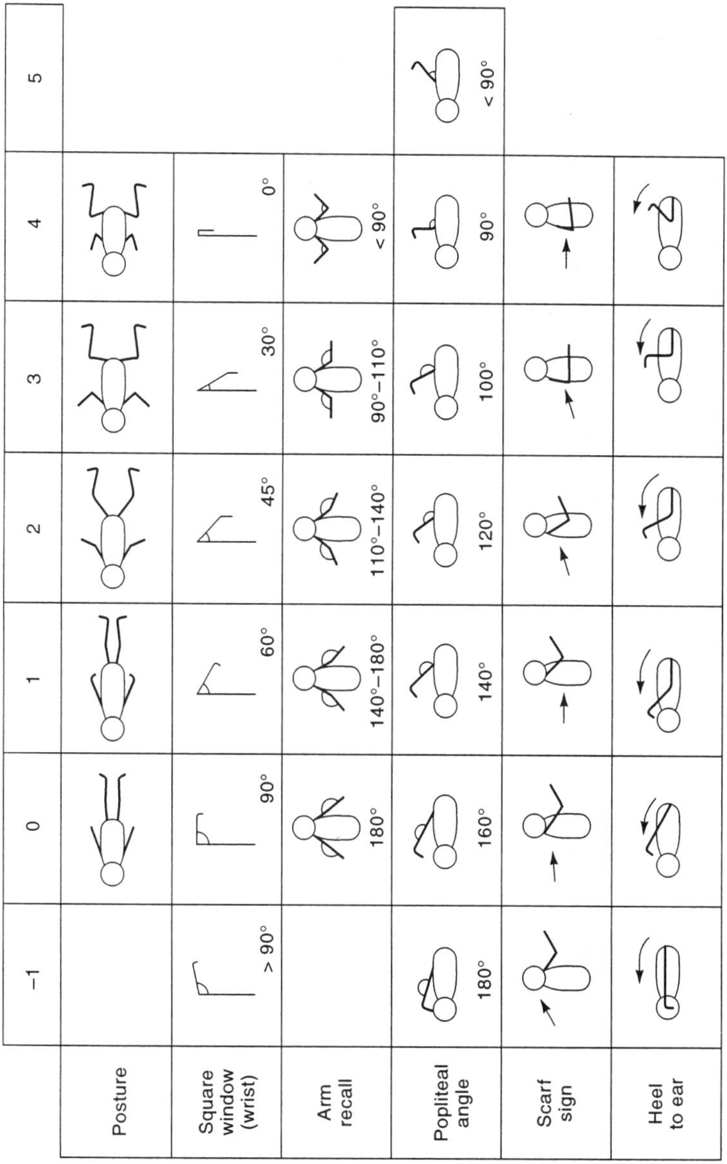

	−1	0	1	2	3	4	5
Posture							
Square window (wrist)	> 90°	90°	60°	45°	30°	0°	
Arm recall		180°	140°–180°	110°–140°	90°–110°	< 90°	
Popliteal angle	180°	160°	140°	120°	100°	90°	< 90°
Scarf sign							
Heel to ear							

Fig. 18-11. *Continued*

    6. Describe the stage of puberty using the Tanner scale.
    7. A pelvic examination should be performed if:
      a. The adolescent is sexually active.
      b. Contraception is to be initiated.
      c. There are signs or symptoms of genitourinary tract disease.
      d. There is primary amenorrhea at age 16 or older.

V. Cardinal Symptoms and Abnormal Findings

  A. Common signs and symptoms of illness

    1. Fever. A child's febrile response to a cause is much higher than an adult's. Chills, delirium, and convulsions often accompany high fever. Infections of the respiratory tract are the most common cause. Prolonged or recurrent fever with no apparent cause may result from neoplasms, leukemia, rheumatoid arthritis, hypersensitive reactions, occult osteomyelitis, and diseases of the central nervous system. Premature and newborn infants may have little or no fever even with severe infections; temperature instability, poor appetite, vomiting, and irritability may be the only symptoms of sepsis.

    2. Abdominal pain.

      a. This pain is often difficult to evaluate in children, because some degree of periumbilical pain is associated with many illnesses not directly involving the gastrointestinal tract. In young children, all abdominal pain tends to localize in the umbilical area. In infants, persistent screaming and crying, flexion of the thighs on the abdomen, grunting respiration, and vomiting are indications of abdominal pain. Associated symptoms of vomiting, diarrhea, or constipation may provide the clue to diagnosis.

      b. Colic, sometimes seen in the first months of life, is characterized by crying and irritability that is often relieved by feeding. The crying tends to recur at the same time of day, usually in the late afternoon and early evening.

      c. Possible causes of abdominal pain in children include appendicitis, intestinal obstruction due to intussusception or volvulus, pancreatitis, peptic ulcer, and urologic diseases (especially infection).

    3. Vomiting.

      a. Gastroesophageal reflux (regurgitation, spitting up) is often seen in early infancy and may persist for 9 to 12 months. Reflux does not usually result in poor growth, and if the child is failing to thrive, he or she must be evaluated to exclude a more serious underlying disorder.

      b. Esophageal atresia (vomiting shortly after birth; large amounts of mucus in the mouth) causing choking and cyanosis indicates aspiration.

      c. Bowel obstruction. In the newborn period, vomiting of bile-containing material always indicates obstruction until proved otherwise.

      d. Pyloric stenosis (nonbilious vomiting associated with visible peristaltic waves in the upper abdomen) becomes increasingly projectile with no nausea (refeeding is easily done).

      e. Central nervous system lesions. Vomiting associated with nausea may be detectable in the very young child only by facial expression or the preceding "stomach cough."

      f. Drugs. Overdose of many drugs, commonly salicylates, produces nausea and vomiting.

      g. Metabolic disturbances. Inborn errors of metabolism may result in hyperammonemia or acidosis, diabetes mellitus with acidosis, galactosemia, adrenogenital syndrome with salt loss, or renal tubular acidosis.

    4. Failure to gain height or weight or loss of weight (failure to thrive). Children normally show a progressive, although variable, weight gain through adolescence. Failure to thrive may be associated with:

a. Malnutrition.
b. Defects in digestion and absorption of food, as in cystic fibrosis and various malabsorption syndromes.
c. Chronic diseases such as infections, heart disease, kidney disease.
d. Hypothyroidism, hypopituitarism, achondroplasia, or hereditary dwarfism.
e. Abuse or emotional neglect. Observation of the mother's handling of the child may be helpful. Careful investigation of the kind and amount of food ingested is important, including analysis of formula preparation and recording a 72-hour diet diary.
f. Eating disorders (in the adolescent) such as anorexia nervosa or bulimia.

5. Stridor. This is a harsh, high-pitched crowing noise most distinct during inspiration. It originates high in the respiratory tract (usually the trachea or larynx) and is due to airway obstruction. Stridor may be combined with cough, dyspnea, hoarseness, retractions of the chest wall with respiration, and tachypnea. In infants, the small size of the airway is conducive to increased frequency and severity of obstruction. Slight stridor with crying is normal in some babies. Stridor may be caused by:
a. Congenital structural abnormalities such as flaccidity of the epiglottis, laryngeal web, cysts, and defects in the tracheal cartilaginous rings (most common cause in newborns).
b. Acute spasmodic laryngitis (croup) with sudden onset, often at night, little or no fever (common cause in the older child).
c. Laryngeal edema due to serum sickness, irritation from smoke or chemicals, or obstruction by a foreign body.
d. Retropharyngeal abscess, tracheitis, or epiglottitis.

6. Dyspnea. Shortness of breath and labored respiration may occur at any age. The differential diagnosis varies according to age. Causes include the following:
a. Premature infants. A periodic pattern of breathing with short periods of apnea is common and gradually disappears. Dyspnea associated with atelectasis or respiratory distress syndrome is seen in premature babies and those born to mothers with diabetes.
b. Newborns. Dyspnea may be associated with aspiration of amniotic fluid, congenital anomalies such as lung cysts and diaphragmatic hernia, and congenital heart disease with or without heart failure.
c. Children. Pulmonary infection and asthma are causes of dyspnea. Dyspnea must be distinguished from hyperventilation, seen in diabetic acidosis, fever, acetylsalicylic acid poisoning, and intracranial lesions.

7. Delayed development (mental retardation). Comparison of a child with other children of the same age and delay in normal achievements in motor development, language skills, adaptive behavior (reaction and manipulation of the environment), and person/social behavior can lead to suspicion of mental retardation. Physical stigmata such as microcephaly, hydrocephaly, and dysmorphic features suggesting chromosomal defects or congenital disorders are important clues.

8. Convulsions.
a. In the newborn, intracranial damage or congenital defects of the brain are nearly always combined with definite neurologic abnormalities.
b. Hypocalcemic tetany may occur in first two months of life and is often accompanied by carpopedal spasms and laryngeal stridor.
c. Generalized epileptic seizures represent over 50% of seizures in children. The seizures are characterized by abrupt onset with loss or alteration of consciousness and variable motor activity.
d. High fever (regardless of cause) is the most common cause of convulsions in children.

    e. Metabolic abnormalities may cause convulsions associated with severe electrolyte imbalances, hypoglycemia, acidosis, or hyperammonemia.

B. Systematic review of abnormal findings

  1. Pulse and respiratory rate

    a. Respiratory rate and depth of breathing may increase with respiratory or metabolic acidosis and are often the initial physical findings of these underlying abnormalities.

    b. Cardiac and pulmonary disease are also reflected by deviations from the normal pulse and respiratory rate.

  2. Skin and subcutaneous tissues

    a. Decreased tissue turgor (skin that remains creased and raised) is an indication of dehydration or undernutrition.

    b. Jaundice that appears during the first 24 hours of life usually indicates hemolytic disease due to maternal antibodies against the infant's red cells. Persistent jaundice that gradually becomes more intense over the first few weeks may indicate congenital anomalies of the biliary tree with obstruction or "neonatal hepatitis."

    c. Seborrheic dermatitis ("cradle cap") in the newborn is a greasy, yellowish scale over the scalp that sometimes involves other areas of the head, especially behind the ears.

    d. Tinea capitis (ringworm of the scalp) presents as edema, reddening, and crusting of an area of the scalp. The hair in involved areas is broken off close to the scalp.

  3. Head

    a. Asymmetry of the head may result from the following:

      (1) Premature closure of some of the sutures

      (2) Flattening of a portion of the cranium, often associated with diseases such as torticollis or mental retardation and due to the tendency to maintain a constant position

    b. Cephalhematoma (in the newborn)

      (1) A swelling resulting from bleeding beneath the periosteum of the cranium and limited to a single cranial bone

      (2) May organize into a clot with a small, firm, elevated margin, which may be palpated; calcification may occur later

      (3) May appear similar to the caput succedaneum but does not cross or overlie suture lines

    c. Increased intracranial pressure

      (1) Separation of sutures that have previously been approximated

      (2) Bulging and tenseness of the anterior fontanelle

    d. Microcephaly

      (1) Head circumference >2 SD below the mean

      (2) Associated with mental retardation with underlying brain defect

      (3) May indicate premature synosteosis

    e. Macrocephaly

      (1) Head circumference >2 SD above the mean

      (2) Associated with hydrocephalus, tumors, or anomalies of the central nervous system; should be evaluated with head ultrasonography, head computed tomography (CT), or magnetic resonance imaging (MRI) scan to visualize the posterior fossa

  4. Eyes

    a. Many neurologic diseases or congenital infections cause chorioretinitis, retinal pigmentary degeneration, or optic atrophy.

    b. Prominent epicanthal fold may be familial, but may also be characteristic of a genetic disorder.

  5. Ear, nose, and throat

    a. Hoarseness is often present with laryngitis, hypothyroidism, tetany, or gastroesophageal reflux.

    b. High-pitched, piercing cry in the infant may indicate increased intracranial pressure or mental retardation.

    c. A nasal quality of speech may be caused by pharyngeal paralysis due to poliomyelitis or diphtheria.

    d. Monotone verbalization may indicate hearing loss.

    e. Acute pharyngitis nearly always involves the tonsils.

    f. A retracted, bulging, or immobile tympanic membrane may indicate acute suppurative otitis media or otitis media with effusion. The eardrum must be carefully examined using the pneumatic otoscope (Fig. 18-12). Tympanometry may be used to diagnose or monitor middle ear disease. Children with suspected hearing loss should have audiometric testing.

6. Chest and lungs

    a. Asymmetry of the chest with bulging over the heart may be present in children with prolonged cardiac enlargement.

    b. Softening of the rib cage due to rickets may cause retraction of the lower ribs from the pull of the diaphragm resulting in Harrison's groove, or there may be enlargement of the costochondral junction, resulting in "beading."

    c. Decreased breath sounds accompanied by wheezing may be due to asthma or airway occlusion by a foreign body.

    d. Infants and children who present with wheezing or difficulty breathing should be evaluated with:

      (1) Pulse oximetry

      (2) Peak flow spirometry

7. Heart

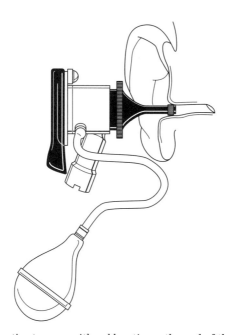

Fig. 18-12. Pneumatic otoscope with rubber tip on the end of the ear speculum to give a better seal in the external auditory canal. (Adapted from Bluestone CD, Klein JO. *Otitis Media in Infants and Children,* 2nd ed. Philadelphia: WB Saunders, 1995 [Fig. 21-4].)

    a. Changes in the second heart sound are similar in adults and children. Wide splitting of the second sound suggests right bundle branch block, pulmonic stenosis, or atrial septal defect.

    b. Murmurs are very common. Most are innocent and not associated with heart disease. There are six distinct types of innocent murmurs diagnosed by specific features (see Table 18-1).

    c. The quality, position, intensity, and radiation of murmurs due to organic heart disease are different. Suspected organic murmurs should be evaluated with an electrocardiogram (EKG) and echocardiography.

8. Abdomen

    a. Hernia and diastasis recti can best be observed when the child is crying.

    b. Umbilical hernia is common in children up to age 5 to 7 years.

    c. Peristaltic waves associated with bowel obstruction may be demonstrated in the infant during feeding. Hypertrophic pyloric stenosis and other tumors can be palpated during feeding.

    d. Enlarged liver or spleen may occur secondary to tumor, leukemia, infiltrative and storage diseases, or portal hypertension and must always be evaluated by abdominal ultrasonography. Doppler ultrasonography may be used to determine the direction of portal blood flow to identify portal hypertension or venous obstruction.

    e. Abdominal masses may be due to tumors (Wilms', neuroblastoma), abscess, or hydronephrosis and should be evaluated by obtaining plain radiographs of the abdomen or abdominal ultrasound.

    f. Tender abdominal masses, particularly in the right lower quadrant, may be due to inflammatory bowel disease and should be evaluated with single- or double-contrast radiography and ultrasonography.

9. Rectum

    a. Skin tags may be seen in children with constipation.

    b. Hemorrhoids are rare in children and should not be confused with perianal fistulas or with other perianal lesions accompanying Crohn's disease.

    c. Rectal masses or obstruction should be evaluated with radiography and ultrasonography or lower endoscopy.

    d. Fecal impaction may occur owing to organic or functional disorders.

    e. A void rectal ampulla in a constipated child strongly suggests Hirschsprung's disease and is an indication to perform a nonprepped barium enema or a suction mucosal biopsy.

10. Secondary sexual development

    a. Precocious appearance of sexual hair may be caused by adrenal lesions, brain lesions, or gonadal tumors.

    b. Enlargement of the penis or clitoris, often accompanied by appearance of pubic hair, is seen as a result of virilizing adrenal lesions or other causes of precocious development.

    c. Delayed appearance or absence of sexual hair may be found in pituitary, thyroid, or gonadal insufficiency and with certain chronic illnesses.

    d. Partial fusion of the labia minora is common in prepubertal girls.

    e. Because of the patency of the inguinal canal and the sensitive cremaster reflex, the testis may appear to be undescended. Several examinations are necessary to confirm that the testes have not descended into the scrotum.

11. Musculoskeletal system

    a. Abnormal positioning of the arm may result from injury of the brachial plexus.

    b. Congenital dislocation of the hip can be diagnosed by using the Barlow and Ortolani maneuvers (see Fig. 18-10).

    c. Tufts of hair over the spine or deep sacral dimpling may indicate an underlying spina bifida.

12. Nervous system

    a. In early infancy, the nervous system may be insufficiently developed to give reliable neurologic signs.

    b. The common signs of meningitis (Brudzinski's or Kernig's signs) may not be seen in children <2 years. Lethargy, anorexia, vomiting, and other less specific signs and symptoms may be the only findings of meningeal irritation.

    c. Increased intracranial pressure may occur as a result of increase in the volume of the brain, blood, or cerebrospinal fluid within the cranial cavity. Increased pressure is itself dangerous. Signs and symptoms of increased intracranial pressure vary with age and include the following:

        (1) Bulging anterior fontanelle

        (2) Separation of the bony plates of the skull

        (3) Visual disturbances, anisocoria, and abnormalities of lateral gaze

        (4) Papilledema

    d. Hypotonia in infants is a common sign of many disorders affecting the brain, spinal cord, and muscles, and it also occurs as a nonspecific sign of systemic illness including sepsis.

    e. Hypertonia indicates a central nervous system disorder.

VI. Abnormal Findings in the Newborn Infant

A. Umbilicus. A single artery may indicate an anomaly of the heart, central nervous system, or gut.

B. Sepsis may occur in premature infants or full-term infants and manifest with the following:

    1. Fever or temperature instability

    2. Poor feeding or vomiting or both

    3. Lethargy, irritability, sepsis, and coma

C. Respiratory system

    1. Premature infants may have brief periods of *apnea* lasting up to 20 seconds.

    2. *Respiratory distress* may be seen as increased rate, grunting, retraction of intercostal and subcostal spaces and suprasternal notch, see-saw sinking of chest with rising abdomen, and flaring of nostrils. It may be due to intrinsic lesions of the lungs; intracranial lesions including anomalies, hemorrhage, damage due to anoxia; congenital heart disease; and diaphragmatic hernia.

    3. *Airway obstruction* may be due to atresia of choanae, syphilis, and atresia of the esophagus (characterized by excessive mucus in the nose and mouth).

D. Liver. Hyperbilirubinemia and jaundice may be physiologic or associated with hemolysis, liver or biliary tract disease, or sepsis.

E. Pancreas. Hypoglycemia may occur in malnourished babies and those born to mothers with diabetes. Unusually large infants (>3800 g) are often born to mothers with diabetes.

F. Oral cavity

    1. Thrush (moniliasis): infection of the mucous membranes with slightly raised dull white patches

    2. Epstein's pearls: pearly white nodules limited to the palate

G. Genitourinary system

    1. Anomalies of the genitalia: hypospadias, hydrocele, hernia, ambiguous development indicating possible abnormal sexual development secondary to endocrine influences

    2. Failure to pass urine within 24 to 48 hours: requires investigation as to cause

H. Gastrointestinal system

1. Failure to pass meconium within 24 to 48 hours requires investigation as to cause including cystic fibrosis, Hirschsprung's disease, and bowel obstruction.
2. Abdominal distention is an emergency and must be evaluated with contrast radiographic studies of the upper or lower gastrointestinal tract.

  I. Nervous system
1. Seizures may be seen with hypoglycemia and hypocalcemia or a central nervous system disorder.
2. Hypotonia must be evaluated.

VII. Available Technology
The techniques and studies used in the diagnosis of pediatric conditions are generally the same as those used for adults.

VIII. Bibliography

Bluestone CD, Klein JO. *Otitis Media in Infants and Children,* 2nd ed. Philadelphia: WB Saunders; 1995.

Markel H, Oski JA, Oski FA, McMillan JA. *The Portable Pediatrician.* Philadelphia: Mosby-YearBook; 1992.

McAnarney ER, Kreipe RE, Orr DP, Comerci GD. *Textbook of Adolescent Medicine,* 2nd ed. Philadelphia: WB Saunders; 1992.

Oski FP. *Principles and Practice of Pediatrics,* 2nd ed. Philadelphia: JB Lippincott; 1993.

Zitelli BJ, Davis HW. *Atlas of Pediatric Physical Diagnosis,* 2nd ed. Singapore: Mosby-Wolfe; 1994.

IX. Key Search Words
The following key words reflect the content of this chapter. They are provided to assist with an on-line search of computer databases, such as MEDLINE, if you wish to pursue the topic of this chapter further.

Adolescence
Apgar score
Cephalometry
Child
Child development
Child, preschool
Infant
Infant, newborn
Physical diagnosis, pediatrics
Physical examination, in adolescence
Physical examination, in infancy and childhood
Puberty

Appendix A. ADAM GOLDSTEIN'S SPEECH

I'd like to introduce myself. I'm Adam Goldstein, and I'm one of the 200-plus University of Michigan Medical School students in the graduating class of 1995.

I would first like to congratulate my classmates for successfully completing probably the most difficult 4-year stretch of your lives. Everyone of us had a slightly different reason for embarking on this long journey, all for the privilege of adding a very important two-letter title to the end of our names: "M.D."

With this new privilege come many new responsibilities. Yesterday—as Mr., Mrs., or Ms.—we had many obligations. First and foremost of these over the past 4 years was being a student, learning all that we could in preparation for our new roles as physicians. Today, as doctors, we accept new responsibilities and obligations, most of which were covered in medical school. But some of these, as I have recently experienced, were not formally introduced in the modern medical school curriculum.

Thinking back, it seems as if it was only yesterday that we uncovered our cadavers in gross anatomy class for the first time. It was not that long ago that we donned those brand-new short white coats, stuffing each pocket as full as possible with pens, note cards, handbooks, and drug-rep paraphernalia. We all experienced many ups and downs and unexpected curves on our paths through medical school. Each of us had a unique experience, a different story to tell—each story culminating here at graduation. My road to graduation was not quite the same as everyone else's here. My road took an unexpected turn in November of our M-4 year.

Many of you know, but some may not know, that I spent the month of November of our M-4 year in the University of Michigan Hospital, not as a medical student but as a patient. I alternated between the Wilson cardiology service, the cardiac intensive care unit, then finally on the hematology/oncology service. I was first diagnosed with what was thought to be a rare cardiac angiosarcoma, which carried a grave prognosis. Three weeks into my hospital stay, upon further testing, on Thanksgiving Day, my diagnosis was changed to a much more favorable diagnosis of non-Hodgkin's lymphoma. I immediately started chemotherapy and was soon discharged. My diagnosis changed once again this past May, to Ewing's sarcoma. My road to recovery is on its way.

I wanted to speak to all of you, not to tell you this story, but to talk to you briefly about some lessons that I learned during my rare experience as a patient during medical school. I wanted to pass on a few of these lessons with some simple yet effective advice, which I hope you will remember throughout your careers as physicians. Some of these lessons were brought to my attention because care was overlooked and therefore bothersome. Other lessons became evident because of the support they provided my family and me and, therefore, comfort. The advice may seem like common sense—much of it is. Some of the concepts are very specific, and others are more general. Many doctors just don't take the time. These lessons and this advice will prove beneficial for both you and your patients.

This speech and these tips were selected from the final chapter of the book that I am currently writing about my experience as a medical student and patient. I named the book, as well as this speech, *Hidden Lessons*. The book has a dual dedication. First, it is dedicated to my wife, Michele, who has provided more support than thought humanly possible. The second dedication is to the University of Michigan Medical School Graduating Class of 1995.

Lesson 1: Pain is real.

Believe your patients when they say they are experiencing pain. You need not instantly prescribe the latest pain medication, but *believe* your patients, show some concern and compassion. I experienced excruciating pain on a few occasions as an inpatient. What I found most comforting was a hand to squeeze and a calm, supporting, consoling voice as I squinted and clenched my teeth in agony. There is nothing worse than being in great pain while those around you whisper to each other—or worse—are silent. I vividly remember my intern telling me to hang in there as I squeezed one of our fellow classmates' hands. They were by far the most comforting figures in my most agonizing moments.

My advice here is not to ignore the situation. Don't be afraid to be the one who lends the hand to squeeze or to be the one with the comforting voice. Let your patient know that he or she is not alone.

Lesson 2: See each patient every day.

Although it is mandatory as an intern or resident to see your patient daily, we will all be attending physicians some day. Whether you are the primary attending or the consulting physician, make it a point to see each patient every day. It's easy to say you are too busy or that you have no new information—therefore why take the time? But that's no excuse. If your patients are sick enough to be in the hospital, you owe them, each of them, the courtesy and human decency of a visit each day. Even if it is just for 1 minute, even if it is just to say, "Hi, there's nothing new, but I was thinking about you. Do you have any questions?" It is simple, and it takes 10 seconds. You would be surprised at the amount of good this visit will do for each of your patients and for your relationships with your patients. There's nothing worse than going 1 or 2 weeks without seeing one of your doctors while you are an inpatient. I know from first-hand experience.

During this short daily visit, take an extra 5 seconds to pull up a chair and sit down—your doctor-patient relationship will be that much stronger. You owe it to every patient.

Lesson 3: Friends, family, and significant others are an important part of the healing process.

Including family and friends in the patient's care is another way that you can assure your patient that he or she is not alone. In medical school we are taught to focus 100% on the patient and his or her ailment. The patient is only one member of the team. Illnesses affect wives, husbands, children, parents, grandchildren, and friends as well. Not only will including others cut down on the amount of confusion among family members, but make everyone feel involved and share some of the responsibilities. The patient's support system wants to help.

My advice is to include family, friends, and others in discussions that include such topics as diagnosis, treatment, and prognosis. Make alternatives clear to everyone. Make every effort to include those close to your patients in the decision-making process. Often your patient is in no position—either mentally or physically—to make important decisions on his or her own. Also, include these persons in certain appropriate parts of your patient's care while in the hospital and after discharge.

Lesson 4: Know what you know, and know what you don't know.

This lesson actually came from the first day of my clinical rotations during my M-3 year, but I was able to experience it during my November hospital stay. Patients appreciate and expect honesty—complete honesty—when it comes to their health care. Today's degree of physician specialization and subspecialization does not allow physicians to be experts in everything. Don't be afraid to say, "I don't know." Don't be afraid to consult with colleagues or refer your patient to the proper specialist, if need be. Medical students go through their educational process, starting at an early age, attempting and expecting to learn and understand everything. It is unnatural and awkward to admit ignorance. I developed more respect for my cardiologist when he admitted he did not completely understand some aspect of my cancer and I respected my oncologist more when he deferred my cardiology-related questions.

Do not be afraid to say, "I don't know." Your patients will respect your honesty.

Lesson 5: Patients express similar illnesses in different ways.

I am not talking about the presentation of the illness that leads one to a diagnosis, although patients do present in unique ways. I am referring to the way patients physically and mentally act and react to their illness and diagnosis. For example, do not pigeon-hole all cancer patients into the category of frail, weak individuals with poor prognoses. Some cancer patients may fit this description; others don't. Some suffer great pain, others suffer multiple treatment side effects, many need emotional support, some need physical assistance. Most patients would like to talk about their problems, whereas others would rather keep silent. The point is that there are as many different presentations of similar illness as there are patients who suffer these illnesses.

My advice is to treat each patient according to his or her needs—not the diagnosis. Make every effort to treat each patient as an individual. You may have 10 patients with the same diagnosis, but you also have 10 patients who require 10 treatments. Paul Pearcell, a famous Detroit-area neuropsychologist, once stated, "it matters less what type of disease the patient has than what type of patient has the disease."

Lesson 6: Investigate each symptom no matter how minor it seems to you or your patient.

This skill goes all the way back to the basics of history-taking. You would be surprised at the subtleties of medicine. Crushing chest pain may indicate a heart attack in one person, whereas mild shortness of breath can indicate the same disease process in another—yet be ignored because of its subtlety. After 2 or 3 weeks in the hospital, I realized a subtle symptom in myself: numbness along an area of skin on my abdomen. I didn't think much of it at the time. Turns out this simple finding, once expressed and taken seriously by my doctors, revealed a new mass, ultimately removing me from the heart transplant list. One wise internist once told me, "Remember, your patients are telling you what is wrong with them; they are the ones with the illness and symptoms; they have all the answers."

Open your ears and mind, not just your mouth, when talking with your patients. They possess all the needed information.

Here are just a few suggestions to improve your relationship and the care of your patients.

1. Pain is real.
2. See each patient every day.
3. Include family and friends.
4. Don't be afraid to say,"I don't know."
5. Treat patients according to their needs, not their diagnosis.
6. Open your ears and mind; you may learn something.

If I must pick a common theme that incorporated these lessons and advice, it would be to treat each patient as an individual, while making them feel as if they are not battling their problems alone. You may have heard these lessons and this advice before, but for the most part they are not taught in medical school. Unfortunately, I learned them as a patient. Now, I will never forget these lessons, as well as many other lessons. I hope you believe me when I say they are simple and straightforward in concept, but take a caring doctor to fulfill. Each of your patients deserves the attention. I know mine will appreciate it.

Good luck to all of you as you embark on your new medical journeys.

Appendix B. COST OF TECHNOLOGY

Technology	Code
SKIN	
Skin biopsy	
Shave biopsy	$$
Punch biopsy	$$
Excisional biopsy	$$
Potassium hydroxide (KOH) examination	$
Microbial culture	$$
Patch test	$$
ENDOCRINE	
Hormone analysis; immunoassays	$$$$
Dynamic testing	
Stimulation testing	$$$$
Suppression testing	$$$$
Imaging studies	
Magnetic resonance imaging (MRI)	$$$$
Thyroid visualization	$$
Ultrasonography	$$
Chest x-ray	$
Computed tomography (CT)—chest	$$$
Pancreatic islet cell anatomy	*
CT—abdomen	$$$
Endoscopic ultrasound	$$$
CT—adrenal	$$$
Radioisotope studies	
Thyroid	$$$$$
Parathyroid	$$$$$
Adrenal scanning	$$$$$$
HEMATOPOIETIC	
Complete blood count (CBC)	$
Examination of bone marrow	$$$
Lymph node biopsy	$$
Positive-pressure test for capillary fragility (Rumpel-Leede phenomenon)	*
Chest x-rays, including lateral views	$
Lymphangiography	$$$$
Nuclear studies	
Gallium scan	$$$$
Liver-spleen scan	$$$$
Positron emission tomography (PET)	$$$$$$
Bone scan	$$$$
Imaging studies	
CT	$$$
Skeletal survey	$
Lymphangiography	$$$$
MRI	$$$$
EYE	
Fluorescein staining	*

Technology	Code
Visual fields	$$
Refraction	$
Biomicroscope (slit-lamp)	*
Exophthalmometer	*
Ophthalmodynamometer	*
Doppler and magnetic resonance angiography	$$$$$
Fluorescein angiography	$$$$$
CT	$$$
MRI	$$$$
Ultrasonography	$$

EAR, NOSE, AND THROAT

Technology	Code
Weber test	$
Rinne test	$
Audiogram	$$
Auditory brainstem response audiometry (ABR)	$$
Caloric test	$$
Sinus x-rays	$
CT	$$$
MRI—head	$$$$

RESPIRATORY

Technology	Code
Chest x-ray	$
CT	$$$
Arterial blood gases	$$
Pulmonary function studies	$$$
Cardiopulmonary exercise testing	$$$
Sputum examination	$
Flexible bronchoscopy	$$$$
Radioisotope ventilation and perfusion lung scans	$$$$
Pulmonary arteriography	$$$$$
Percutaneous needle lung biopsy	$

CARDIOVASCULAR

Technology	Code
Electrocardiogram (ECG)	$
Chest x-ray	$
2-D-Echocardiogram with Doppler	$$
Transesophageal echocardiogram	$$$
Standard stress test	$$
Stress test with imaging	
Thallium preferred	$$$$$
Echo preferred	$$$
Pharmacologic stress testing	
Adenosine especially useful	$$$$
Dobutamine especially useful	$$$$
24 hr ambulatory ECG (Holter)	$$
Event recorder	$$
CT—chest	$$$
MRI—chest	$$$

Technology	Code
Left heart catheterization and coronary angiogram	$$$$$
Right heart catheterization (Swan-Ganz)	$$$$
Electrophysiologic testing	$$$$$
Cardiac biopsy	$$$$
GASTROINTESTINAL	
Esophagogastroduodenoscopy (EGD)	$$$
Anoscopy	$
Sigmoidoscopy	$$
Colonoscopy	$$$$
Endoscopic retrograde cholangiopancreatography (ERCP)	$$$$
Ultrasonography	
Real-time	$$
Doppler	$$$
Endoscopic	$$$$
Imaging studies	
Abdominal x-rays; supine view (flat plate), upright view	$$
Upper GI with small-bowel follow-through	$$$
Barium enema	$$$
CT—abdomen	$$$
MRI—liver	$$$$
Angiography	$$$$$
Nuclear studies	
Liver-spleen scan	*
HIDA scan	$$$$
Tagged RBC bleeding scan	$$$$$
Gastric emptying studies	$$$$
Esophageal pH monitoring	$$
Esophageal manometry	$$$
Liver chemistries: serum transaminases, aspartate transaminase (AST) and alanine transaminase (ALT), serum bilirubin, and alkaline phosphatase, prothrombin time (PT)	$$
Liver biopsy	$$
ACUTE ABDOMEN	
Routine tests and studies	
Complete blood count (CBC)	$
Urinalysis	$
Pregnancy test	$
Liver panel, amylase, lipase, protime	$$
Admitting panel	$$
Blood type and crossmatch	$$
Abdominal x-rays: supine view (flat plate), upright view	$$
Other diagnostic procedures	
Hematologic studies	$$
Biochemical studies	$$
Serologic analyses	$$
Imaging studies (for selected cases)	
Abdominal and pelvic ultrasonography	$$
CT	$$$
Intravenous urogram (IVU)	$$$
Angiography	$$$
Peritoneal lavage	$$$
Culdocentesis	$$$$

Technology	Code
Laparoscopic evaluation	$$$$
Endoscopy	$$$
GENITOURINARY	
Urinalysis, not by dipstick	$
Ultrasonography	$$
Plain x-ray of the abdomen	$$
Intravenous urogram	$$$
Cystogram	$$$
Cystoscopy	$$
Retrograde urography	$$$
CT	$$$
MRI	$$$$
Radionuclide studies	$$$$$
Renal arteriography	$$$$$
HERNIA	
Ultrasonography	$$
CT	$$$$
Herniography	*
FEMALE REPRODUCTION	
Ultrasonography	$$
Doppler uterine artery blood flow	$$
Tumor blood flow patterns	$$
Nuclear magnetic resonance studies of tumors	$$$$$
BREAST	
Mammography	$$
Ultrasonography	$$
MRI	$$$$
Positron emission tomography (PET)	$$$$$$
NERVOUS SYSTEM	
CT	$$$
MRI	$$$$
Magnetic resonance angiography (MRA)	$$$$$
Carotid duplex studies	$$
Transcranial Doppler	$$
Transesophageal echocardiography	$$$
Angiography	$$$$$
Neuropsychometrics (IQ/memory testing)	$$
Genetic testing	*
Lumbar puncture	$$$
Myelography	$$$$
Electroencephalography	$$$
Electromyography	$$$$
Evoked potential electrophysiologic studies	$$$
Polysomnography/multiple sleep latency tests	$$$$
Intracarotid amobarbital procedure	$$$$$
Corticography	$$$$$$

Technology	Code
Single photon emission tomography/positron emission tomography	$$$$$
Functional MRI	*
Autonomic function testing	$$$
Cisternography	$$$$$
MUSCULOSKELETAL	
X-ray (plain films)	$$
Arthrocentesis	$$
Doppler arterial wave analysis	$$
Bone scan	$$$$
Ultrasonography	$$
MRI	$$$$
CT	$$$
Electromyography	$$
Arthrography	$$$
Myelography	$$$
Arthroscopy	$$$$
Synovial biopsy	$$$$
Compartment pressures	*
Intraosseous pressures	*
Arthroplasty	*
ACUTE INJURY	
Chest x-ray	$
Abdominal x-ray	$
Abdominal ultrasonography	$$
Diagnostic peritoneal lavage	$$$$
CT—head	$$$
CT—abdomen	$$$
MRI	$$$$
Intravenous pyelogram	$$$
Angiography	$$$$$
Cystogram	$$$
Retrograde urethrogram	$$$
Intracompartmental pressure measurement	*

$ = $0–$50; $$ = $50–$100; $$$ = $100–$200; $$$$ = $200–$500; $$$$$ = $500–$1000; $$$$$$ = >$1000; * = highly variable or not available.

Appendix C. POCKET PRIMER

PLAN

Write down when (date/time) the history was taken.
Note the source of the information and an assessment of the reliability of the source.
Your defined database will have four parts:

- Patient profile
- History
- Physical examination
- Laboratory examination

Take shorthand notes. Study and rearrange data later, then compose written record.
Avoid composing history as you go, using medical or complicated terms, asking too many direct or leading questions.

PATIENT PROFILE

Chat for a moment—take this opportunity to start your patient profile:

Name	Age
Occupation	Marital status/ children
Past health, general	Religious/educational factors (optional)

How is the patient feeling at the moment? OK? Then start.

HISTORY

Chief Complaint
"What is troubling you?" or "Tell me about your problem," or use your own words.
Avoid medical terminology; use the patient's own wording to record. Include age, race, sex, and give description and duration of the chief complaint.

Present Illness

Date of onset	Associated complaints
Any and all precipitating factors	All pertinent negatives in system(s)
Severity and character of major symptoms	Known laboratory and treatment
Chronologic sequence and progression	information and sources of these data

Past Medical History
Major childhood illnesses: e.g., measles, mumps, chickenpox, rheumatic fever, frequent throat infections, earaches.

Major adult illnesses: e.g., diabetes, high blood pressure, infections (scarlet fever, pneumonia, veneral, tuberculosis), arthritis, jaundice, kidney or heart trouble, cancer, stroke, ulcer, phlebitis, anemia.

Immunizations: DPT, mumps, rubella, polio, tetanus antitoxin, influenza.

Operations: Date and where performed.

Accidents: Any residual defects or limitations?

Allergies: Drug, food, contact, asthma.

Personal and Social History
Life history: Birthplace, socioeconomic status, education, jobs.

Marital: Spouse's occupation.

Occupational: Present work, hazards, stresses.

Financial: How will this illness affect the patient and family?

Personal: Self-appraisal (e.g., worrier, easygoing)

Habits: Diet, sleep, exercise, tobacco, alcohol, coffee, special drugs (laxatives, sedatives, psychotropics).

Religion: Particularly any health-related tenets.

Travel: Particularly outside the continental United States.

Family History
Status: Of all members.

Pedigree: Diagram, if indicated.

Special diseases: Diabetes, tuberculosis, cancer, stroke, hypertension, renal diseases, deafness, gout/arthritis, heart trouble, mental problems, allergies, anemia, known inherited diseases.

Systems Review
General: Weakness, fatigue, change in weight, appetite, sleeping habits, chills, fever, night sweats.

Skin: Color changes, pruritus, nevus, infections, tumor (benign/malignant), dermatoses, hair changes, nail changes, bruising.

Eyes: Acuity, glasses/contact lenses, blurring, pain, discharge, diplopia.

Ears: Tinnitus, deafness, discharge, pain.

Nose, throat, sinuses: Epistaxis, discharge, sinusitis, hoarseness, sore tongue.

Breasts: Masses, discharge, pain. Self-exam?

Respiratory: Cough (productive/nonproductive), change in cough, amount and character of sputum, chest pain, dyspnea, pack-years of tobacco usage, wheezing, hemoptysis, recurrent respiratory tract infections. Tuberculin test: positive? Last chest x-ray: normal?

Cardiovascular: Chest pain, typical angina pectoris, dyspnea on exertion, orthopnea, paroxysmal nocturnal dyspnea, peripheral edema, palpitations, varicosities, thrombophlebitis, claudication, Raynaud's phenomenon, syncope, near-syncope; past history of murmur or heart attack.

Gastrointestinal: Appetite, nausea, vomiting, diarrhea, constipation, melena, hematemesis, rectal bleeding, change in bowel habits, hemorrhoids, dysphagia, food intolerances, excessive gas or indigestion, abdominal pain, jaundice, use of antacids or laxatives.

Hematopoietic: Anemia, abnormal bleeding, adenopathy, excessive bruising.

Urinary tract: Dysuria, hematuria, frequency and volume, polyuria, urgency, hesitancy, incontinence, renal stones, nocturia, infections.

Male reproductive: Penile discharge, lesion, history of venereal disease, testicular pain, testicular mass, infertility, impotence, libido, hernia.

Female reproductive: Gynecologic history (age of menarche, last menstrual period, age at menopause, postmenopausal bleeding, abnormal menses, amount of bleeding, intermenstrual bleeding, postcoital bleeding), vaginal discharge, pruritus, history of venereal disease, last Pap smear, obstetric history (full-term deliveries, pregnancies, abortions, living children, complications of pregnancies), infertility, libido, methods of contraception.

Musculoskeletal: Joints (pain, edema, heat, redness, stiffness, deformity), muscles (pain, tenderness, weakness, atrophy).

Endocrine: Goiter, heat intolerance, cold intolerance, change in voice, polyuria, polydipsia, polyphagia, change in hair distribution, known thyroid disease.

Neurologic: Headache, syncope, seizures, vertigo, ataxia, amaurosis, diplopia, scotoma, paralysis/paresis, muscle weakness, tremor, dysesthesia.

Mental status: Attention and orientation, language, memory, affect; nervousness, depression, insomnia, nightmares.

PHYSICAL EXAMINATION
Prepare patient and environment. Remove distractions. Wash. Don't rush. Don't cause discomfort (unless absolutely necessary).

Proceed
Vital signs: Pulse, blood pressure (position), respirations, temperature (oral/rectal), height, weight.

General appearance: Nutrition, habitus, apparent age, obvious mental disease; striking findings such as pallor, constant coughing, respiratory distress, voice abnormality, or cyanosis.

Skin: Color, texture, moisture, temperature. Amount, texture, and distribution of hair. Surgical or traumatic scars. Describe any lesions, eruptions, abnormal pigmentations, skin tumors, nail changes, purpura.

Lymph nodes: (Examine by region.) Enlargement, consistency, mobility, tenderness. Record approximate size of nodes in centimeters, if enlarged.

Head: Size, shape, contour, symmetry, tenderness over sinuses or mastoids. Any bruits?

Eyes: Conjunctivae, sclerae, pupillary size and reaction; protrusion, ptosis, arcus senilis; gross visual acuity; extraocular movements; gross visual fields; ophthalmoscopic examination (disks, vessels, hemorrhages, exudates, microaneurysms).

Ears: Tophi, discharge, hearing acuity, description of drums.

Nose: Septal deviation, airway obstruction, discharge, condition of mucosa, enlargement of turbinates, polyps. When sinus disease is suspected, record results of transillumination of sinuses.

Mouth and throat: Odor of breath; color and appearance of lips, tongue, gums; condition of teeth; dentures; appearance of mucosa, palate, uvula, tonsils, and posterior pharynx. When indicated, record findings of examination of nasopharynx and larynx.

Neck: Rigidity or limitation of motion, abnormal pulsations, scars, masses, enlarged salivary glands or lymph nodes. Describe the thyroid gland and the position of trachea. Note carotid and jugular pulses.

Back: Mobility, kyphosis, scoliosis, lordosis; tenderness on palpation or percussion; sacral edema, costovertebral angle tenderness.

Thorax: Configuration, symmetry, respiratory movements. Estimate tactile fremitus. Percuss the chest, front and back. Percuss excursion of diaphragm. Characterize breath sounds, voice sounds; note rales, ronchi, wheezes, rubs, if present.

Breasts: Size, consistency, symmetry, tenderness, palpable masses, discharge from nipples, gynecomastia.

Heart: Inspect precordium; define heart size by percussion. Palpate entire precordium systematically for impulses, shocks, thrills and rubs, noting their location and timing. Localize apical impulse; determine selective ventricular enlargement. Auscultate systematically, especially at valve areas, characterizing rate, rhythm, quality of sounds, extra sounds, murmurs, and rubs, in that order.

Abdomen: Appearance, distention, retraction, symmetry, local prominences. Describe any intrinsic movements. Note dilated vessels, scars, pulsations, hair distribution. Palpate, noting tenderness, rigidity, hyperesthesia, guarding, masses, fluid. Palpate kidneys. Note size of liver and spleen. Use percussion and auscultation when indicated. Inguinal nodes, femoral pulses, bruits.

Extremities and orthopedic: Swelling, tenderness, redness, heat, deformity, and limitation of motion of joints; edema (if present, grade 1+ through 4+); color and temperature of skin of legs, calf tenderness, muscle weakness, tenderness, atrophy, swelling, trophic changes or ulcerations.

Neurologic: Cerebral (alert, lethargic, stuporous, comatose), mental, cranial nerves, sensory (pain, temperature, light, touch, vibratory, two-point, stereognosis), associative functions (speech, writing, reading, apraxia, agnosia), motor (true mass, strength, fasciculation, tremor), reflexes (diagram Bi, Tri, Br, K, A, Abd, Babinski's, Hoffman's, cremasteric; grade 0 through 4+). Gait, Romberg's, cerebellar.

Male genitalia: Penis, scrotum, testes, epididymis, masses, transilluminate scrotal enlargements. Check for hernia.

Female genitalia: External (labia, clitoris, introitus, urethra, perineum), internal (vagina, cervix, adnexa, *cul-de-sac,* discharge), Pap smears, rectal, rectovaginal. Check for hernia.

Rectum: Sphincter tone, hemorrhoids, masses. In male, describe size, consistency of prostate, and any nodules.

SUMMARY STATEMENT
LABORATORY VALUES AND TESTS
SYNTHESIS
Preliminary impressions:
Problem list:
Diagnostic plan:
Therapeutic plan:

Index

Index

Page numbers followed by *f* indicate illustrations; *t* following a page number indicates tabular material; *g* following a page number indicates a glossary entry.

acute injury to, 330
common clinical disorders of, 216–217
examination of, 211–212, 212*f*
pain originating in, 215–216
Knee, 309, 313–314
KOH (potassium hydroxide) examination,
22–23
Krönig's isthmus, 106*f*
Kyphosis, 92*g*, 99, 100*f*, 293*g*

Labia, 241*f*
lesions of, 242*f*–243*f*
Laboratory data, write-up of, 6
Lacerations, pulmonary, 326–327
Lachman's test, 295–296
Lacrimal apparatus, 56, 57*f*, 67
Lactation, mastitis associated with, 267
Landau reflex, 348
Laryngitis, 86–87
Laryngopharynx, 73*g*. *See also* Upper
respiratory and auditory system
cardinal symptoms and abnormal find-
ings in, 86–87
in child, 354–355
examination of, 80–81, 82*f*
Laryngoscopy, indirect, 80–81, 82*f*
Larynx. *See also* Laryngopharynx; Upper
respiratory and auditory system
sounds transmitted from, 115
Lasègue's sign, 296, 312
LCIS (lobular carcinoma in situ),
253*g*–254*g*
Left atrial pressure, 128, 130*f*
Left heart catheterization, 173, 174
Left ventricle, surface landmarks for, 125
Left ventricular dilatation, 157, 158*f*
Left ventricular hypertrophy, 157, 158*f*
Left ventricular pressure, 128, 130*f*
Lens, 57, 67
in elderly person, 69
Lentiginous melanoma, acral, 20
Lentigo, 7*g*
Lentigo maligna melanoma, 20
Leopold's maneuvers, 248–250, 249*f*
Leriche's syndrome, 153*t*
Leukemia, 41*g*, 44–45, 46
Leukocytosis, 41*g*
Leukopenia, 41*g*
Leukoplakia, cervical, 246*f*
Level of consciousness, 320, 322, 322*t*
Lhermitte's sign, 296
Lichen planus, 15
Lifestyle risk factors, 2*t*, 4
Light-headedness, in endocrine disorders,
32
Lingual tonsils. *See* Tonsils; Upper respi-
ratory and auditory system
Lips, 78–79, 84–85
Littre's hernia, 224*g*

Liver. *See also* Gastrointestinal system
abnormal findings, in newborn, 357
acute injury to, 328
common clinical disorders, 192–193
palpation of, 181–182, 181*f*, 189
in child, 345
Liver biopsy, 196, 197
Liver chemistry tests, 196, 197
Liver-spleen scan, 49, 50, 195, 197
Lobular carcinoma in situ (LCIS),
253*g*–254*g*
Louis' angle, 93, 93*f*
Lovibond's angle, 148*f*, 149
Lower motor neurons, 274*g*
Lumbar hernias, 224*g*, 234
Lumbar puncture, 290, 291, 292
Lumbar spine, 307–308, 312
Lung(s). *See also* Pulmonary *entries*;
Respiratory system
acute injury to, 326–327
collapse of, 91*g*
compression of, 91*g*, 118
consolidation of, 91*g*, 118
parenchymal diseases of, 118–119
segmental anatomy of, 95*f*–98*f*
ventilation and perfusion scans of, 121,
122
Lung biopsy, 121, 122
Lymphadenitis, 41*g*
Lymphadenopathy, 41*g*, 45–46
Lymphangiography, 49, 50
Lymph node(s), 44*f*
abnormal findings, 45–46
in breast examination, 262, 264
axillary
cancer in, in absence of palpable
breast mass, 269
palpation of, 42–43, 45*f*, 257–259,
260*f*
examination techniques, 41–43, 42*f*,
43*f*, 45*f*, 46*f*
in child, 342
intramammary, 253*g*
in leukemias and lymphomas, 45, 46
Lymph node biopsy, 49, 50
Lymphogranuloma venereum, 219
Lymphoma, 41*g*, 44–45, 46

Macrocephaly, 354
Macroglossia, 86
Macule, 7*g*, 11, 14*f*
Magnesium-based antacids, 178
Magnetic resonance angiography (MRA)
in neurologic disorders, 289, 291, 292
retinal, 70, 71
Magnetic resonance imaging (MRI)
in acute injury, 332, 333
in breast evaluation, 271, 272
in cardiovascular diagnosis, 173, 174

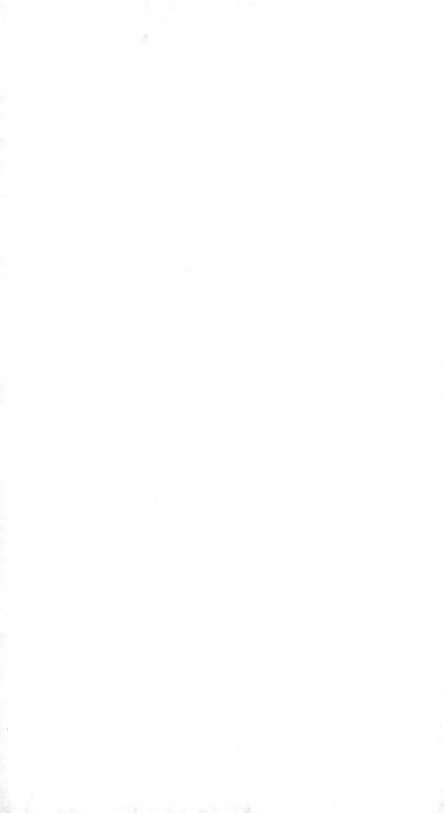